A SEAT ON THE AISLE, PLEASE!

A SEAT ON THE AISLE, PLEASE!

The Essential Guide to Urinary Tract Problems in Women

ELIZABETH KAVALER, M.D.

COPERNICUS BOOKS

AN IMPRINT OF SPRINGER SCIENCE+BUSINESS MEDIA

Published in the United States by Copernicus Books, an imprint of Springer Science+Business Media.

Copernicus Books
Springer Science+Business Media
233 Spring Street
New York, NY 10013
springer.com

Library of Congress Control Number:
2005932045

Manufactured in the United States of America.
Printed on acid-free paper.

9 8 7 6 5 4 3 2 1

ISBN-10: 0-387-95509-7
ISBN-13: 978-0387-95509-4

To my daughter, Sonia, and my parents, Marylou and Franklin.

Acknowledgments

I would like to thank three groups of people who have helped me get to the point where I was able to know enough to write this book: the physicians who trained me, the group that gave me the chance to hone my skills in practice, and the people in the publishing world who brought the concept to fruition.

I am grateful to Dr. Richard Macchia at Downstate for not laughing at me when, as a naïve medical student, I told him that I wanted to go into urology. Without Dr. Michael Droller, who took a risk and accepted a woman into his residency at Mount Sinai Medical Center, I would not be a urologist today. Dr. Shlomo Raz taught me everything I know about female urology and pelvic floor surgery, in addition to showing me how to be a compassionate, patient, and thoughtful physician.

Drs. John Fracchia, Jon Reckler, Edward Muecke, Noel Armenakas, Eli Lizza, and Ernie Sosa took a chance on hiring me to join them in practice. Thank you for trusting your reputation and patients with me. Without the opportunity you offered me to specialize in my area of interest, I would not have the knowledge and experience to write this book. The residents at Lenox Hill Hospital challenge me to think about what I do, and push me to be a better physician. They are Drs. David Hochberg, Jay Bassilote, Arnold Rivera, Gyan Parekh, Dan Kellner, Ginger Isom-Batz, Jamie Bruno, Eric Kwon, and Jennifer Hill. Thank you for taking care of my patients with skill and empathy.

Finally, I want to acknowledge those people who turned this idea into a book. Michael Hennelly called me after receiving my query letter and offered to help me get the book published. Although I am grateful for his help, I am more appreciative of his friendship. He and his wife, Michelle Kling, have become valued friends. Marie Dauenheimer is a gifted artist who was able to spin my descriptions of anatomy and surgery into beautiful illustrations. She has also become a friend. Paul Farrell, Matt Giannotti, Paul Manning, and Michael Koy at Springer publishing inherited the manuscript and artfully turned it into a book. Thank you for the respectful way you worked with me as a new author. Finally, I want to thank my very good friends Amy and Richard Hutchings for the glamorous photograph they took of me for the cover.

Contents

Acknowledgments   vii

Introduction   xi

THE BASICS

CHAPTER 1
*The Nuts and Bolts of the Female Pelvis: Normal Anatomy
and Physiology*   3

CHAPTER 2
*What Can Go Wrong? Pelvic-Floor Problems: Symptoms
and Solutions*   15

CHAPTER 3
*Picking a Doctor: Gynecology versus Urology: Who Treats
Bladder Problems?*   45

URINARY LEAKAGE AND INCONTINENCE

CHAPTER 4
Stress Urinary Incontinence   63

CHAPTER 5
Urinary Urge Incontinence: Overactive Bladder Syndrome   101

CHAPTER 6
The Golden Years: Incontinence in the Elderly   131

DROPPED ORGANS: PELVIC-FLOOR PROLAPSE

CHAPTER 7
Pelvic-Floor Prolapse   177

THE PAINFUL BLADDER

CHAPTER 8
Urinary Tract Infections 225

CHAPTER 9
Interstitial Cystitis and Pelvic Pain Syndromes 271

RELATED ISSUES

CHAPTER 10
Menopause, Hormones, and the Development of Female Pelvic Problems 311

CHAPTER 11
Anesthesia for Surgery and a Crash Course in Pain Medications 335

CHAPTER 12
A Visit to the Urologist's Office: Definitions and Explanations of the Diagnostic Procedures 355

CHAPTER 13
Safety in Numbers: The Epidemiology of Urinary Incontinence 381

Glossary 391
Index 397

Introduction

Hardly a glamorous subject, urinary tract problems in women have become my life's work. But how did I arrive at this decision? Unlike Aphrodite, I did not emerge from the medical school clamshell as a urological surgeon and author. Some autobiographical background is called for.

I grew up in one of the few major cities in America that still has a single-sex public high school for girls. Before attending the Philadelphia High School for Girls, I attended a private all-girls grade school in the suburbs. I transferred to public school in the ninth grade, where I was one of 550 girls in my year. Everyone was female, including the president of the student body, the varsity athletes, the entire marching band, the first chair of the orchestra, the valedictorian, and the editor of the school newspaper.

After graduation, I attended Barnard College, the women's college of Columbia University. Although men attend classes in Barnard and the athletic programs are integrated, Barnard has a distinct place within the University. I had many female professors and advisors. My female classmates majored in physics as readily as they did in economics or English. We had a large number of premedical students with a well-structured mentoring program of women doctors who had all graduated from Barnard. My desire to become a doctor did not surprise my friends or family.

The first coeducational institution that I attended was the medical school of the State University of New York in Brooklyn. Nearly 40 percent of my class was female, and for the first two years, no perceptible differences between the education of the male and female students existed. During the third year, like all American medical students, we spent time in the hospital learning to evaluate and treat patients. The year is divided into specialties, such as internal medicine, surgery, and obstetrics and gynecology. At that time, general surgery tended to be a boys' club. Long, grueling hours spent with the same group of eight or ten students, mostly men, created strong bonds that tended to exclude the few women on the service. Urology, a surgical subspecialty, was a male bastion.

During my fourth year of medical school, I spent a month on the urology service at the Mayo Clinic, in Rochester, Minnesota. While there, I learned about the urological problems suffered by women. I also became aware that there were very few women urologists. No specialty within the medical profession has fewer women practitioners than does urology. Less than 1 percent of urologists in the United States are women.

I realized that it is a field in strong need of well-informed female physicians. I had found my field: I would go into urology, and focus on women's urological problems. Ironically, the next time I dealt with urological issues specific to women was during my fellowship at UCLA Medical Center seven years later. During my six years of residency, I rarely treated a woman who suffered with one of the problems discussed in this book, but not because female patients did not have these conditions. They did, and still do. Rather, the majority of male urologists in practice did not focus on women's urological conditions.

I was the second woman accepted into the urological training program at Mount Sinai Medical Center in New York City in the history of the department. The first woman completed her residency about eight years before I began. She has never practiced urology. Upon completion of her training, she did a second residency in pathology and became a city Medical Examiner. I had no women role models from whom to learn. No women attending physicians trained me, either during my clinical work or my laboratory experience. I was the only woman in every conference and presentation, unless one of the radiologists attended.

Because of this isolation, I became acutely aware of the difficulties that women face when they are seen by male urologists, who traditionally treat male problems. Of course, most physicians, urologists included, are compassionate and interested in giving their patients excellent care. After all, their wives and daughters are women. But most male urologists do not make an effort to learn and understand female urological disorders. Unless special interest is taken to think about them, little progress will be made on either an individual or a scientific level. That is why specialty training is so important. It is not just the experience that one gets from it, but the focus of one's thoughts and ideas in one specific area.

Upon completion of my chief residency year in urology, I pursued a fellowship in pelvic surgery at UCLA, where I learned about female pelvic-floor problems and was exposed to the creative and complicated reconstructive surgery that can be done to correct these problems. I also realized how desperate our patients are; desperate for information, for answers, and for education. They flew to Los Angeles from around the world because access to physicians experienced in this speciality was not available near their homes. My choice of medical specialty was validated by the fellowship. During that year, I decided that a book on this subject, written by a committed medical professional, would be helpful to many women.

Over the past 20 years, tremendous social and financial resources have been put into research on cancer and heart disease. As a result of the scientific advances in these areas, people are living longer. Older Americans expect to lead active lives playing golf, traveling, and continuing to engage in sexual relations later in life. Quality of life has taken on new meaning in the recent decade. Male impotence, once rarely discussed or acknowledged as a medical issue, is now taken seriously and treated effectively. With more women physicians treating women patients, we, too, are acknowledging the importance of lifestyle problems in our patients.

This book serves as a guide for women who are seeking treatment for the debilitating problems of the urinary tract for their family members. It touches on disorders that affect millions of women, most of whom have no idea where to turn for help. In many cases, physicians themselves are not familiar with the problems from which many of you suffer. As a clinician and a surgeon, I am committed to understanding my patients' problems and applying the optimal treatment available in order to ease and cure their urinary tract problems. No book addresses urinary tract problems in women exclusively. It is my great hope that this book will enlighten women to better understand their problems and help to ease their embarrassment, anxiety, and suffering. As more women become assertive in discussing their concerns in this medical field, more physicians will respond effectively and, one hopes, empathetically.

I have divided the book into five sections, each of which focuses on one aspect of the urinary tract. The first section reviews terminology and anatomy, as well as which medical specialty to turn to for help for your problems. The second section addresses urinary leakage, of which two main types occur in women: stress incontinence and urge incontinence. Stress incontinence occurs when mechanical stress, or pressure, such as laughing, coughing, or sneezing, causes urine to squirt out of the urethra. The second type of incontinence, and the cause of much embarrassment, anxiety, and discomfort for women who are so afflicted, occurs when the urge to urinate results in leakage before you can get to the bathroom.

The third section deals with pelvic organ prolapse, a condition in which the bladder, rectum, small intestine, or uterus falls into the vaginal canal. The fourth section reviews the causes and treatments of the painful bladder, including urinary tract infections and interstitial cystitis. The fifth section looks at the effects menopause can have on urological symptoms. Anesthesia and pain control for urological surgery are also reviewed. Finally, a glossary provides easy-to-understand explanations for the technical and medical terms discussed throughout the text.

PART ONE

THE BASICS

CHAPTER 1

The Nuts and Bolts of the Female Pelvis

Normal Anatomy and Physiology

In women, the urinary tract is composed of four organs. From top to bottom, these include the kidneys, the ureters, the bladder, and the urethra. The **kidneys** sit under the ribs in the back. Isolated from the organs of the abdomen, the kidneys are covered in fat and muscle. They filter the blood, reabsorbing the red blood cells and eliminating toxins into the urine. Also producing agents that help with the metabolism of calcium and the production of red blood cells, the kidneys are vital structures. Fortunately, most of us have two of them but we can live normally with only one. If one kidney becomes diseased, it can be removed without any negative impact, as long as the other one is normal.

When kidneys become inflamed, they cause severe back pain and fever. Infections of the kidneys start either in the bladder and ascend into the kidneys, or they begin in the blood and seed the kidneys. Kidney infections are serious. They cause high fevers and require long-term antibiotics for eradication. Fortunately, only 1 percent of bladder infections in women ascend the urinary tract and affect the kidneys. The kidneys are very resilient organs. In an anatomically normal woman, even a severe kidney infection will not cause permanent damage.

After filtering the blood, the kidneys eliminate toxins from the body through tiny tubes called **ureters**. The ureters are conduits through which the urine passes on its way into the bladder. If there is a blockage below the kidneys, the ureters will become dilated and will fill with water. As anyone who has had a kidney stone can attest to when the ureters become dilated, it is excruciatingly painful. A blocked ureter will cause severe, colicky back pain. The most common cause of urethral obstruction is a stone that forms in the kidney, gets washed into the ureter, and becomes stuck in the small-caliber tube.

If the process causing the blockage is slow-growing, the dilation of the ureter may not be painful. If the ureters are blocked by a prolapsed

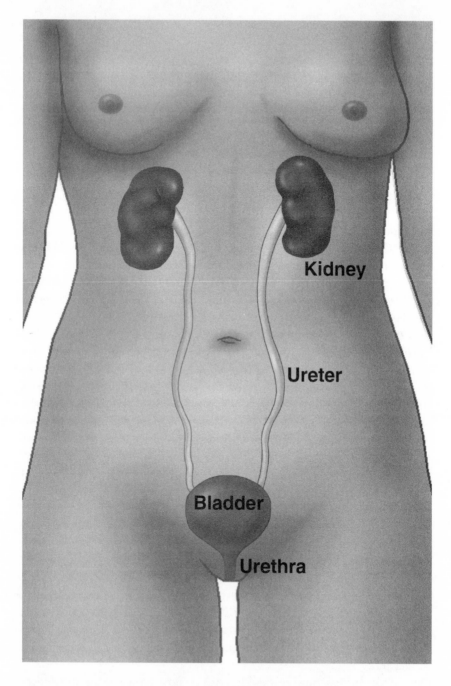

FIGURE 1. *Female Urinary Tract.*

bladder or a mass growing into the ureters, you will not feel pain despite the obstruction. Without special testing, the blockage could go unrecognized. If it is a long-standing obstruction, even with elimination of the causative factor, the ureter will remain dilated. As long as the urine is passing from the kidneys into the bladder, the way the ureter looks is not important.

Finally, the urine enters the **bladder**, where it sits until it is eliminated. Urologists used to think that the bladder was an inactive organ that served only as a holding vessel. However, with more attention being paid to conditions that cause bladder pain, researchers are finding that the bladder is a vital, active organ, with a complex neurological and vascular system.

The urinary bladder (we are not talking about the gall bladder, which is a small sac that sits under the liver and can fill with stones and cause pain) is composed of four distinct layers. The lining is called the **mucosa**. A watertight system, it protects the inner layers from the toxins that enter the organ. This active layer of cells gets replaced by new cells on a regular basis. Defects in the lining that allow urine to penetrate into the deep recesses of the bladder can cause pain, irritability of the bladder, and frequent urination. Recurrent infections and chronic pain syndromes may possibly be caused by these defects.

The next layer is called the **submucosa** ("under the mucosa"). It is a thin, indistinct layer through which the blood vessels and nerve endings enter and supply the other layers. One can see that if the mucosal layer is imperfect, the urine can easily affect the nerve and blood supply to the bladder since that is the next layer of exposure.

The third layer of the bladder is the real business end of the organ. It is the muscle layer, and is formally called the **detrusor**. The exact character of the muscle is not known, but it does get thick and muscular when it works hard to empty against a resistance, just like the biceps muscle gets larger from weight lifting. However, voluntary control of the detrusor does not seem possible in the same way that we can control our biceps muscle. There is a direct, although subconscious, effect that our brains have on the bladder. In women with certain types of bladder control problems, the detrusor will contract and cause uncontrollable loss of urine if the brain senses cold, anxiety, or proximity to a bathroom. As many of you know, suppression of these impulses is very difficult, making the reaction involuntary but certainly under some sort of conscious control.

The complex detrusor muscle is different from any other muscle in the body in that it can expand to huge proportions (like the uterus) and deflate within seconds (unlike the uterus). It can be controlled by the brain

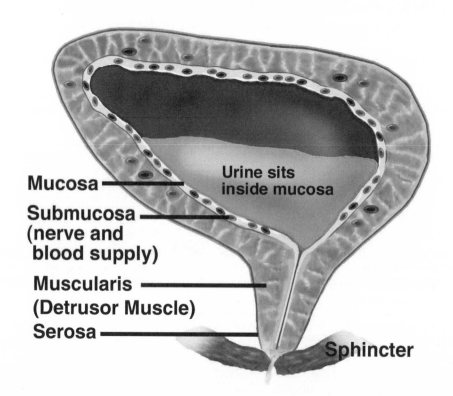

FIGURE 2. *The Layers of the Bladder.*

(voluntary urination) or escape the normal suppressive channels (resulting in leakage). It can thicken due to pushing against a resistance (like the biceps muscle) or it can be thin and paper-like, with no change in symptoms. It can be overdistended and lose its ability to function for weeks or months on end, only to become decompressed and return to normal activity within days. In short, it is quite a resilient muscle that is at the root of many urination problems among men and women.

In women, the detrusor muscle tends to be thin and floppy. Because women don't have prostates to block the flow of urine, they never develop the thick-walled muscle from which men with enlarged prostates suffer. Women suffer from the opposite problem; as a woman ages, her urinary sphincter becomes less efficient, creating less resistance to outflow, often resulting in incontinence. In older women, nothing exists between the bladder and the outside except a very inefficient valve. This is one reason why women suffer from incontinence more than men.

The second reason that men don't develop incontinence is also related to differences in their anatomy. Men have a prostate that supports the bladder (the prostate provides the juice in which the sperm swim around in the ejaculate). Because of that support, and the fact that no empty cavity sits under the bladder (in women, that would be the vagina), a man cannot suffer from a "fallen bladder" (more about that later). So, anatomically, men and women are very different in this area, resulting in different problems requiring different treatments.

The final path of the urine as it leaves the urinary bladder is through the **urethra**. In women, the urethra is only 3 cm long (about $1\frac{1}{2}$ inches); whereas in men, it is about 15 cm long (about 8 inches). This tiny tube sits above the vagina inside the labia. Many women do not realize that the urine comes out of a separate opening. Women have three openings: the urethra, through which urine passes; the vagina, through which a baby passes; and the anus, through which stool passes. Men only have two openings: one at the tip of the penis, the urethra, for both urine and semen; and one behind, the anus, for stool.

The urinary sphincter comprises about one-half the length of the urethra in women. As a muscle, the function of the urinary sphincter is to hold urine in the bladder while the bladder is filling without letting a drop come out. During voluntary urination, the urinary sphincter opens and lets the urine pass out into the toilet. It clamps shut when the bladder is empty in order to allow for bladder filling to resume. It is always contracted and closed, except for the few seconds each day that it relaxes in order for the bladder to empty.

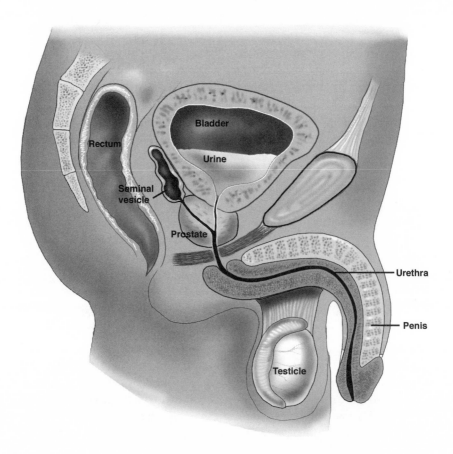

FIGURE 3. *Normal Anatomy of the Male Pelvis.*

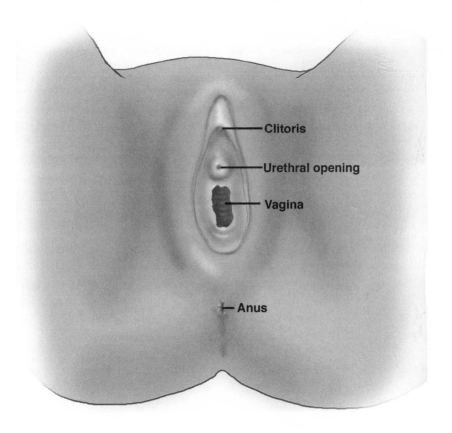

FIGURE 4. *View of the Perineum.*

On a microscopic level (see Figure 5), the fibers that make up the urinary sphincter are organized in a circle. The circle is even, so that when it is contracted, the walls on each side come together and act as a closed, watertight seal, preventing leakage of fluid. Only the urinary sphincter, this wonderful muscle, maintains dryness in the female urinary tract. Damage to the sphincter will result in leakage.

In summary, the female urinary tract comprises four main organs: the kidneys, the ureters, the bladder, and the urethra. But no discussion of the urological conditions in the woman would be complete without reviewing the location of the genital organs in relation to the urinary tract, since these structures play a vital role in urinary health as well (see Figure 6).

The vagina is a muscular canal that sits between the urethra and the anus. The uterus is connected to the vagina through the cervix, which is the passage through which menstrual blood, and, during vaginal delivery, a baby, can pass out of the uterus, into the vagina, and finally out of the body. The uterus is held in place with flexible ligaments that can expand and contract with its changing size due to pregnancy. As the uterus enlarges, the ligaments stretch, and sometimes they become loose. The uterus can lose its supportive tissues and slide into the vaginal canal.

If you are looking from the outside into the pelvis, the bladder sits on top of the uterus. First, you have the pubic bone, then the bladder, and finally the uterus. The two structures, the bladder and the uterus, are separated by a tiny layer of tissue. Their proximity to one another means that they can affect each other. They share some of the same blood and nerve supply. Any of us who experiences frequency of urination and bloating during menstruation knows how much these two organs interact on one another.

The fallopian tubes, which bring the egg from the ovary into the uterus, are connected to and are a part of the uterus. On the other hand, the ovaries are not part of any other organs. They are distinct structures that sit inside the abdominal cavity, which the bladder, the uterus, and the fallopian tubes do not. In order to access the ovaries, the abdomen, which contains the intestines, has to be opened. In addition, the ovaries have a different blood and nerve supply than the uterus and the bladder. The ovaries cannot collapse into the vaginal canal the way the uterus and the bladder can.

If the uterus is removed, the space where the uterus was is filled with loops of the small intestine. No space remains vacant in the human body when an organ is removed. The endless tubes of intestine will find their way into the pelvis, sitting on the top of the vagina. This is important in understanding why some of these organs can wind up in funny places in our bodies.

Normal　　　　**Post-trauma**

OPEN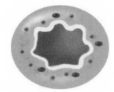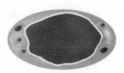

CLOSED

FIGURE 5. *Normal and Post-Traumatic Urethra.*

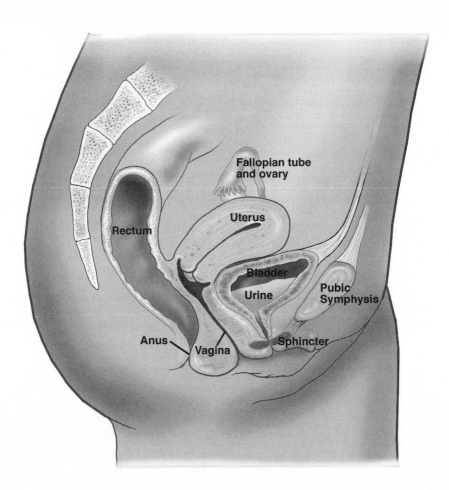

FIGURE 6. *Normal Female Anatomy: Side View.*

Sitting under the vaginal canal is the rectum. If the back wall of the vagina is weak, the rectum can bulge, causing constipation.

To review the anatomy, the vaginal canal is surrounded by three structures: the bladder on the top, the uterus at the end, and the rectum underneath. If you have had a hysterectomy, the uterus is not longer at the end of the vagina; small intestine has moved into its place.

SUMMARY

This discussion lays the foundation for understanding the causes and treatments of the conditions that are discussed later in the book. The four organs of the urinary tract and the uterus and rectum are the main structures that we are discussing. The interaction of these organs with one another will help you to get a sense of what problems we can be faced with and why the symptoms present as they do.

CHAPTER 2

What Can Go Wrong?
Pelvic-Floor Problems: Symptoms and Solutions

I recently had a woman come into the office who was having problems with her bladder since the delivery of her last child. When M.R. was in her thirties and forties, she did not find the problem too bothersome. Mostly, she would have to go to the bathroom frequently, and she couldn't hold it very well when she had the urge to go. Occasionally, she would leak a tiny bit when she laughed hard. Nothing too drastic; she could manage it. Then came menopause and things began to get out of control.

Instead of the occasional accident, M.R. began to have accidents on a regular basis. She would cough and squirt. She would sneeze and squirt. She would get up from a chair and squirt. Sometimes, she would laugh, and not squirt; she would actually pee *in her pants! She really didn't have to laugh that hard.*

She brought it up with her gynecologist on her yearly examination. He referred her to me. When I examined her lying down, I asked her to cough and she leaked. I noted that her bladder was falling slightly into her vagina, which she could feel at times, although she didn't realize that it was her bladder that was falling down. With a mirror, I pointed out the anatomy so that she could see the problem and understand the proposed treatment.

M.R. had surgery to repair the leakage and the bladder descent. Done vaginally under general anesthesia, the surgery took about an hour to complete. When it was over, she awakened in the operating room, and was transferred to the recovery room with a catheter coming out of her bladder and a packing in her vagina.

The following morning, the catheter and the packing were removed, and she was able to get out of bed and move around. She urinated without difficulty and was discharged home. She felt wonderful that the leakage had resolved completely. She doesn't wear pads anymore, she can hold her urine longer than she could before the surgery, and she does not get up at night to urinate.

She is pleased with the outcome, and only wishes that she had known that this problem could be solved sooner.

M.R.'s story is typical of women with urinary problems. She had lived with her problem for years before discussing it with a medical professional. Once she brought it up, however, she was directed to a source that could help her, and she was treated effectively. The conditions that are discussed in this book are more common than diabetes, heart disease, and high cholesterol, yet most of us don't know where to turn for help. Many of you don't know what is considered "normal" bladder behavior for someone in your age group, or you have been too embarrassed to ask your physician or even your friends. Therefore, we tend not to report on many of the symptoms discussed in this chapter because we don't realize that these symptoms can be treated or cured.

This chapter is set up to help you "diagnose" your condition in order to learn about the problem from which you are suffering. It is divided into three main categories: painful problems, causes of urinary leakage or incontinence, and symptoms due to pelvic organ prolapse. If you look through the chapter and find the list of symptoms that you have, you can give the condition a name and skip to that chapter directly. In some cases, the presenting complaints are not so straightforward, or perhaps a few different problems are occurring at the same time. A quick overview of all of the urinary tract disorders discussed in the book may also help those of you who are in this category.

CATEGORIES OF UROLOGIC CONDITIONS

- **Painful Bladder Conditions**
- **Urinary Incontinence**
- **Pelvic Floor Prolapse**

CAUSES OF PAIN

PAINFUL UROLOGICAL PROBLEMS

Urinary Tract Infections
Pelvic Floor Spasms

PAINFUL UROLOGICAL PROBLEMS—continued

Interstitial Cystitis
Radiation Cystitis
Non-bacterial Cystitis
Autoimmune Cystitis
Gynecological causes
    Endometriosis
    Uterine Fibroids
    Ovarian Cysts
    Pelvic Inflammatory Disease

Pain is one of the most difficult problems for both patients and doctors to manage. For patients, the frustration of not being understood or taken seriously is unmatched by any other complaint. In many cases, the cause of the pain is not readily identified by objective, conventional, diagnostic methods, so no "physical" abnormalities can be seen. For this reason, many physicians do not acknowledge the pain, further alienating the patient. Therefore, it is impossible to know if any progress is being made in the treatment, except for the patient's word. You may continue to feel badly, and the doctor just can't explain why.

In urology, pelvic pain generally results from urinary tract infections, pelvic-floor spasms, interstitial cystitis, post-radiation effects, or gynecological problems, such as endometriosis, fibroids, ovarian cysts, and pelvic inflammatory disease.

Urinary Tract Infections

URINARY TRACT INFECTIONS

(Also called cystitis or bladder infections)
Pain in the pelvis
Frequent urination
Urgency of urination
Burning with urination
Occasionally, blood in the urine
Cloudy urine
Foul odor in the urine

Over 80 percent of you will experience a urinary tract infection at some time during your lifetime. In many cases sexual activity will be the precipitating factor, but even if you are not sexually active, you can still get them. The symptoms include burning, frequency of urination, back pain, urgency of urination, bloody urine, and, occasionally, leakage of urine. Not all of the symptoms will occur in all women who get cystitis. A diagnosis is made through a urine test which can be done at a local laboratory or at the doctor's office. Most doctors prefer to collect a urine sample before prescribing antibiotics to be sure that the you are really suffering from a urinary tract infection. Usually, antibiotics are given for a week to ten days and the symptoms disappear. Many of you suffer from recurrent infections, which are defined as more than three infections in a year. If this is the case, you may need to see a urologist to be sure that no abnormalities within the urinary tract are causing the problem.

Red flags that we look for to suggest that further testing is needed include the following:

1. Infections that began during childhood, before the onset of sexual activity.
2. Infections that result in fevers over 101.5°F.
3. A personal history of kidney stones.
4. A personal history of urinary tract surgery or abnormalities.

Childhood Urological Infections

Infections that began before the onset of sexual activity suggest that an anatomical defect may be present that predisposes you to infections. Usually, if a child develops a urinary tract infection, her pediatrician will refer her to a pediatric urologist for testing. If you remember getting infections as a child, but you have never seen a urologist (an experience that most children remember), it is worth consulting with one now to check things out. The evaluation is usually simple. A kidney ultrasound (sonogram— same test) is done to evaluate the kidneys. This is a painless, noninvasive test that looks at the structure of the kidney. Kidney stones, masses, tumors, cysts, and the absence of a kidney can be detected by ultrasound. The function of the kidneys cannot be assessed, but as a screening test, the ultrasound is the best place to start.

Fevers with Infections

Infections that result in fevers over 101.5°F indicate that one or both of the kidneys may be infected as well the bladder. Most run-of-the-mill urinary tract infections do not migrate up the urinary tract and settle into the kidneys. Even though women with cystitis often suffer from low back pain, the infection remains contained within the bladder. The low back pain is secondary to inflammation and spasm of the pelvic-floor muscles on which the infected bladder sits. Kidney infections cause pain in the mid-back and flank, immediately under the ribs. In a healthy young woman who is not immunosuppressed, a kidney infection nearly always results in a fever over 101.5°F. Radiographic imaging and a visit to the urologist are warranted if a urinary tract infection results in a fever.

Kidney Stones

If a woman with a history of kidney stones gets a urinary tract infection, an evaluation should be done to be sure that no new stones have grown that have led to the infection. There is a 50 percent chance that any given person will get another kidney stone if she had one previously. Fortunately, however, the second stone tends to occur 8 to 10 years after the original stone. You can have a stone sitting up in the kidney without feeling it. It is only when they pass out of the kidney and get stuck in the small-caliber ureter that intense pain results. Stones can complicate matters because they are usually infected and because they can block the outflow of urine. If a woman with recurrent urinary tract infections has a stone sitting in the urinary tract, it should be removed in order to reduce the risk of getting more infections and to prevent the excruciating pain that can result from the spontaneous passage of the stone. All kidney stones harbor infection. However, not all stone patients suffer from infections and not all infections in stone patients come from the kidney stone. It is wise to get rid of the stone in case it is the cause of the infection. With the sophisticated, noninvasive techniques that we have available now to remove kidney stones, it is a good idea to remove them if they are found.

Surgery

If you had surgery as child to correct an abnormality of the urinary tract, it is a good idea to see a urologist if you are getting recurrent infections. One or two infections per year are not harmful, but more than that suggests that something may not be right. A urologist will order some radiological studies to evaluate the kidneys. The study that is ordered depends on what abnormality you suffered from originally. Often, these x-rays can be difficult to read if the person reading them is not familiar with the defect and its correction. That is where the urologist comes in. The urologist can tell if an abnormal-looking x-ray is within the normal limits of a corrected problem. Many radiologists are experienced in genitourinary radiology and can read these x-rays quite well, but corroborating information between the two specialists is helpful. In addition, the urologist can determine whether or not the original problem has recurred, progressed, or remained stable. Treatment can then ensue from there.

Pelvic-Floor Spasms

PELVIC MUSCLE SPASMS

Frequency of urination
Sense of incomplete bladder emptying
Urgency of urination
Getting up at night to urinate
Burning after urination
Crampy discomfort in the pelvis

VERSUS URINARY TRACT INFECTIONS

UTI causes burning with urination
UTI causes foul-smelling urine
Must do urine culture to distinguish diagnosis

Pain secondary to pelvic-floor spasms is a common occurrence that many of you will experience at some time during your lifetime. It frequently goes unrecognized by both physicians and patients. The pelvis is a bony structure whose floor is covered in slings of muscle. This muscular floor prevents the pelvic organs from falling onto the ground, just like the abdominal wall muscle holds the intestines inside the body. The bladder, uterus, and rectum sit on the pelvic-floor muscles. Three structures pass through these muscles. They are the urethra (which drains the bladder), the vagina (which is attached to the uterus), and the anal canal.

Just like other muscles in the body, the pelvic-floor muscles can go into spasm. Muscle spasms occur when a muscle contracts without conscious control. The most familiar spasms occur in the lower back. For those of you who have suffered from low back pain, you know that you can bend over in a certain way and cause an injury that results in a muscle spasm. The first line of treatment is usually bed rest to relax the muscle, combined with anti-inflammatory agents, and occasionally steroid therapy. The pelvic-floor muscles can go into spasm in much the same way. The causative event may be subtle, resulting in irritation of the muscles, which then go into spasm.

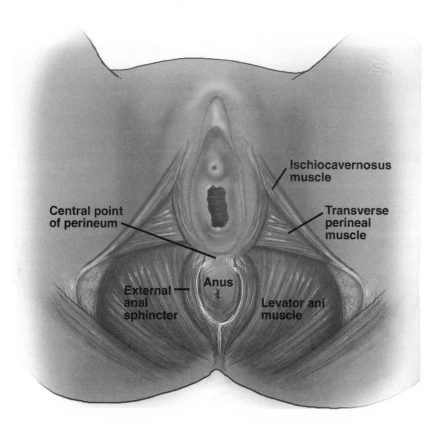

FIGURE 1. *Pelvic-Floor Muscles.*

In young women, pelvic-floor spasms can be caused by a urinary tract infection, a back condition, trauma, or stress. A urinary tract infection will cause inflammation and irritation of the bladder wall, producing pain and discomfort, especially with urination. In response to the burning, you may clench and tighten the pelvic floor while trying to empty your bladder. Bladder emptying requires *relaxation* of the pelvic floor in order to open the normally closed urinary sphincter, or muscle. The muscles subsequently go into spasm.

The spasms produce symptoms similar to those caused by an infection. They include frequency of urination and pelvic pressure, but two very important symptoms are not seen in pelvic-floor spasms but are present with a urinary tract infection. With pelvic muscle spasms, there is no burning *with* urination and the urine is not foul-smelling. Often a course of antibiotics is prescribed, even when the urine tests are negative for a urinary tract infection. There may be slight improvement of the symptoms, but they persist or come back after the antibiotics have been discontinued. Often, a second or even third course of antibiotics is prescribed. The antibiotics, themselves, can cause further bladder irritation and inflammation. The cycle is perpetuated.

Pelvic muscle spasms result in women with low back problems because the pelvic muscles are recruited to help support the weakened back. The increased weight and demand on these muscles can throw them into spasm, resulting in the symptoms described above.

Stress can also cause spasms of the pelvic floor. Different people manifest different problems when they are under stress. Some women get headaches, some people clench their jaws and can develop tempero-mandibular joint pain (TMJ), some patients develop back spasms, while others get pelvic-floor spasms. During stress, you may tighten your pelvic floor muscles without realizing it. The muscles go into spasm from the repeated tightening. It is difficult to identify the cause of the discomfort as a muscle spasm because it is an unfamiliar sensation. There is no inhibition of movement as one would experience with a low back spasm. It is mostly a burning feeling as if the muscle has been fatigued by overexercise and lactic acid has built up. Some of you also have problems with bladder emptying because the muscles don't relax to allow the urine to flow. As a result, frequency ensues, as does pelvic pressure. Many of you have to awaken from sleep to empty the bladder, resulting in disrupted sleep, growing fatigue, and a worsening of the condition.

Treatment goes from the conservative to the more involved. The first line of treatment is exercise, warm baths, fluid reduction, and antiinflammatory agents, such as ibuprofen. The next step is muscle relaxants, which are taken by mouth. Finally, pelvic-floor physical therapy can be instituted to relieve the spastic muscles.

Interstitial Cystitis

INTERSTITIAL CYSTITIS

Pain all of the time
Frequency every five minutes
Pain relieved with urination
No odor in urine
Persistent symptoms for six months or more

Interstitial cystitis is a pain syndrome that involves the entire pelvic floor. A mysterious disease, the number one complaint is pain, whereas for pelvic muscle spasms and urinary tract infections, the predominant symptoms are frequency and urgency. The cause(s) of interstitial cystitis is not known, although many theories have been proposed. Some etiologies, or causes, include infections, autoimmune diseases, parasites, nerve damage, and vascular problems. Most of the sufferers are young women in their early 20s or 30s. It has been recognized in children and in men, although these cases are rare.

Many of you who have this condition have previously suffered from a series of urinary tract infections that were treated aggressively with antibiotics. The symptoms then begin to occur without any evidence of infection and the antibiotics no longer take away the burning and pain. Many women describe the pain as feeling like the worst urinary tract infection that they have ever had without any relief of the symptoms. The only relief they get is the few tenths of a second that they are on the toilet urinating. Because they get relief with urinating, many women spend most of their time on the toilet. Some patients even sleep on the toilet. They feel that as long as they are up 15 to 20 times per night going to the bathroom, they may as well just sleep there. Because they are so sleep deprived, many of these women cannot function. They cannot work or carry on relationships with other people. Their entire lives are consumed with relieving this pain. The entire pelvic area feels inflamed and sore, so sexual relations are out of the question. Some patients need to be placed on disability.

Recent widespread recognition of this disease has led to more research into treatments. Most cases resolve spontaneously or, at least, improve, over time. Some women have periods of remission interspersed with episodes of exacerbation. Some unfortunate patients continue to have progression of the disease. For a short time, urologists were removing the bladders of some of these desperate women. The thought was that if the source of the pain was removed, the patient would at least get some relief. The bladder was replaced with a strip of bowel that was configured into a sphere and connected to the ureters for the kidneys to drain urine. The results were disastrous. The pain did not go away with the removal of the bladder. This experience was a hard way to learn that the disease is not only a bladder problem, but related to the muscles and the nerves of the pelvic floor.

Medications are available to help alleviate some of the terrible symptoms. No cure is available yet, although I suspect that once the cause is found, the cure will not be far behind.

Radiation Cystitis

RADIATION CYSTITIS

Bloody urine
Pain with urination
Frequency
Urgency
History of radiation to the pelvis

Radiation cystitis is inflammation of the bladder caused by radiation injury to the bladder. Luckily, these women usually only suffer for a short period of time. Symptoms usually occur at the middle or the end of the treatment, when the dose of radiation has accumulated over time. Occasionally, bleeding can ensue, resulting in what is called **hemorrhagic cystitis.** This is very uncomfortable because blood clots can block the outflow of urine. Sometimes, a catheter has to be inserted into the bladder to evacuate the clots and restore normal urine flow. If the bleeding does not stop, agents may need to be instilled into the bladder to coagulate the vessels of the bladder wall. These instillations can be painful and usually must be done under anesthesia. Eventually, the bladder heals and the bleeding and symptoms all resolve without consequences.

Most of the more-modern protocols for treating cancerous tumors with radiation do not result in permanent problems. Sophisticated planning systems and more finely tuned and aimed dosage protocols have resulted in excellent cancer control with fewer side effects from the radiation treatments.

Nonbacterial Cystitis

NONBACTERIAL CYSTITIS

Same symptoms as urinary tract infection
No bacterial growth on urine culture
History of autoimmune illness
Recent viral syndrome, like the flu

What most patients and doctors call urinary tract infections are caused by bacteria. However, viruses can also infect the urine, causing inflammation of the bladder wall and symptoms typical of a urinary tract infection. The urine culture will not grow bacteria because bacteria are not causing the problem; a virus is. Viruses cannot be cultured as easily as bacteria can. No simple test can be performed to diagnose **viral cystitis**. Usually, there will be signs of a systemic viral syndrome, such as the flu, as well as the urgency, frequency, and burning with urination. These systemic symptoms include fever, malaise, and achiness. Flu-like symptoms coupled with bladder symptoms usually means viral cystitis. The bladder symptoms may take a day or two longer to resolve than the systemic symptoms. Only supportive interventions will help, such as nonsteroidal medications (ibuprofen) and rest. Viruses have to run their course.

Autoimmune cystitis is seen in patients who suffer from autoimmune diseases, such as lupus, Sjögren's syndrome, rheumatoid arthritis, and fibromyalgias. Autoimmune disorders cause the immune system to overreact to irritants, some of which are native to the patient. In other words, the patient's immune system begins to attack her native tissues. During exacerbation of an autoimmune episode, the bladder may become a target of the attack. The bladder becomes inflamed and irritated for no reason. The symptoms mimic bacterial cystitis. Usually, other symptoms related to the autoimmune disorder are present at the same time. One's whole system is out of whack. Treatment is supportive until the underlying autoimmune disorder can be controlled.

Gynecological Disorders

GYNECOLOGICAL CONDITIONS

Pelvic pain
Vaginal bleeding
No urinary symptoms
Bloating
Cramping
Occasionally constipation

The most common gynecological conditions that can present as pelvic pain include endometriosis, uterine fibroids, ovarian cysts, and pelvic inflammatory disease.

Endometriosis

Endometriosis is a benign (noncancerous) condition. Deposits of tissue that resemble the lining of the uterus, called the endometrium, spot the pelvis. They can be found near the ovaries, on or in the bladder, in the pelvic cavity, and in the abdomen. Endometriomas, as these deposits are called when they fill with blood, can be found anywhere in the body. These tissue deposits respond to hormonal fluctuations just like the lining of the uterus does. During certain times of the month, the endometriomas become symptomatic, causing cramping, bloating, and pain.

Uterine Fibroids

Uterine fibroids are noncancerous growths on the uterus. They can grow on the outside or inside of the uterus. If they grow on the inside of the uterus, they tend to cause excessive bleeding during menstruation. If they grow on the outside, they usually do not cause symptoms, unless they grow very large. When they do grow quite large, you can see a bulge in the abdominal wall where the fibroid is bulging out. It looks like you are pregnant. On examination, the gynecologist will describe the size of the fibroid by how "pregnant" the uterus feels. For example, the doctor may say that you have a 12- or a 16-week size uterus. A pelvic or transvaginal ultrasound (where the probe is inserted into the vagina), is the best way to determine the size of the uterus.

Uterine fibroids are not cancerous and do not become cancerous. They are only treated if they are causing symptoms, such as excessive vaginal bleeding, cramping, and/or pelvic pain. Women as well as physicians frequently ask me if fibroids can press on the urinary bladder and cause problems with urination, such as frequency, urgency, and incontinence. No studies have actually proven one way or another that fibroids can affect the bladder. However, after treatment of the fibroids many patients are not any better from a urological standpoint. In healthy young women, the urinary bladder is a very pliant structure. If something is in its way, it will fill around the uterus. If you take an x-ray of a bladder being filled with a large uterus sitting on top of it, the bladder will take on a funny shape, but it will still fill. Fibroids should not be removed solely with the hope of improving bladder function. If a woman has bladder issues and a large fibroid (which is not bleeding or causing other symptoms, such as pain), I would first deal with the bladder issues to see if satisfactory treatment can be obtained without removing the fibroid. Usually, the bladder problems can be treated successfully.

Ovarian Cysts

Ovarian cysts are ubiquitous, and are frequently the cause of pelvic pain, especially in young women who still ovulate. Girls are born with all the eggs that they will produce in their lifetimes already intact. Beginning in puberty, one egg will be released each month by one of the two ovaries. Before the egg is released, it undergoes changes within a cyst that forms on the ovary. When the cyst ruptures, the egg is released, where it travels down the fallopian tube and implants into the uterine wall. If fertilization is to occur, it will happen during the decent down the fallopian tube. Every month, when the cyst matures and ruptures, releasing the egg, ovulation is occurring. This event it called *mittelschmerz*. Many women feel the cyst rupturing. Sometimes uncomfortable, it is rarely painful. These events are all normal and healthy. No treatment is usually needed when you suffer from discomfort due to mittelschmerz.

If you have complaints of pelvic pain and a transvaginal ultrasound is performed, a cyst may be seen on the ovary. If the ultrasound is performed around the time of ovulation, it may be difficult to determine whether or not the cyst is a functional cyst; that is, a cyst due to the impending release of an egg, or if it is due to another cause. Often, the doctor will suggest that the ultrasound be repeated during a different phase of the menstrual cycle to see if the cyst changes or disappears. A functional cyst disappears after the egg is released. Other cysts do not. If the cyst grows, changes shape, or looks like it has material inside of it, the gynecologist will often suggest that it be removed. Ovarian cysts are usually benign, but not always. Distinguishing benign from malignant cysts can be difficult on ultrasound, computed tomography (CT), and magnetic resonance imaging (MRI). Most physicians recommend removing suspicious ovarian cysts whenever there is doubt.

Pelvic Inflammatory Disease

A condition that causes excruciating pelvic pain, pelvic inflammatory disease (PID) is an infectious process that comes from sexual activity. It is rare now that antibiotics are available to treat most of these infections. However, it does occur and should be considered if severe pelvic pain is encountered.

Chlamydia and gonorrhea are the two most common causes of PID. Routine visits to the gynecologist's office include culturing for these two bacteria. Usually, women suffering from these infections have a thick yellowish vaginal discharge, accompanied with pelvic pain and fevers. During examination, the woman will nearly jump off the table with pain when the doctor touches the cervix. This is called the chandelier sign, because she nearly hits the chandelier when she flies off the table in pain.

If the condition progresses, it can travel up the cervix, through the uterus, and into the tubes. The body will then wall off the infection as it enters the abdominal cavity, where the intestines lie. This walled-off infection involving the affected tube and ovary is called a tubo-ovarian abscess. Diagnosis is suspected on physical examination and confirmed with either an ultrasound or CT scan. Now that powerful antibiotics are available, intravenous antibiotics alone may be enough to treat the condition. Occasionally, surgery will need to be done to clean out the infection.

CAUSES OF URINARY INCONTINENCE

Urinary incontinence is the involuntary loss of urine. It can involve small amounts or an entire bladder volume. Some women wear pads to manage the problem, some wear diapers, and some women wear nothing. Some women urinate frequently in order to reduce the amount of leakage. Some women change their underpants instead of wearing pads. Self-management of urinary incontinence is very individual and no conclusions regarding the degree of leakage can be drawn regarding the number of pads that someone wears in any given day.

The reason we distinguish among the four types of urinary incontinence is because the treatments differ dramatically. Stress incontinence is mainly a surgical problem. Urge incontinence is treated with medication. Overflow and total incontinence are treated based on the underlying condition.

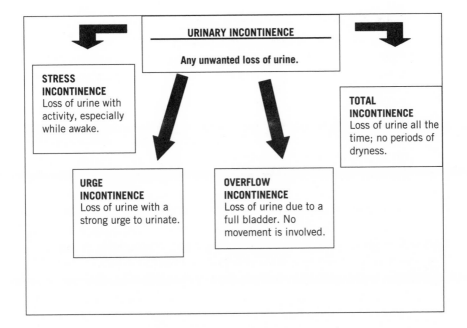

Stress Urinary Incontinence

STRESS URINARY INCONTINENCE

Loss of urine with activity: cough, laugh, sneeze, run
Occurs almost only during the day
No frequency
No urgency
No pain
No getting up at night to urinate

Stress incontinence occurs when a woman coughs, laughs, sneezes, changes position, runs, or stands up, and looses urine. Activities that physically (not emotionally) stress, or push down on the bladder, resulting in squirting of urine, cause stress incontinence. If you are sitting still or sleeping, no leakage occurs. Generally, women report wearing pads during the day, but not at night. If you leak at night, it only happens during movement between the bedroom and the bathroom. The amount of leakage caused by stress incontinence varies from small drops to large volumes of leakage. Only the event that causes the leakage defines the type of incontinence, not the amount of urine that is lost.

Stress incontinence is caused by a weakening of the pelvic-floor muscles, which the urethra relies on for support. The weakness beneath the urethra does not provide strong support during increases in pressure, such as coughing or laughing. Instead of the forces pushing on the urethra resulting in the urethra collapsing onto a backboard of muscle and squeezing closed, it just falls against nothing. Without that support, the urethra remains open, and urine leaks out. Sometimes this problem is referred to as anatomic incontinence because the problem is due to a change in the physical structure, or anatomy, of the pelvic floor (see Diagram).

Stress urinary incontinence is mostly seen in women who have endured vaginal deliveries or have had a hysterectomy. Usually, some damage to the pelvic floor predisposes you to stress incontinence. This is not to say that *every* woman who has delivered a baby vaginally or who has had a hysterectomy will suffer from stress incontinence. These occurrences are just predisposing factors that put you at risk for developing a problem.

The reason that stress incontinence occurs after vaginal deliveries is that the vaginal tissues are stretched during the delivery, creating weakness in the middle of muscles that surround the vagina and support the urethra. Postpartum, the presence of estrogen in the system maintains the elasticity of the weakened tissue. The bladder and the urethra may be more mobile than before delivery, but the integrity of the tissues is intact, so some support is still present.

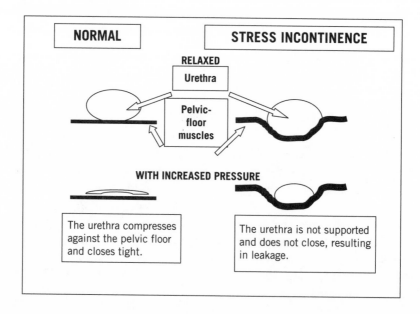

NORMAL	STRESS INCONTINENCE

RELAXED

Urethra

Pelvic-floor muscles

WITH INCREASED PRESSURE

The urethra compresses against the pelvic floor and closes tight.

The urethra is not supported and does not close, resulting in leakage.

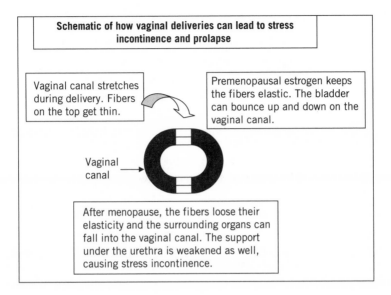

Schematic of how vaginal deliveries can lead to stress incontinence and prolapse

Vaginal canal stretches during delivery. Fibers on the top get thin.

Premenopausal estrogen keeps the fibers elastic. The bladder can bounce up and down on the vaginal canal.

Vaginal canal →

After menopause, the fibers loose their elasticity and the surrounding organs can fall into the vaginal canal. The support under the urethra is weakened as well, causing stress incontinence.

After menopause, the loss of estrogen results in the loss of the elasticity of the weakened fibers. The fibers become weaker and thinner. Very little support remains and the tissues loose their ability to support the urethra. Usually, stress incontinence worsens after menopause. Before menopause, many women notice the beginning of leakage, especially during exercise. Often, but not always, it is not until you are well into your 50s and 60s that you develop a problem requiring pad use, or a problem that interferes with your quality of life.

Urinary Urge Incontinence

URINARY URGE INCONTINENCE AND OVERACTIVE BLADDER

Frequency
Urgency } Overactive bladder
Getting up at night to urinate

Leakage with the urge to urinate
Awakens wet at night } with urge incontinence
Can be large volume or small drops

Urge incontinence is defined as the loss of urine that is preceded by a sudden urge to urinate. Urgency, without incontinence, is when someone gets the sudden urge to empty her bladder and has to run to the toilet but does not leak urine. If leakage ensues, it is called urge incontinence. Urge incontinence is not due to changes in the anatomy of the pelvic floor, at least not on any visible level. Microscopic changes within the bladder and its nerve and blood supply may be the cause of the problem, but as of now, the cause of urge incontinence is not known.

Postmenopausal women tend to develop urgency and urge incontinence. These problems are considered part of the aging process and are not considered abnormal, but should still be treated. When you go to the doctor complaining of sudden urges to urinate without being able to control the outflow, neither you nor the doctor should be concerned that a more ominous problem is present. As long as the examination and the urine analysis are normal, no further testing is necessary before treatment can be started. If the treatment fails, more extensive diagnostic tests can be done to see if other problems, such as stress incontinence, are contributing to the problem.

Although these problems are not as common as they are in older women, premenopausal women can develop urgency and urge incontinence as well. Especially after childbirth, the changes in the pelvic floor can result in urgency symptoms. Women are often concerned that their symptoms will worsen as they get older. Young women with urgency and urge incontinence do not always develop more severe problems as they age. Only time will tell what the future will hold. Many factors go into the development of urinary problems in the elderly. If the problem is mild in a young woman, I recommend dealing only with the symptoms that are present at that time. We can always revisit the problem in the future if it gets worse.

If you have neurological problems, further testing should be done before any medication is started. Strokes, multiple sclerosis, Parkinson's disease, and seizure disorders can all affect urination. Urodynamic testing (described in the Glossary) will help guide treatment. Sometimes changes in urination precede other neurological changes, indicating a worsening of a previously stable neurological problem. For example, a person with multiple sclerosis, which has been stable for a number of years, suddenly develops urinary incontinence with a precipitating urge. Urodynamic studies may help determine if the multiple sclerosis has progressed, and if so, a follow-up appointment with a neurologist will need to be arranged. Urodynamic testing cannot determine what neurological condition is causing the leakage. Rather, it can only show that something abnormal is going on with the nerve supply to the bladder.

Any disorder that affects the brain or the spinal cord can cause urinary changes. In young women (pre-menopausal) who present with urge incontinence (not just urgency), a full neurological history should be taken by the urologist or gynecologist. Questions that will be asked include a history of headaches, head trauma, such as in a car accident or a fall, blurry vision, weakness or tingling in the hands or feet, low back pain, or a history of spinal or disc surgeries. If the answer is yes to any of these questions, then a urodynamic study should be done to determine if the bladder appears to be neurologically impaired. If the answer is no to all of the questions, then it is up to both the patient and the physician regarding the need for further testing. Often, women are concerned about the cause of their symptoms and want information regarding the etiology, or origin, of the symptoms. Urodynamic testing will rule out neurological disorders.

Overflow Incontinence

OVERFLOW INCONTINENCE

Leakage all of the time
Recurrent urinary tract infections
History of neurological disease, diabetes, or pelvic surgery, such as
    hysterectomy or bowel resection

Overflow incontinence is the result of leakage due to a full bladder. If the bladder is always full, any further addition of liquid that is added by the kidneys will result in "overflow" and leakage. Overflow incontinence is rare in women. It is usually the consequence of another problem that needs to be addressed first in order to allow the bladder to empty. Causes of overflow incontinence include diabetes mellitus, neurological conditions that affect the bladder, and previous bladder or pelvic surgery.

Diabetes mellitus is a common condition affecting the entire body in which the sugar cannot be processed correctly. There are two main causes, both of which result in the same consequences. The first type of diabetes (which used be called juvenile diabetes, but is now called type 1 diabetes) occurs when the pancreas, which produces insulin, is destroyed by a virus, thus eliminating the body's only source of insulin. In type 2 diabetes (formerly referred to as adult-onset diabetes), the pancreas produces insulin but the insulin cannot attach itself to the sugar molecules circulating in the bloodstream because the insulin receptors are blocked. Without functioning insulin, sugar cannot be adequately digested by the body. The excess sugar circulating in the bloodstream gets stuck in the tiniest blood vessels in the body, blocking the blood flow to these tissues. Without blood flow, the tissues cannot get oxygen and nutrients, so they die. The tissues at risk include the eyes, the kidneys, and the nerves. The results are vision disturbances, kidney failure, and numbness in the hands and legs. The nerve damage translates to the vital organs as well, including the heart and the bladder. Many diabetics suffer from heart attacks, but never feel it. These are called "silent heart attacks" because they go unnoticed. Pain is an important alert to danger.

Just like in the heart, sensation in the bladder is lost in diabetic patients. As the bladder fills, the diabetic woman may not feel the urge to empty. The bladder continues to fill beyond its intended capacity. Over time, usually years, the bladder loses its elasticity because it gets stretched out of shape. The result is poor emptying and overfilling. Eventually, the bladder can overflow, resulting in leakage. If diabetes is identified early and controlled with diet and medication, some of the disastrous consequences of this pervasive disease can be prevented.

CAUSES OF OVERFLOW INCONTINENCE

Diabetes mellitis
Neurological conditions
Stroke
Multiple sclerosis
Parkinson's disease
Brain injury
Spinal cord injury
Previous bladder surgery
Previous pelvic surgery
Colon surgery
Gynecological surgery

Neurological disorders can also cause overflow incontinence. These include spinal cord injuries, brain injuries, strokes, and multiple sclerosis. If the nerve supply to the bladder is damaged, the bladder will not contract correctly. With each failed attempt at emptying the bladder, more and more urine builds up, resulting in a high residual volume after voiding. Eventually, the residual urine gets so high that no more urine can enter the bladder without it overflowing. The result is overflow incontinence. Because there is nerve damage, the sensation of the incomplete emptying is not noticeable. Sometimes women notice that their clothing is getting tight around the middle, or they may feel bloated. They have no sense that the bladder is overfilled, except for the leakage.

If you undergo bladder surgery that inadvertently results in obstruction of urine flow, over time you may develop overflow incontinence. A mechanical blockage of the outflow of urine results in incomplete emptying. If the urethra is kinked by an operation, to correct prolapse, for example, each time that you urinate, the bladder will have to work very hard to overcome the obstruction to empty. Eventually, the bladder will deteriorate and stop emptying completely. The amount of residual urine accumulates with each void. The end result is leakage. Onset of this problem is so slow and insidious that you may not even notice it until the leakage begins.

Pelvic surgery, such as colon surgery or gynecological surgery, can result in damage to the nerves that supply the bladder. As the nerves leave the spinal cord, they traverse the pelvis and enter the bladder. During their course through the pelvic floor, they can be injured when a section of the intestine is being removed or the uterus is being taken out. Cancer surgeries, in which the nerve and blood supply to the diseased organ must be widely excised to cure the patient, are the most common operations in which nerve injury can ensue. Occasionally, diverticulosis of the colon (small bulges in the colon caused by low-fiber diet and age) results in severe inflammation of the pelvic floor that results in nerve damage.

When the nerves that supply the bladder are injured, the bladder loses its ability to sense fullness, as well as its ability to contract and empty. This condition is called a flaccid bladder. Again, no pain is involved in identifying the problem. You show up at your doctor's office complaining of incontinence and have a history of pelvic surgery. Inability to empty the bladder confirms the diagnosis.

Overflow incontinence is easy to diagnose. First, a thorough history will reveal a risk factor for developing incontinence, such as diabetes or previous surgery. You would describe either frequent urination with small volumes of output, or you may only void once or twice per day. A good history will certainly point the physician in the direction of considering overflow incontinence as a possible cause for your leakage. You will be sent to the bathroom to empty your bladder as thoroughly as possible, and then you will be examined. Usually, on physical exam, your bladder can be felt to be distended all the way up to the bellybutton. When empty, it should be tucked behind the pubic bone, deep in the pelvis. If there is any question, a catheter can be inserted into your bladder and the volume of output measured. A less invasive method of measuring the output is through an ultrasound, which most gynecologists and urologists have in their offices. No exact definition of overflow incontinence exists, but if your bladder has over 400 cc (normal bladder volume at full capacity) or 13 ounces of urine in it *after* you void, you are most likely in overflow. If you are walking around with a bladder full of urine without noticing it, you have a very abnormal bladder.

Total Incontinence

TOTAL INCONTINENCE

Leakage all of the time, day and night
No dry times at all
No urge to urinate, except occasionally in the morning

Total incontinence is a rare condition in which the sufferer leaks urine constantly. If you have total incontinence the cause is nearly always a hole between your bladder and your vagina. The urine leaks out through this hole, bypassing the urethra and the urinary sphincter. In medical terminology, this hole is called a **fistula.** A fistula is an unnatural connection between two organs or a connection between two organs that should not be connected. A fistula between the bladder and the vagina is called a vesicovaginal fistula (vesico-means bladder).

The hole is the result of obstetrical trauma, gynecological surgery, or radiation therapy. It does not happen spontaneously. Without one of these prior events, you cannot have a fistula. In developing countries, obstetric trauma is the leading cause of vesicovaginal fistulas. A temporary loss of the blood supply to the uterus and its neighboring organs as well as ripping of the tissues due to prolonged labor will result in the hole. In many of these countries, young girls undergo circumcision which partially closes the vagina. As the baby's head comes through the canal, uncontrolled ripping occurs. Often, holes between the bladder and the vagina will result. In the United States, vesicovaginal fistulas are more commonly caused by gynecological surgery or radiation therapy. During gynecological surgery, bleeding will be controlled by inadvertently clamping blood vessels to neighboring tissues, which then become oxygen deprived and die. A hole will be left in its place. Radiation therapy for cervical or uterine cancer will cause shrinking of blood vessels. Loss of blood supply causes tissues to die, leaving a hole through which urine passes.

Women with total incontinence and women with overflow incontinence often present the same way—they have a constant spillage of urine. There is no difference in output between daytime and night. They wear pads at all times. In both cases, they rarely go to the bathroom normally. They rarely get the urge to urinate, but for different reasons. In overflow incontinence, the bladder is so deteriorated that it never contracts to try to empty, so the woman doesn't get the urge to go. In total incontinence, the bladder never fills because urine in draining constantly from the hole in the bladder. Again, you have no urge to go because the bladder never fills completely. They are distinguished by measuring the amount of urine left in the bladder after urinating. In overflow incontinence, the bladder is full; in total incontinence, it is empty.

PELVIC-FLOOR PROLAPSE

PELVIC-FLOOR PROLAPSE

(Also called pelvic organ prolapse)
Pressure or pulling sensation in the pelvis
Feeling of something in the vagina or protruding
through the opening in the vagina
Sensation of sitting on something
Constipation

Pelvic-floor prolapse is a fancy way of describing the collapse of the support structures of the pelvic floor resulting in the bladder and other pelvic organs dropping into the vagina. Women have no idea what organs are coming out of the vaginal canal. They just feel that the vagina has something in it. Symptoms include pelvic pressure and pulling, back pain, and a mass effect in the vagina. If it is really bad, you can barely walk because something is hanging between your legs.

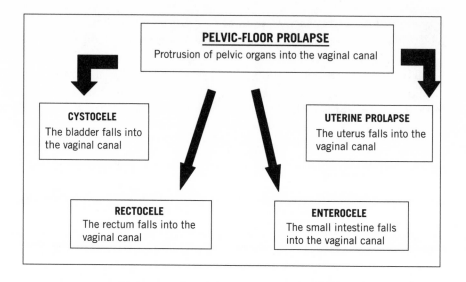

Four organs can fall into the vagina: the bladder, the uterus, the small intestine, and the rectum. Bladder prolapse is the most common type of pelvic-floor prolapse (pelvic-floor and pelvic-organ prolapse are the same term and are used interchangeably). Another word for bladder prolapse is a **cystocele**: "cyst" means bladder and "cele" means hernia. It is a hernia of the bladder. A hernia is a weakening in muscle through which an organ can protrude. Any muscle can result in a hernia. The most common hernias occur in the abdominal wall muscles, like the groin (inguinal hernia) and the belly button (umbilical hernia).

Bladder prolapse results when the pelvic muscles that support the pelvic floor weaken and the bladder falls through the weakened muscle. The bladder is covered by vaginal tissue as it falls into the canal. So, when the doctor looks into your vagina, he does not see exposed bladder. He sees the bladder, covered with vaginal skin, falling into the canal. The cervix, or neck of the uterus, can also descend into the vaginal canal. When the cervix slides into the vaginal canal, a small, round, firm ball of tissue with a tiny slit in the center of it can be seen peeking through the vaginal opening. The process of the descent may be slow, in which case the cervix gradually falls into the vagina. Perhaps no symptoms are noticed by the woman for many years. Eventually, as it falls further, a firm ball of tissue can be felt during activity or during urination. Many women will feel it when they wipe after voiding. In some cases, the descent is rapid. All of a sudden, she will notice this thing coming out of her vagina. It can be very disturbing, even if it is

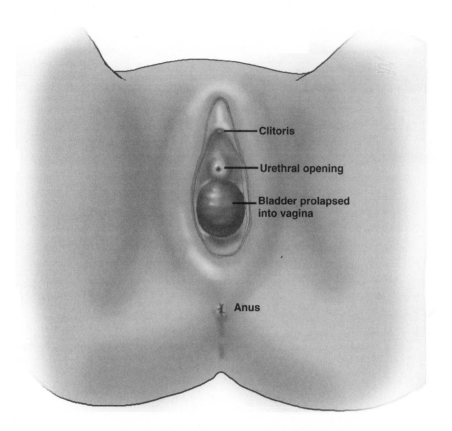

Figure 2. *Bladder Prolapsed into Vagina.*

Uterine Prolapse

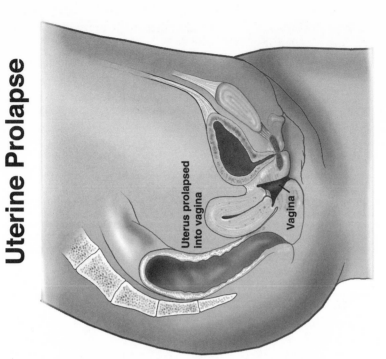

Uterus prolapsed into vagina

Vagina

Normal Anatomy

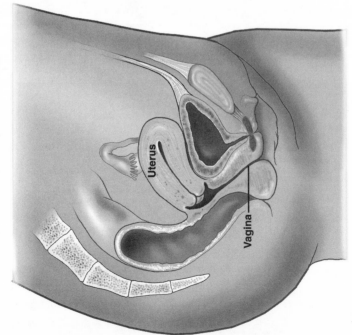

Uterus

Vagina

FIGURE 3.

not painful or bothersome. Just the idea that one's organs are moving around can be very alarming.

Besides the bladder and the uterus, the rectum can also fall into the vagina. This defect is called a **rectocele**. The bladder falls from above into the vagina, whereas the rectum pushes up from below and creates a bulge in the floor of the vagina. The bulge that the rectum causes creates a pocket in the rectal wall in which stool can sit. The fullness from the stool in the vault will give you the urge to defecate, but when you try to go, it takes a tremendous amount of pressure to empty the pouch.

The two most common symptoms of a rectocele are a bulge in the vagina and constipation. Most women do not realize what is bulging through the vagina. They just feel the ball when they go to wipe themselves. Unlike bladder conditions, rectoceles do not cause urinary symptoms. So, if a woman has a bulge with no frequency, urgency, or urinary leakage, she may have a rectocele as opposed to a bladder prolapse. Constipation results because stool gets caught in the pouch before it leaves the anal canal. A great deal of force is required to empty this pouch. Sometimes women have to push on the vaginal bulge in order to evacuate their bowels.

The final defect that can create a bulge in the vagina is a weakening in the top of the vagina, allowing the small intestine to fall down. This problem can only happen in patients who have already had a hysterectomy. After the uterus is removed, the top of the vagina is sewn closed. The space which the uterus took up is now filled with small intestine. The intestines float around inside the abdominal cavity and fill any spaces that are created. If the top of the vagina becomes weak, the intestines that are sitting on top of it will begin to fall into the canal. The result is called an **enterocele.** "Entero" means small intestine and "cele" means hernia, or muscle weakening. Thus, an enterocele is a weakening of the vaginal muscle, resulting in the small intestines coming through. Of course the small intestines are not exposed. When the doctor examines you, she can see vagina tissue covering the small intestine. Often, the examining physician cannot tell what organ lies behind the protruding vaginal skin. It is possible to have a good idea based on the location and shape of the defect. Some physicians will order tests, such as CT scans or MRIs to get a better sense of the structures that lie behind the prolapsed tissue. Other physicians operate without knowing for sure what is there. They will correct whatever defects they can find.

Many women with enteroceles notice that their vaginas are shorter than they used to be. As the top of the vagina is pushed in by the intestines, the canal becomes shorter. Sexual relations can become difficult. If you are not sexually active, you may not realize the change in vaginal depth. Part of

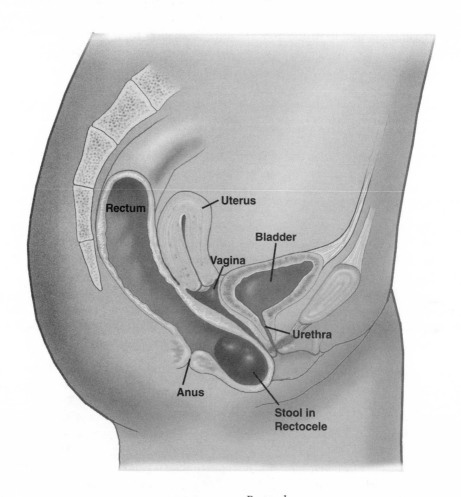

FIGURE 4. *Rectocele.*

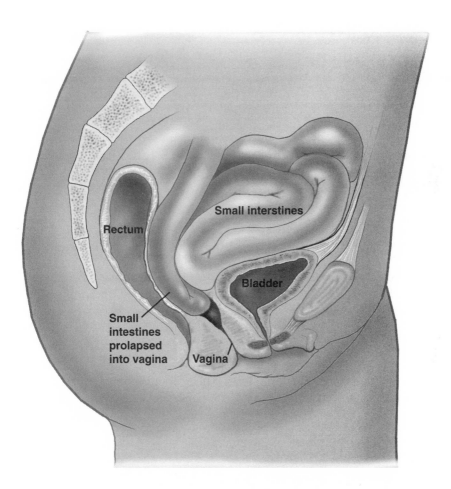

FIGURE 5. *Enterocele.*

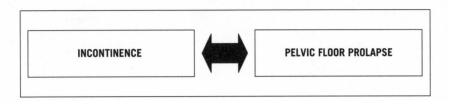

repairing an enterocele involves replacing the top of the vagina back where it belongs so that vaginal depth is maintained. Again, enteroceles are only found in women who have had a hysterectomy.

Many of you with incontinence do not have prolapse, but enough of you do so that the physician must examine you for pelvic-floor weakening before any treatment plan can be initiated. Prolapse and incontinence often go together.

SUMMARY

This chapter offered an overview of the urinary tract disorders from which women can suffer. Some women have straightforward problems that are easily addressed in a few visits, while other women have multiple issues that need time and patience to sort out. Urinary tract infections, pelvic pain conditions, incontinence, and pelvic-floor prolapse are interrelated entities. After all, they all share the same organs of origin, all of which lie close together and are interconnected. Often, treatment of one problem will unmask another. At other times, multiple problems are treated with a single intervention. Whatever the problem, patience and thoughtful evaluation will uncover solutions that are both efficacious and agreeable.

CHAPTER 3

Picking a Doctor

Gynecology versus Urology:
Who Treats Bladder Problems?

A local urologist referred one of his patients to me who was having a difficult urinary incontinence problem. On recounting her history, J., the patient, disclosed to me that she feels as if she lives in the bathroom. It has become somewhat of a joke among her friends that she will need to use the bathroom no matter where she is. Lately, however, it's not so funny because it is getting worse. She hardly drinks any fluids because if she does, she will be in the bathroom for the rest of the day. Forget coffee, alcohol, or soda. Drinking the slightest amount of any of those liquids will just ruin her day.

J.'s urinary problems began in her 20s with urinary tract infections, a "honeymoon cystitis" kind of problem. It resolved a few years after she got married, but left her with frequency and urgency of urination. She mentioned these symptoms to her gynecologist during a routine visit. He checked her urine for infection and blood, and examined her. Everything was normal, so he reassured her.

After menopause, the problem got really bad. J. began to get the urge to go so suddenly that she sometimes didn't make it to the bathroom. She began to wear panty-liners, then graduated to pads. Now, she wears pull-up diapers like her grandchildren, especially at night when she can't control her bladder. While getting a family history, she told me that her mother had a similar problem. She remembers that her mother went to the bathroom frequently when J. was a child. J. asked her mother about it once, but her mother did not want to discuss it.

She still sees the same gynecologist. He is a wonderful doctor; he delivered both of her children and is a patient listener. But, he doesn't know too much about how to treat these urinary problems. He recommended that she see a urologist.

Not knowing much about urology, she went to her husband's doctor. The urologist's waiting room was very busy. It was filled mostly with men, and their wives. The doctor was very pleasant and thorough in his exam. He prescribed some medication after reassuring her that her problem was not "serious." Urinary leakage problems were not his area of specialization. He suggested that if the medication did not work, that she consult with me since that is my area of particular interest.

J. did see me, and after an examination and some routine testing, we were able to combine medications with behavioral strategies to bring J.'s condition under control. The need to visit so many doctors' offices to find the right one to treat her problem surprised J., as it does many women. How do you go about finding a specialist? So what exactly does specialization mean? How do we become specialists? Why is knowing this information important in choosing a doctor? These are essential questions that every woman should know the answers to.

Medicine has become so specialized; patients often don't know whom to see for what problem. If the right big toe hurts, they need to find a specialist in the right big toe, not the left big toe, and certainly not a foot doctor. He knows nothing about right big toes! The fragmentation of medicine has many advantages, the obvious one being that once you find the right doctor, you can be reasonably sure that you are getting the best care available. The disadvantage is that it can require a different doctor's visit for every organ in your body.

The following chapter takes you through the process through which a college graduate becomes a doctor, and eventually a candidate for board certification in one of the major fields in medicine. I then focus on the differences between urologists and gynecologists in order to guide you in choosing a physician to treat your particular urinary tract problem. Finally, I review the different types of hospitals we have in this country to help you understand the philosophy behind the care they offer. No matter what a physician's training or hospital's origin, excellent care can be found in every category. No judgments are being made by raising the differences. I am only trying to clarify the perspective from which you are getting your advice.

FROM COLLEGE GRADUATE TO MEDICAL DOCTOR

After completing college, a prospective physician must complete four years of medical school. Graduates earn Medical Degrees, or M.D.s, immediately upon completion and can officially be called "doctor." Residency is the practical arm of medical training that begins immediately after medical school. The first year of residency is called the "internship" and takes place in a teaching hospital.

Upon completion of a residency, a doctor is eligible to become certified to practice in his or her field by a nationally recognized board. This recognition is termed *board certification* and signifies a basic competence in the field in which the certification was granted. Board certification is not required to practice in this country, but is becoming more and more important for obtaining hospital privileges and insurance contracts. You cannot assume that a physician is board-certified. If you want to know, you have to ask.

Younger physicians should all be board-certified. If they are not, you need to know why. You may want to ask. Older physicians have more leeway since this credential was not as necessary 20 or 30 years ago. The American Medical Association (AMA) publishes a listing of all of the practicing physicians in the United States and their certification status. Most libraries have the reference books put out by the AMA, or the AMA web site (www.ama-assn.org) will provide the phone number to call for the information. HealthGrades.com is one of the many websites that will give the full training record of any physician for a fee. Most of these sites charge anywhere from $5 to $15 for the information. It is considered public information, even if may be difficult to obtain.

After residency has been completed, a physician has the option to enter practice immediately or pursue specialized training through either research or further work with patients. These special areas of interest are called *sub-specialties* and the extra period of training is called a *fellowship*. If you run into a *fellow* during your medical experience, you will know that he or she (the term *fellow* is no longer gender-specific and is now used interchangeably) is more experienced than the residents, but not yet a fully independent practitioner. Fellowships are offered in every medical and surgical specialty. Not every physician elects to do a fellowship. Those who do, spend an extra year or two focusing on a particular aspect of their field, allowing them to become an expert. When new techniques are being developed or research is being carried out, the fellows are usually involved with a senior physician. This specialty training can be either accredited or not. If the specialty field is well established, accredited fellowships are usually available. Sometimes, a specialty field is very new, so no accreditation efforts have been instituted. *Fellowship accreditation is not nearly as important as residency accreditation.*

Not all sub-specialists complete fellowships. If a physician becomes interested in a particular field during his training, he may choose to focus his practice on that area. His experience will make him an expert without having done a fellowship.

After residency and fellowship, the physician passes her examinations to become board-certified. Now an *attending physician*, she is able to admit patients to the hospital on her own. Again, not all attending physicians have specialty training, but nearly all are board-certified to practice within their given field.

Urology versus Gynecology

I want to provide a framework to help you to get a perspective on how these two fields are divided. The entire medical field is subdivided into two main areas: *medical* specialties and *surgical* specialties. Certain fields in medicine do not fit into a neat category of medicine or surgery. These fields include obstetrics and gynecology, neurology, radiology, pathology, dermatology, anesthesiology, and pediatrics. Generally, medical doctors (in the old days, these doctors were called physicians) as opposed to surgeons, treat problems with medication, while surgeons treat problems with surgery. The boundaries between the two groups have blurred because of technology and the development of less invasive treatments that both surgeons and medical doctors learn to use. But, generally, medical specialists complete a residency in internal medicine (general medicine) and can then become board certified in internal medicine.

Medical Specialties	Surgical Specialties	Other
General/internal medicine	General surgery	Obstetrics and gynecology
Cardiology	Urology	Anesthesology
Gastroenterology	Opthomology	Radiology
Pulmonary/critical care medicine	Ear, nose, and throat	Pediatrics
	Orthopedics	Neurology
Endocrinology	Neurosurgery	Psychiatry
Nephrology	*Cardiothoracic	Pathology
Infectious disease	*Colorectal	Dermatology
Rheumatology	*Head and Neck	
Hematology/oncology	*Plastic	
Gerontology	*Surgical oncology	

* Must complete most or all of general surgery training.

After the three years in a medical residency, an internist has the option of specializing in one of the subspecialities of medicine. Each specialty has a board that approves training programs and offers credentialing to its trainees. These include gastroenterology, cardiology, pulmonology, rheumatology, infectious diseases, hematology (blood diseases), oncology (cancer), endocrinology (specialists in the glands—thyroid, pancreas, adrenal, and others), gerontology (medical problems specific to the elderly), and nephrology (kidneys). Nephrologists are kidney specialists with a medical background, whereas urologists are surgeons who treat kidney problems.

Urology

Within the division of surgery, however, the training is somewhat different. The surgical specialties include ophthalmology, neurosurgery, otolaryngology (ear, nose, and throat), urology, and orthopedics. Within general surgery, physicians can subspecialize further after completing a full general surgical training program. These areas of interest include cardiothoracic surgery, colorectal surgery, plastic surgery, surgical oncology, and head and neck surgery. General surgeons complete training in general surgery, which can range from five to eight years after medical school. The specialties within general surgery require completion of either one or two years of general surgery before entering the specific area. Unlike in medicine, where the specialists can sit for the internal medicine boards, the specialists in surgery cannot sit for the general surgery boards. Once a doctor enters his chosen specialty, he finishes that program and becomes eligible for board certification in his specialty. He can then receive further training if he wants within that field, thus becoming more specialized.

Traditionally, urologists focused on the urinary tract of both men and women, as well as the male genital organs. The problems that urologists are most well-known for treating include prostate disease, kidney stones, erectile dysfunction making fertility and testicular, bladder and kidney cancer. Recent advances in training programs and demands by women patients have led many urologists to start focusing on problems specific to women. Urinary incontinence as well as urinary tract infections and pelvic pain syndromes have come under the domain of the urologist. Some urologists are particularly interested in treating problems specific to women, while others don't feel as comfortable in that area. Most large groups or practices will have one or two physicians who have completed a fellowship in *female urology* (usually one or two years of training in addition to the five or six years of urology residency) or who, through their own experience, have become expert in this particular area of female urology.

Female urologists are not the same as *women* urologists. Female urologists specialize in problems specific to women. Women urologists are women who go into urology. There is no additional accreditation for urologists in the specialty field of female urology.

A small number of urologists will treat pelvic organ prolapse in addition to incontinence. This area of the female anatomy can come under the auspices of either obstetrics and gynecology or urology, depending on the training of the physicians in your area. If you have a problem involving incontinence and pelvic organ prolapse, the urologist and the gynecologist may work together, or one may treat both problems.

Obstetrics and Gynecology

In order to become an obstetrician/gynecologist, a medical student applies to a residency that begins immediately after graduating from medical school. Most programs are four years in length and combine obstetrical with gynecological training. Obstetrical training revolves around the treatment of pregnant women. Both the fetus and the mother are patients of the obstetrician. Gynecological training includes learning about the medical and surgical management of women's genital problems. Gynecology is not a surgical subspecialty, in that trainees do not officially spend time in general surgical training. However, gynecologists are trained to perform surgery as part of their general training. After four years of residency at an accredited program, graduates are eligible to sit for the obstetrics and gynecology (ob/gyn) boards examinations and practice general ob/gyn.

As in all fields in medicine, specialty areas have developed in ob/gyn. A resident may spend time with a faculty member in her program and decide that she especially likes one aspect of the field. After completing the preliminary four years of general ob/gyn training, she can enter a fellowship. Fellowship areas in obstetrics include maternal/fetal medicine and high-risk obstetrics. Areas of concentration in gynecology include reproductive medicine, advanced laparoscopy, oncology (cancer), and urogynecology. Most of these programs require an extra two or three years of training above and beyond the general residency in ob/gyn. Unlike urology, ob/gyn offers further formal accreditation for the subspecialty areas.

Urogynecologists learn about the surgical and medical management of urological problems in women. In other words, they manage problems with the bladder and with the female genital organs. This combination makes perfect sense. After all, as I illustrated in the anatomy section, all of these organs are very close together. Without the extra training in urogynecology, many ob/gyns are not comfortable managing urinary problems in women. You have to ask your doctor what his or her comfort level is managing your particular condition.

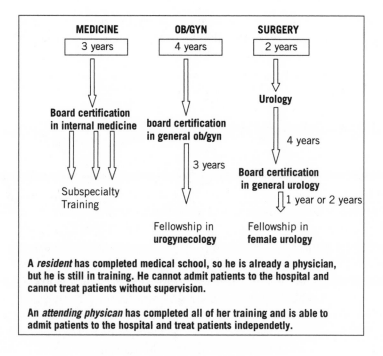

A *resident* has completed medical school, so he is already a physician, but he is still in training. He cannot admit patients to the hospital and cannot treat patients without supervision.

An *attending physican* has completed all of her training and is able to admit patients to the hospital and treat patients independetly.

HOW DO YOU CHOOSE A DOCTOR FOR YOUR PROBLEM?

How do you determine how qualified any given physician is to manage your problem? What does it mean to be a specialist, and is it necessary to have a specialist treat you? The definition of a specialist is nebulous. Anyone can call themselves a specialist. No piece of paper will determine that a particular doctor is really good at what he does. Many patients come to my office and claim that they saw a "specialist," the premiere physician in their area on the subject of female pelvic-floor problems. *And*, he is the director of the "incontinence center." All of these claims may be legitimate. But, what do they mean, and how do you know if the guy really knows what he is doing?

There are several essential questions you must ask the doctor:

- How did he or she *become* a specialist?
- Did he take a course to learn a few surgical techniques and now has opened an "incontinence center"? (not good)
- Did he spend three years in the lab doing research on animal bladders and now understands as much as anyone does about the physiology of the bladder? (very good)

- Did he spend a year studying with a preeminent expert in the field and is now performing the techniques that he learned during that year? (good)
- Did he spend four months as a resident with an attending physician who had a focused interest in the field? (may be good)
- Has he been in practice for 10 years, focusing his interests in one particular field? (very good)

Many specialties today were not recognized 10, or even, 5 years ago. Fellowship directors often became experts on their own. They read extensively on the subject, practiced techniques on cadavers or animals, and eventually translated that information to patient care. Many years of learning and practice have led to their specialization. These physicians become the "grandfathers" of their field, paving the way for younger doctors to take their knowledge and move it to the next level. A fellowship serves as a year of concentrated study in which the fellow (yes, they are called fellows) learns as much as possible from those physicians who came before him. It brings the fellow up to speed in that field and saves years of time gaining experience in that field. Most well-recognized fellowships are directed by the originators of accepted ideas and practices within the field.

As a result of the confusion that many patients experience over choosing a qualified doctor, as well as an effort to share information, the American Board of Urology and the American Board of Obstetrics and Gynecology have attempted to merge the fellowship training for female pelvic disorders. The fellowship would be offered to both urology and ob/gyn residents who have completed a training program, According to the latest plan, the urology residents would complete two years of fellowship training and the ob/gyn residents would complete three years of training. Each combined fellowship would be directed by both a urologist and a gynecologist. A certificate will be awarded to those physicians who have completed the combined program.

The idea sounds good. However, the implementation of the combined program will be very difficult. First, gynecologists and urologists come to fellowships with a very different residency experience. Urologists are trained as surgeons and gynecologists learn about the medical and surgical management of women, as well as obstetrics. Secondly, urologists have six years of residency before they can begin a fellowship. Gynecologists have four years of training. Thirdly, those of us in female urology and urogynecology who have trained before the combined program are not going to support a system of training that does not recognize our expertise as well. So the problems are both practical and political. But, theoretically, the idea is quite good.

Choosing a Doctor

Now the questions are: How do you choose a physician for your urinary problem? And, how do you know that that physician knows what he is doing? What I advise is for you to combine the facts I have outlined above with your intuition. The first consideration, before you get to surgical skills and effective treatment options, is: Does the physician have the interpersonal skills that suit your personality and needs? You need a physician whom you can trust with the most intimate details of your life. You want the physician to respect you enough to listen and validate your complaints. *No matter how well a physician is trained, if he denies that your problem exists, he will not be able to help you.*

Secondly, she should have the time to spend with you in order to understand what the problem is. Many patients still think that the busier the physician, the better he is. If you can't get an appointment for three months, she must be a *really* great doctor. Alas, by the time you get seen and tested, your condition may have worsened.

A clean office and courteous staff are obviously necessary. A thorough and meticulous diagnostic evaluation is imperative. After you give your history, the physician, *not* his nurse, nurse practitioner, or physician assistant, should examine you. If you are going to be seen by a nurse practitioner, you should be told that at the time that you call. If you expect to see a physician, then that is whom you should see.

Finally, she should speak to you about her impression of the problem and what her proposed plan of treatment is. The first visit is an information-gathering visit. You are paying for advice from your doctor regarding your problem. If she is not communicative or can't articulate her assessment, if she is brusque, hurried or inattentive, then she may not be the physician for you. Different physicians have different styles. If her style does not match your personality, then you may want to switch doctors.

After the first visit, you find that you like the doctor. She has been forthcoming with information and was thorough with the evaluation. Now the question is: Is she as capable as she sounds? Does she know what she is talking about? This is where credentials and reputation come in. First, how did this doctor become a specialist in her area? As I discussed above, it is important to have some sense of what the doctor's experience has been. Probably the best validation of a physician's competence is a recommendation from another patient. If another patient reports to you that this doctor was wonderful and attentive, and available throughout the whole treatment process, then that is a pretty good endorsement. However, just because one patient likes a doctor does not mean another patient will. Patient endorsements let you know that you are dealing with someone who has served another person well. You will not know if her style will work for you until you actually meet her.

If surgery is part of the treatment plan, the choice of physician may change. Although bedside manner is important, *surgical skill is paramount in selecting a surgeon.* In this case, patient endorsement is very important. If you know someone who has been operated on by a particular surgeon and the outcome was good, then she is probably a competent surgeon. In selecting a surgeon, it is also important to find someone who is accessible if things don't go as planned. *I always tell patients to choose a surgeon for how she handles complications, not for the cases that go smoothly.*

A surgeon who handles complications efficiently, correctly, and with candor is the type of doctor you want taking care of you. During the first visit with the surgeon, ask him what the possible complications of the proposed surgery are and what he does if he encounters one. All experienced surgeons have had misadventures. If he tells you that there are no complications with this procedure or that he has not had any, he is either not being honest or he hasn't done enough of them. If he tells you that he has been doing his procedure every week for the last 10 years and has seen every possible problem that can occur, he is probably the kind of guy you want operating on you.

In pelvic surgery, postoperative care can be complicated. The availability of the surgeon or one of his staff is crucial. If you have questions or problems, you need to know that the surgeon will answer your questions in a timely fashion, whether it is during business hours, on the weekend, or the middle of the night. A perfect operation can be destroyed by postoperative problems that are not recognized and dealt with expeditiously. Written postoperative instructions are helpful for patients. If a physician gives you written information with all your required prescriptions and dressings preoperatively, he is, most likely, an organized, thorough, and experienced surgeon.

So, now you have found a doctor with whom you can communicate and you feel that you can trust. Is he qualified? If he has met the specifications that I discussed above in terms of training and experience, you are in good hands. Or at least, you have done as much as you can to protect yourself, whether he is a urogynecologist or a urologist.

Background Checks

A cross-check worth mentioning is the databank of physician lawsuits. Available on the internet is a website that informs the public of physicians who have had law suits end in an unfavorable direction. Cases that are settled between a physician and a patient are not made public. Only suits in which a jury decided against a physician are posted on the site. However, just because a physician lost a case does not mean that he is not a competent doctor or surgeon. The information offers another piece of data in your assessment.

A word of caution in using this website information: many physicians who wind up in court are doctors who take on difficult cases—cases in which patients have been operated on multiple times or who have very complex problems. These types of problems may result in poor outcomes. Even though the patient was informed of the difficulty of their case and the possible poor outcome, they may still sue and win. Judgments against physicians in many cases are not a condemnation of their ability as much as their lack of communication with the patient or the patient's own lack of understanding of the potential outcome.

Second Opinions

Second opinions are another way of reinforcing the opinion of a doctor. A good physician will welcome the request for a second opinion. Ask for your records and the results of all of your tests before meeting the second doctor. There is no need to repeat the testing because it will only waste time. If a doctor gets angry at the request for records to be sent to another doctor's office, he may not be the doctor for you. If you like the second guy better than the first, it is perfectly acceptable to transfer your care to the second doctor. *You do not owe anyone anything. You are dealing with your body and your health.* You need to feel confident in the choices that you make in taking care of yourself. I tell my patients that if, for some reason, something goes wrong and you are lying in the hospital, you need to think to yourself: "I needed to do this and I feel confident that my doctor is taking care of me as well as any doctor would." If you can't see yourself feeling that way, don't put yourself in that person's hands. As a realist in cases of surgery or intensive medical treatments, I believe that one should prepare for the worst.

THE LOWDOWN ON HOSPITALS

Now, a few words are in order on the choice of hospital. Hospitals differ all over the country, as does the quality of the ancillary staff, such as the nurses, the orderlies, the social workers, and the food. Although good hospital care can make the difference between a pleasant and unpleasant experience, the physician is the person who is going to either make you better or not. *You choose the hospital for the physician, not the physician for the hospital.* If Doctor X only works out of Hospital Y, then you will go to Hospital Y. It would be foolish to tell Doctor X that you can't have him operate on you because you heard that Hospital Y was not a good hospital. Of course, if someone close to you died at that hospital and you have bad associations with that hospital, you may ask him if he has privileges elsewhere as well. Many doctors will have admitting privileges at more than one hospital, especially if they practice in a well-populated area.

Many different types of hospital exist in the United States. There are *private, for-profit* hospitals that serve a community and attempt to make money in the process. There are hospitals that are associated with a *religious* group, such as Catholic or Jewish hospitals. These hospitals may get some of their support from the affiliated religious group, but not always. Some hospitals will have started out as part of a religious group but then became independent. Just because a hospital sounds like it is affiliated with a religious group does not mean that it is, or that you need to have some association with that religion to be a patient. The relationship is usually just financial, if anything. *Public* hospitals still exist in some parts of the country, such as New York, Los Angeles, and Chicago. These hospitals serve all patients who enter, no matter what the insurance or immigrant status of the patient is. Each hospital is supported by the city or county in which it is located. These hospitals serve as excellent training facilities because they are very busy and the pathology is so varied. Unfortunately, they are usually underbudgeted and in dire financial straits, resulting in cutbacks in staff and supplies. *University* hospitals are affiliated with a medical school that is usually on the same campus as the hospital. The physicians that staff these hospitals usually have teaching responsibilities for both medical students and residents. These are centers of research in both basic science and clinical medicine.

The type of hospital that a physician works in used to be an indicator of the type of practice he runs. For example, physicians that worked in university hospitals were thought to be involved in research and innovative medicine, whereas physicians who practiced in small community hospitals were less up on the newest technology. That is no longer true. Some of the most advanced techniques come out of community environments. University hospitals still tend to appeal to physicians who want to participate in research. However, the lines between all the different types of practice have become finer and finer.

The issue of resident and medical school student involvement in patient care often comes up. Recent attention has been paid to overzealous residents and under-involved attending staff, especially in the operating room. Although some of the stories are probably true, most physicians supervise the residents closely during both surgery and the hospital course. Residents can be assets during your hospital stay. They serve as another set of eyes and ears for the attending physician (that is the official name of the doctor under whose name you are admitted and who is primarily responsible for your care during your hospital stay). If the attending physician is in the operating room or in the office all day, the residents can help to expedite discharges, answer questions, write medication orders, attend to emergencies, order tests, and generally act as a go-between for the patient and her doctor. Generally, they are young, energetic, bright, and eager to learn. Many of them are knowledgeable and quite experienced. In most states, work hours for residents have been curtailed by law, so they no longer work the 100+ week that they used to. They also tend to pass information along from physician to physician. If a new doctor has just joined the staff from another state or medical school and he does a procedure differently, the residents will pass that information around the department. In this way, new techniques get introduced.

Residents also attend meetings and do research projects in many programs. New ideas get disseminated through their efforts and travel. Most training programs in all areas of the country and all specialties require weekly conferences in which cases are reviewed by the entire resident and attending staff of that hospital within that specialty. These conferences are called *grand rounds*. They offer a forum in which literature can be reviewed and different approaches to problems can be discussed. Many hospitals that don't have residents also offer conferences for the attending staff. The requirements for attending involvement in research and academic training are not as rigorous, however, in non-resident hospitals.

HOSPITAL	PHYSICIAN
Academic (medical school)	*Solo practice
Religious	*Multi-specialty group
Community	*Single specialty group
Teaching (with residents)	Hospital-based
Public	
	*Indicates private practice

Finally, the difference between *private practice* and *hospital-based* practice should be discussed. A physician who operates his own office, pays his own overhead, and receives payment directly from his patients or their insurance company is a private practitioner. A physician who gets paid by the hospital is hospital-based. A physician will choose one or the other for a number of reasons. Hospital-based practices used to allow physicians to schedule time for research and academic interests. Part of their salary line was used to pay for non–revenue-producing activities, such as teaching or basic science research. Private practitioners usually choose to be independent of the hospital because they want to control their finances. If they work harder, they can make more money.

However, recent fiscal difficulties within large academic medical centers have shifted the focus for many hospital-based physicians. They have now become responsible for bringing in revenue in order to support their salaries. Many private practitioners have become involved in research, especially clinical research, often through pharmaceutical company funding. Because private offices generate large patient numbers, they are fertile ground in which to conduct research projects. For these reasons, the differences between the two traditional types of practices have narrowed. Frankly, I don't think it matters what kind of practice your physician works in as long as it is clean, the staff is courteous, and the doctor is available when you need her.

Some of the newer types of practices that have emerged include multi-specialty groups and large physician groups. Multi-specialty practices are made up of physicians of all different specialties. They share overhead, and often profits. The advantage of this type of set-up for the patient is that you get one-stop shopping. You can see the internist, the gynecologist and the urologist in the same place, perhaps even on the same day and most tests can be conducted on-site. Charts are usually shared, so information is easily transferred among each of the specialties.

Large physician groups within one specialty have also become common. These large groups allow the physicians within them to specialize in one specific area of practice within the general field. For example, in urology, a large group may have a laparoscopist, a stone specialist, a female urologist, an infertility doctor, and an oncologist, as well as general urologists. The physicians refer patients to one another depending on the problem that the patient has, and the specialist needed. This set-up allows patients to get the most advanced care within a single practice.

SUMMARY

Although the choices seem overwhelming, the truth is that it all comes down to the person sitting across the desk from you and how *you* relate to her. The more confident you are in the information that you are getting from your doctor, the more you can trust him or her. Trust and confidence in your physician are absolutely imperative to the therapeutic process. If you don't believe in your doctor, you cannot have a positive relationship. You don't have to like her, but you do have to trust her. The best way of assessing your physician is intuition, but intuition bolstered by understanding her background and training for your particular medical problem.

PART TWO

URINARY LEAKAGE AND INCONTINENCE

CHAPTER 4

Stress Urinary Incontinence

Leakage with activity: cough, laugh, sneeze, run
Occurs during the day
No frequency
No urgency ⎫ **If you have these as**
No pain ⎬ **well, you may have**
No getting up at night to urinate ⎭ **mixed incontinence,**
                                                   so read Chapters 6 and 7.

A woman, J., came to see me and told a fairly typical story regarding her problem with incontinence. Two years ago, at the age of 55, J. developed urinary leaking. It began gradually with coughing, laughing, sneezing, or exercise. She simply changed her underwear when necessary or wore a thin pad for protection. She thought nothing of it. During her annual visit to the gynecologist for a PAP test, she mentioned the problem to the doctor, who suggested that she have surgery to correct the problem. The doctor explained that her uterus was pushing on the bladder, causing the leakage, so a hysterectomy and bladder lift would solve her problem. After discussing it with her husband, she consented to the operation; after all, it made sense. She couldn't have any more children, and the leakage was annoying.

The surgery seemed to go well. She had her uterus removed and her bladder lifted, all through a small bikini incision in her abdomen. She remained in the hospital for five days before returning home. It took her about a month to recover her strength and return to work. She felt great, but the leakage resumed almost immediately after the surgery. Her gynecologist felt that further scar tissue formation may take care of the leakage.

Six months after the surgery, her leakage was worsening. She tried medications, but they did nothing, except dry out her mouth. Jan was now in minipads, and was ready to get another opinion.

When I saw her, she had healed well from the hysterectomy. She brought the operative reports of her previous surgery with her so that I could see what her gynecologist had done. I realized that, although her bladder was well supported, he did not put any support under her urethra. The weakened muscles that resulted, most likely, from her vaginal deliveries were not reinforced, resulting in continuation of her leakage. Although easily corrected, this problem is not going to respond to medication. She would need another operation to insert a pubovaginal sling under her urethra. The vaginal operation would take about 30 minutes to perform and could be done outpatient or with a short overnight stay. Anesthesia would be required.

No waiting period due to her recent surgery was necessary. She consented immediately because she wanted to get on with her life. The surgery was performed on a Wednesday, she went home on Thursday morning, and returned to work the following Tuesday. J. is now dry, wears no pads, and is very satisfied with the results.

Jan suffered from stress incontinence, which is the involuntary loss of urine during activity. Nothing to do with emotional stress, stress incontinence refers to leakage during *physical* pressure that is exerted on the bladder resulting in squirting urine through the urethra. The most common causes of leakage include coughing, sneezing, laughing, exercise, and sudden movements. Accidents involve losses of varying amounts of urine at frequent intervals, regardless of the fullness of the bladder. Women with pure stress urinary incontinence report leakage during the day, primarily. Some women will wear pads at night as well. When asked, they report squirting urine when they turn over in bed or when they get up in the middle of the night to use the bathroom, as opposed to *awakening* from sleep with a wet pad or nightgown.

In contrast, urge incontinence is the involuntary loss of urine without a precipitating event. Some women will report leakage when they get an urge to urinate (thus, the name "urge" incontinence), while others will wet without warning. Urge incontinence occurs without rhyme or reason; a woman can be sitting in her chair and just begin to leak. Generally, urge incontinence is accompanied by urgency to urinate, frequency of urination, and awaking at night to urinate. **We distinguish among all of the different types of incontinence because the treatments differ.**

These two types of urinary incontinence are the most common leakage problems suffered by women. Total incontinence and overflow incontinence are less common, but need to be ruled out before successful treatment can ensue. Understanding the different types of incontinence is easier when they are compared with one another. To complicate matters, most women, especially those in their postmenopausal years, suffer from some combination of incontinence.

Stress incontinence and *urge incontinence* are the most common types of urinary leakage suffered by healthy women who have not had surgery, or who have no neurological problems. Distinguishing between these two types of leakage is very important because the treatments are vastly different. Stress incontinence is mostly a surgical problem, while urge incontinence is treated more with behavior modification and medication. If a woman has primarily urge incontinence, surgery will not correct her problem. Before we had medications to offer patients, surgery was done more often because we had no other options available to patients. Many women did not get better in spite of the surgery because many of them had urge incontinence. The operations got a bad reputation because of these failures. Now, we have more sophisticated diagnostic tests to help clarify the cause of the leakage, as well as directed treatment options. Surgical failures have diminished in number as a result.

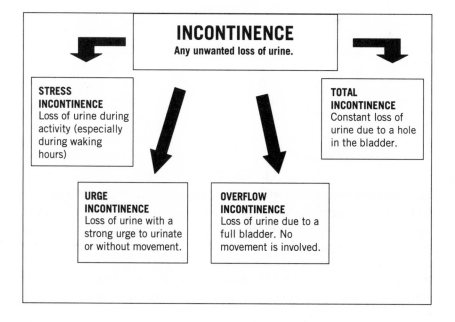

INCONTINENCE
Any unwanted loss of urine.

STRESS INCONTINENCE
Loss of urine during activity (especially during waking hours)

TOTAL INCONTINENCE
Constant loss of urine due to a hole in the bladder.

URGE INCONTINENCE
Loss of urine with a strong urge to urinate or without movement.

OVERFLOW INCONTINENCE
Loss of urine due to a full bladder. No movement is involved.

Although the distinction between the two types of incontinence seems fairly straightforward, many women suffer from a subtle combination of both. Usually, by the time a woman comes in to see me for her urinary leakage, she is so fed up with it that she doesn't know when it happens or why it happens. She only knows that she leaks and she can't stand it anymore. A few simple questions on my part usually can determine which type if incontinence is likely to be more prominent. Physical examination and testing will sort out which direction we will go in order to get some relief.

	Stress Incontinence	Urge Incontinence
Characteristics		
Cause of Leakage	Activity	Urge to urinate, or nothing
Time of Leakage	Day	Day and night
Risk factors for developing leakage	Vaginal childbirth Hysterectomy	Age-related—older Neurological problems
Pathology	Weak urethral support Normal bladder	Bladder spasms Normal urethra
Treatment	Exercises Surgery	Behavior modification Exercises Medication Nerve stimulators
Associated problems	Bladder Uterine Intestinal Rectal } Prolapse	Stroke Multiple sclerosis Back injury

CAUSES AND RISK FACTORS OF STRESS INCONTINENCE

Stress incontinence occurs when the urinary sphincter is not able to close tight enough to prevent the leakage of urine through the urethra during increases in bladder pressure. It is called "stress" incontinence because mechanical pressure, or stress, needs to be exerted on the bladder in order for the leakage to occur. The "stress" may be very mild, like leaning over, or it may be great, such as with high-impact aerobics. Whenever direct mechanical pressure on the bladder results in urinary leakage, you are said to have "stress incontinence."

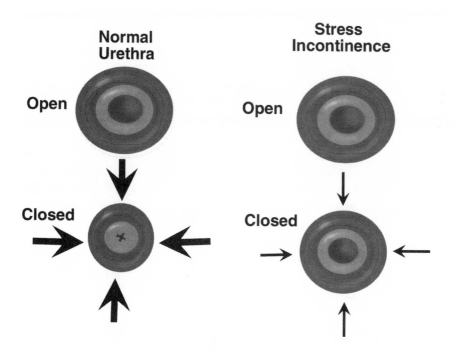

FIGURE 1.

The reason that the urine leaks has nothing to do with the bladder. In pure stress incontinence, the bladder is totally normal. The problem is with the urinary sphincter or the muscles surrounding the urinary sphincter. The urinary sphincter is a ring of spongy tissue that lines the inside of the urethra, the tube that brings urine from the bladder to the outside. That ring of spongy tissue is sealed closed during resting position. During urination, the walls will fall away from one another and allow the urine to drain. If the walls are damaged, during the trauma of childbirth or surgery, they will not seal closed in the resting position. The small breaks in the seal will allow urine to exit if pressure is exerted on the bladder walls.

The muscles that support the urethra play an important role in maintaining continence. When you move from, say, a sitting to a standing position, the urethra presses down on those supporting muscles. In a continent patient, the muscles stay fixed during movement, allowing the urethra to compress against the backboard of muscle and remain closed. If those muscles are weak, as a result of childbirth, surgery, or hereditary misfortune, the urethra will descend with movement and not remain sealed.

In summary, damage to the urinary sphincter or to the muscles that support the urethra will lead to stress incontinence. If only one area is damaged, you can still suffer from leakage. The degree of leakage does not correspond to which area is involved. We used to make a distinction between the two areas of damage and treat the patient accordingly. However, we no longer determine where the problem lies: the sphincter or the muscles. We treat both problems the same way.

CAUSES OF STRESS INCONTINENCE

Defect in the urinary sphincter
Weakened pelvic floor muscles

Stress urinary incontinence will generally begin after a vaginal delivery. Typically, the leaking will begin toward the end of the pregnancy, and will continue during the first few months of the post-partum period before resolving. Occasionally, there will be squirts of urine into your underpants with bursts of activity, such as playing tennis or swinging a golf club. Over the ensuing years, the leakage may worsen, requiring you to wear a minipad. As menopause approaches, the leakage will get worse. The minipad will now need to be replaced many times during the day, until finally, a larger pad is

Normal   **Post-trauma**

Open

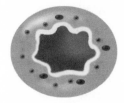
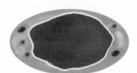

Closed

FIGURE 2.

needed. The problem is not so bad at night. As a matter of fact, no pads are required at night.

In some cases, the incontinence will continue and not improve with time. If the delivery was particularly difficult, if forceps or a vacuum extractor was used, or if the baby came out breech, then the stress incontinence may not improve. It is wise to wait a few months postpartum to see where the symptoms finally settle out. It is impossible to predict how you will do and how anyone will heal after a vaginal delivery. For this reason, no immediate decisions should be made regarding treatment.

The teaching has always been that a woman with stress incontinence has to have had either a vaginal delivery or a hysterectomy. If she has not had either risk factor, then she cannot have stress incontinence. However, my experience has shown that that is not always the case. There are women who have had no pelvic disorder or traditionally recognized risk factors but may still have pure stress incontinence. Family history turns out to be an important consideration in these women. Upon questioning, many of you will remember that your mother had some sort of problem with her bladder. In many cases, nothing was done, and certainly, your mother may not have felt comfortable discussing it openly with family members. The details are not always available, but family history generally can be found in many women with stress incontinence.

RISK FACTORS FOR STRESS INCONTINENCE

Vaginal delivery
Family History
Age

Age plays a role in the manifestation of stress incontinence as well. Older women tend to display symptoms more often than younger women. Many women with mild symptoms of stress incontinence in their 30s and 40s will have worsening of their symptoms as they go through menopause. Many women with no problems in their childbearing years begin to have problems during menopause and after. The exact effect(s) that hormonal changes have on the bladder, the urinary sphincter, and the muscles of the pelvic floor is not yet fully known; however, there appears to be some impact. (see Chapter 10) Most of the surgeries that are done for stress urinary incontinence are done on postmenopausal women.

EVALUATION FOR STRESS URINARY INCONTINENCE

Evaluation of the stress-incontinent woman includes a thorough history, physical examination, urine studies, and, in some cases, more invasive testing to rule out other problems. The history is the most important aspect of the assessment. Listening carefully to the woman's symptoms will usually identify where the problem lies. In many cases, more than one type of incontinence problem exists in the same person. This dual diagnosis is called *mixed incontinence*. Because mixed incontinence is so common, many clinicians will do more extensive testing in most patients to be sure they do not miss anything before treatment begins.

OFFICE EVALUATION FOR PATIENTS WITH STRESS INCONTINENCE

Thorough history
Physical examination
Urine analysis
Urine culture
Optional:
    Post-void residual urine volume
    Voiding diary
    Cystoscopy
    Urodynamics

History

The history begins with a description of the problem. Questions that your physician will want to know include:

1. *What Causes You to Leak?*
   - Is it precipitated by a sudden urge to urinate?
   - Does it happen with activity, like walking or running? Or while coughing, sneezing, or laughing?

Determining the cause of the leakage from a medical history is one of the most important factors in determining from which type of incontinence you are suffering. If you leak with activity or coughing, then you have, at least, some component of stress incontinence. The answer to this one simple question will make at least part of the diagnosis. Every activity may not cause leakage, and the amount of leakage may not be the same every day, but if any degree of activity causes a squirt of urine, then stress incontinence can be diagnosed. But keep in mind, not every diagnosis needs a treatment, and just because a little leakage occurs with activity does not mean that it needs to be treated or that it is the only source of the problem.

2. Do You Leak at Night or during the Day? Which Is More of a Problem?

Women, who leak only during the day, with no leakage at night unless they get up to go to the bathroom in the middle of the night, usually have stress incontinence. Since stress incontinence is caused by activity, sleeping will not cause leakage. Most women with pure stress incontinence do not leak unless they are standing. Even sitting will not cause leakage, although moving from a sitting to standing position may.

3. Do You Feel the Leakage?

Some women do not know when they are wetting. They may notice that the pad is wet when they get to the bathroom to pull down their pants or they may feel the urine run down their legs. In many cases, the actual squirt of urine can be felt as it leaves the urethra, but it cannot be prevented or controlled. Most patients with pure stress incontinence can feel the leakage as it is happening.

4. Do You Wear Pads? How Thick Are They—Minipad or Diaper?

Wearing pads is a very difficult reality for many women to accept. In some cases, a woman will not "succumb" to wearing a pad because she feels like it represents a lack of control, another index of aging, a diminishing of self that most of us are loath to acknowledge. She will not allow herself to "go there." I hear this self-blame on a daily basis when discussing incontinence with women. Quantification of pads is helpful in objectively determining how bad the problem is. If you are soaking three or four large pads every day versus a small minipad once per day, then the interventions may be different. However, each person's experience is her own. So, if you get a spot of urine on a minipad once a day and it really upsets you, then that cannot be minimized. But all the information together helps the doctor get an idea of the whole picture.

Since many women do not wear pads, further questioning may be needed to get a good sense of how bad the problem is. Some of you will carry extra underwear and change as needed. Some fold up toilet paper and layer it in your underpants. All of these maneuvers give the clinician some sense of how problematic the leakage is and how much it inhibits your activities. Often those of you who refuse to wear pads are the most bothered by the problem.

5. Do You Urinate Frequently—More Than Every Two Hours?

If you go often, is that because you have an urge, or is it because you don't want to leak? Frequency of urination can often give clues to the type of incontinence a woman has. If a woman has a strong urge to urinate every hour or two during the day and two to three times per night, she may have problems with her bladder that do not have anything to do with the stress incontinence. Women with pure stress incontinence generally do not have urinary frequency and do not get up to go to the bathroom more than once or twice per night. Urgency and frequency can be related to urinary tract infections and urge incontinence. This finding on history should alert the practitioner to look at the bladder more closely.

Some women with stress incontinence try to limit the amount of leakage by urinating more often. The less full the bladder, the less they will leak. If the frequency is not related to a strong urge, or if you can sleep through the night without getting up, then your bladder is probably not the source of the frequency. The frequency is more of a behavioral method to limit the amount of leakage.

6. Can You Hold It If You Get an Urge or Will You Leak on the Way to the Toilet?

If you have stress incontinence, you do not leak with an urge to urinate. You may leak on the way to the bathroom with an urge to void, but if you are sitting in a chair and get an urge to void, you will not start to leak into your underpants while sitting. When moving from a sitting to a standing position, the leakage may begin, and continue on the way to the bathroom. Although these details seem petty, they can be very helpful in sorting out where the main problem lies.

7. Do You Wake Up at Night Because You Have to Go to the Bathroom?

This can be a tough question to answer since so many people have sleep problems. If you wake up in the middle of the night for any reason, you will most likely go to the bathroom, whether the urge is there or not. If the urge to urinate is so strong that it awakens you from sleep, then that is significant in determining the problem. Women with pure stress incontinence usually do not wake up more than once or twice because they have to urinate.

8. Do You Drink More Than Four Glasses of Fluid per Day? What Do You Drink, How Quickly, and When Do You Do Most of Your Drinking?
The answer to each of these questions will help determine what type of incontinence the patient is experiencing and whether or not behavioral changes can be helpful in reducing the amount of leakage. The eight-glasses-of-water-a-day recommendation by many physicians and nutritionists does nothing for women who are constantly in the bathroom. Eight glasses of water in addition to coffee, tea, wine with dinner, and all the water in the foods we eat can throw any borderline bladder into complete disarray. If a woman with any urinary leakage, or urinary frequency, tells me that she is drinking over four glasses of water per day in addition to her baseline coffee, etc., I tell her to first cut down on the fluids before undergoing any further evaluation or treatment. Surprisingly, many women are resistant to changing their fluid intake. They are convinced that the water helps keep their skin smooth and hydrated, and contributes to overall health. Of course that may be true, but the downside of all that fluid is that it is destroying their quality of life. Moreover, all that water is going through their system and is not being absorbed by the skin and hair. If it were, they would not be in the bathroom all the time!

Too much water can actually wash out the concentration gradient of the kidneys. The more a person drinks, the less likely the kidneys are to reabsorb the excess water. The kidneys get lazy because they expect that the water will continue to be replenished. The kidneys do not need to chase after the water that comes through them and recapture it. For this reason, it may take a few days for the output to slow down after the water consumption stops. In addition, you will feel thirsty because water is being depleted and not replenished. The kidneys will recover and the urine will start to turn more yellow, but the change may not be noticeable immediately. If you sip instead of chugging water throughout the day, your system will recover and the thirst will resolve. Often simple lifestyle changes can improve matters enough that major interventions are not necessary.

STRESS INCONTINENCE BY HISTORY

1. Activity, coughing, laughing, sneezing causes incontinence.
2. Worse during the day than at night.
3. Leakage can be felt as it is happening.
4. Uses anywhere from no pads to multiple diapers in one day.
5. Frequent urination is not a problem.

STRESS INCONTINENCE BY HISTORY—continued

6. No leakage with a strong urge to urinate.
7. Getting up at night to urinate is not common.
8. Limits water intake to reduce leakage.

Once you give a good description of the leakage to your doctor information regarding the risk factors for the development of incontinence needs to be reviewed. History of vaginal deliveries and the nature of those deliveries may be important. If forceps or a vacuum extraction device was used, that may indicate trauma to the pelvic muscles during the delivery. Protracted labor or a large baby can strain the muscles surrounding the vagina. Past history of a hysterectomy needs to be discussed. The reason for the surgery plays a role.

Family history of incontinence may have some impact. It seems that stress incontinence, as well as pelvic floor prolapse, runs in families. Among elderly women, especially in previous generations, the affected family member did not want to discuss her urological problems with others. The family may know that a problem was present, but the details were never discussed. The more information that can be obtained, the better it is for the physician.

Physical Examination
After the history, the physical examination may be the most important aspect of the evaluation of the incontinent woman. The clinician will ask you to remove your clothes, including your underpants, and wait for her on the examining table. A pelvic exam will be performed, during which you will be asked to cough while the doctor observes the urethra and pelvic floor. If you squirt urine through the urethra while lying down with an empty bladder (patients usually empty their bladders and give a urine sample upon entering the office), then you have stress incontinence. Not all women with stress incontinence will leak at this time, but if leakage occurs, the diagnosis is made.

If no leakage occurs, the practitioner may ask you to stand up and cough. If no leakage occurs at that time, he may choose to fill your bladder with water about one-third to one-half of its capacity (100 to 150 cc, or 4 to 6 ounces of water) to see if leakage will result with a partially full bladder. If this is done, a catheter will need to be inserted in order to fill the bladder. She will ask your permission to insert the catheter since it is a mildly invasive procedure. It is slightly uncomfortable, but is usually not painful, especially if lubricant is used generously.

The physician will need to do an internal examination of the vagina and the pelvic organs. She needs to identify masses in the pelvic area. Bladder masses can be felt in the middle of the pelvis behind the pubic bone. A mass in this area is considered bladder cancer until that diagnosis can be eliminated by tests. X-rays and cystoscopy will readily make a diagnosis. Masses on the uterus are usually fibroids, benign growths on the uterine wall. Fibroids can enlarge and fill up the entire pelvic region. Generally, fibroids do not create enough pressure on the bladder, which sits in front of the uterus, to cause leakage. Occasionally, I will be asked to determine whether a fibroid is causing bladder problems. The answer is nearly always that it is not. A fluid organ, the bladder will fill in any direction in which it can take up space. If that means that it fills the left side of the pelvis as urine collects and not the right side, then it will shift in that direction. So, a fibroid would need to fill the entire pelvic cavity before it would begin to hamper bladder function.

Ovarian masses, such as cysts, adenomas, and tumors, do not usually present with bladder symptoms. The ovaries sit on the sides of the pelvis inside the abdominal cavity, far away from the bladder. However, if a physician finds a mass on the ovary during an examination for stress incontinence, that finding becomes a priority. It must be evaluated and managed before stress incontinence treatment is initiated.

The physical examination will also identify bladder prolapse, uterine prolapse, vaginal cuff prolapse, and rectal prolapse, all of which can coexist in a woman with stress incontinence. Pelvic-floor prolapse occurs when the organs of the pelvis fall into the vaginal canal because the support of the vagina is weak and cannot suspend the structures that surround it. Stress incontinence is one of the earliest presentations of pelvic floor muscle weakness. With stress incontinence, the tissues that support the urethra are weak, resulting in leakage when pressure is exerted on the bladder.

A woman may not be aware of the presence of a prolapse because it is not always symptomatic. Depending on the degree to which the organ droops into the canal, the sufferer may or may not feel the mass between her legs. Just with a physical examination, the examiner, however, should be able to assess the presence of a prolapse easily, which is important to be aware of when treatments are discussed.

Laboratory Tests

After the physical exam is completed, the clinician will review the urine studies. The urine analysis can be done with a dip stick in the office. It will show if there is blood, white blood cells, protein, or sugar in the urine. The color and the clarity of the urine can be assessed as well. Any abnormality on the urine analysis should be addressed before definitive treatment for the incontinence is discussed. Some physicians will spin the urine down in a centrifuge and look at the cells through a microscope. Bacteria can be seen, as well as red and white blood cells. If an infection is suspected by the urine analysis or the microscopic exam, then the specimen will be sent for culture to define what bacteria is growing and which antibiotics will eradicate it.

If an infection is suspected, it must be treated before the incontinence can be properly diagnosed. Infections alone can be a cause of incontinence. If the infection is treated, the incontinence may go away or improve. Blood in the urine can indicate the presence of a kidney stone or a growth in the bladder. Kidney stones do not usually cause stress incontinence, but they can cause severe pain as they travel down the urinary tract from the kidney to the bladder. Bladder polyps and tumors can cause incontinence, as well as other problems. Both will need to be removed before any other treatment is discussed.

If blood is seen on the urine specimen, a CT scan or ultrasound (a sonogram is the same test) will need to be done to look at the kidneys. A cystoscopy needs to be performed to evaluate the bladder lining. A cystoscopy is a procedure in which a scope is inserted through the urethra into the bladder to visualize the walls of the bladder. A growth on the bladder wall will be easily identified this way.

Many urologists and urogynecologists will want to know if your bladder is emptying well. An office ultrasound can determine if the bladder is empty. In this test, a small probe is rubbed over the skin of the pelvis. An image is transmitted onto a screen that displays the structures under the skin. No radiation is used. The big advantage to ultrasound is that bladder volume can be measured without having to insert a catheter into the urethra. This measurement is not essential but may be useful for some physicians.

Some doctors like to use voiding diaries to get an idea of the frequency of urination and the degree of leakage throughout the average day for the woman suffering from incontinence. A three-day record is kept that includes the volume of fluid taken in, the number of times you urinate, the volume emptied with each visit to the bathroom, and a record of the leakage. Some physicians want the amount of leakage estimated. Although it is a cumbersome task, the voiding diary can be an excellent tool for communicating the degree of the problem and assessing the success of therapy.

In many cases, no further testing is done and the treatment options are discussed with you. If any concern arises over other bladder issues elucidated by the voiding diary, the history, or the physical exam, then urodynamic studies (also called cystometrics) should be done (see Chapter 12 and the Glossary).

Aspects of urinary behavior can be gleaned from the history that indicate further testing is warranted. Those of you who wake up more than twice per night or who cannot hold it during the day for more than two hours at a time may have problems with the functioning of the bladder itself, not just with the supportive structures that surround the bladder. Those of you who leak with an urge to urinate, or when sitting in a chair, have urge incontinence. Urge incontinence is treated very differently from stress incontinence. If any question regarding bladder function exists, then urodynamic studies should be done before any definitive treatment is offered.

The information obtained from urodynamic testing can be extremely useful and may help prevent unexpected outcomes, especially if surgery is being considered as an option. Over 60% of women with incontinence suffer from a combination of urge and stress incontinence, which we label *mixed incontinence.* They will leak with movement (stress incontinence) and they will not always make it to the toilet before they lose a few drops of urine (urge incontinence). The problem that bothers you the most should be treated first. Urge incontinence is mostly treated with medications, whereas stress incontinence is treated with surgery. Many women prefer to try the medication first to see if the urge component can be controlled. The leftover leakage that comes from the stress incontinence may not bother you enough to undergo surgery. If the stress incontinence component is bothersome, then you need to be aware of the fact that you may need medication after surgery to control the urgency and urge incontinence if it persists.

Now that the evaluation is over, treatment options can be discussed. Just remember, time is on your side. You do not need to make any quick decisions. Research, second opinions, and just plain old pondering the options cannot hurt before any decisions are made.

TREATMENT OPTIONS FOR STRESS URINARY INCONTINENCE

Behavioral Modification
Fluid restriction
Timed voiding
Kegel exercises
Biofeedback

TREATMENT OPTIONS FOR STRESS URINARY
INCONTINENCE—continued

Medication
  Pseudophed
  Imiprimine
  Estrogen
  Duloxetine
Injection Therapy
  Collogen
  Durasphere®
Surgery
  Sling
  Abdominal surgery
  Laparoscopic surgery

TREATMENT OPTIONS FOR STRESS INCONTINENCE

Stress incontinence remains primarily a surgical problem. Although other options for control of the leakage are available, the best chance of cure lies with surgery. New treatment options lie on the horizon, but as of now, none of them offer the same chance of cure as surgery does. Other interventions can reduce the amount of leakage, which may be all that is necessary for some of you. Small degrees of leakage can be minimally bothersome to some women but horrible to others. Less-invasive options should be explored before taking the surgical plunge.

Behavior Modification
Fluid Reduction
Behavioral modification is often implemented by women reflexively. The most common coping strategies include reduction in water and fluid consumption, frequent bladder emptying, and the use of protective pads. The less fluid that you consume, the slower the bladder fills, and the longer one can go between episodes of leakage. Of course, many women are told to drink water for overall health reasons or to lose weight. The reduction in fluid intake is counter to all the advice that most of us are used to getting. Eight glasses of water per day may be healthful for other organs, but it can wreak havoc for the incontinent woman. Each person has to come to a reasonable compromise between water consumption and restriction. All I can

say is that if you are suffering from urinary incontinence and you are drinking eight cups of fluid per day, you may get tremendous relief just from reducing fluids.

Many women think that their urine should be clear. I actually get patients who call and tell me that their urine has turned a very concentrated yellow color. That is the color that urine is supposed to be! If your water consumption results in clear urine, then you are probably drinking a bit too much. Reducing your fluid consumption is the first step.

Timed Voiding

Frequent bladder emptying is another adaptive behavior. Keeping the bladder empty will reduce the amount of leakage that results with each cough, laugh or sneeze. The reality is that the bladder is never *totally* empty, but the less fluid in the bladder, the less there is to leak out. No matter how often one goes to the bathroom, there will always be a little bit of urine left in the bladder.

Timed voiding is the term we use when a person urinates at regular intervals as opposed to when she has the urge to go. Some women will use the bathroom every two hours, for example, to keep the volume of fluid in the bladder down. The result is that when she leaks, a smaller amount of urine will be expelled. Although this adaptive behavior can be effective, it can also be inconvenient. It is not harmful to the bladder and will not result in the development of a "small" bladder. If the bladder never fills to capacity, it does not mean that the bladder will shrink in size and lose its ability to expand.

Kegel Exercises

These exercises were introduced over 50 years ago by a gynecologist who described an intensive program of exercises to help build up the strength of the muscles that surround the urethra and bladder base. The pubococcygeus is the most important muscle that is targeted by the exercise. This muscle supports the pelvic organs and increases the tone of the urinary sphincter. The effectiveness of the exercises lies primarily in their proper instruction and implementation.

Teaching proper technique is the first obstacle to performing the exercises. I find the best way to explain how to tighten the pubococcygeal muscle is to tell women to try to stop the flow of urine during urination. Most people cannot actually stop the flow, but it helps identify the muscles that we are targeting. Once the attempt is made, you finish emptying. When you are doing other activities, like watching TV or driving in your car, you can do the exercises during a commercial break or at a traffic light. No one can see when the exercises are being done because the muscles are contracted internally. Ten contractions can be done at a time. One set is done quickly; the next step is done slowly, counting to five while holding the contraction. Over time, the muscles will begin to tighten noticeably. During sexual relations, your partner may feel you squeezing with your pubococcygeusal muscle, or a physician can feel the contraction during vaginal examination.

Progress with pelvic muscle exercises is slow, so patience is essential. It can take many months of regular exercise before any noticeable change is made. The real test of the effectiveness of the exercises lies in how well it protects you against leakage. The idea behind the technique is that you squeeze your muscles when you cough, laugh, or sneeze. If you are in good pelvic muscle shape, you may be able to prevent or, at least, reduce the amount of leakage.

Biofeedback

More sophisticated muscle training includes the use of biofeedback. Biofeedback involves exercise therapy while being hooked up to a machine that measures the strength and effectiveness of the muscle contraction. Wires are snapped onto sticky pads that are applied to the buttock and inner thigh. These wires are hooked up to a computer with a needle that will deflect according to the success of the contraction. In this way, you will get a response regarding the effectiveness of your effort.

Biofeedback can be taught by anyone who is trained in the technique. The practitioner does not need to be a medical person as long as she knows how to apply the pads and set up the machine. In some cases, you can take the machine home and use it yourself. Many urologists and gynecologists have trained personnel in their offices who will work with motivated women.

The success of pelvic muscle exercises and biofeedback in the treatment of stress incontinence is very difficult to measure. Many women will get better, but not be perfect, and that may be enough for them. Other women will not be happy until they are completely dry. Women who leak at night while moving during sleep cannot implement the contractions and will not get better. Other women who leak with coughing or laughing may get excellent results. Kegel, himself, reported a 90% improvement among the women he worked with who had pure stress incontinence. These impressive results have not been reproduced by other skilled practitioners.

Physical Therapy

A specialization of physical therapy has been developed that deals with exercises to reduce leakage due to stress incontinence. Working with patients on a weekly or biweekly basis, the physical therapist develops the tone of the pelvic-floor muscles. The one-on-one attention ensures that you are exercising your muscles effectively. Different techniques are employed by the therapist to target the weak areas. Skilled practitioners are difficult to find, but the field is growing in response to the rising demand by patients. Medical insurance does not routinely pay for this type of physical therapy, so out-of-pocket expenses can be high. However, between the physician, the physical therapist, and the patient, coverage for the therapy can often be obtained.

In my experience, Kegel exercises are worth a try. They are easy to do, do not interfere with possible future treatments, and are useful for sexual activity even if they do not satisfy in terms of stress incontinence.

Medication
Medical therapy for stress incontinence has proven to be elusive. No medications alone will cure stress incontinence. As with exercise therapy, medication serves as a temporizing measure until the problem becomes bothersome enough for surgery. The original medical treatment for stress incontinence was a class of medications called α-*adrenergic agonists*. This class of drug acts to increase the resistance of the urethra and the bladder neck so that urine will not sneak through. A form of these medications can be bought over-the-counter for use as cold remedies. The most commonly known type is pseudoephedrine (Sudafed®).

MEDICATIONS FOR STRESS INCONTINENCE

Alpha-agonists
Imipramine
Estrogen
Duloxetine

Alpha-Agonists
The theory behind using these medications sounds good, but the results are poor. First of all, the studies that led to the use of alpha, or α,-agonists, in women were done in men. Men have a large number of α-receptors in the bladder neck, urethra, and prostate. Because of enlargement of the prostate, men can develop the opposite problem that women have: they cannot urinate at all. The initial treatment for men with outlet *obstruction* is an α-*blocker*, which is the opposite of an agonist. The α-blocker relaxes

the bladder neck, the urethra, and the prostate, allowing the man to urinate more effectively. These medications have revolutionized the treatment of benign prostate disease, reducing the number of surgeries per year to one-tenth of what they were 15 years ago.

The results of these studies were applied to the treatment of female incontinence. If α-blockers relax the prostate, urethra, and bladder neck in men, then they must do the same in women. Therefore, if we give women the opposite treatment, they should stop leaking because the urethra and bladder neck will be tighter as opposed to looser. That all sounds well and good, except that studies did not confirm the importance of these receptors in female continence. These receptors are present in women, just like they are in men, but probably not in the same quantity and with the same responsiveness seen in men. Besides, women do not have prostates, which is the most important target organ for these medications.

Imipramine

Another medication that was thought to help strengthen the urethra but actually produced disappointing results is *imipramine*. Imipramine is an antidepressant (in the class of tricyclic antidepressants) that relaxes the bladder and tightens the urinary sphincter in low doses. At higher doses, it acts as an antidepressant. The reason it came into effect is that depressed patients were noticing that their urinary problems were improving while they were on this medication. In reality, imipramine is more effective in treating urge incontinence than in treating stress incontinence. The bladder-relaxing effects are stronger than the sphincter-strengthening effects. The main side effect of imipramine is drowsiness, so it is better taken at night.

Estrogen

The benefit of estrogen in the treatment of stress urinary incontinence is not well characterized. Although estrogen receptors have been isolated in the urethra, the bladder neck, and the body of the bladder, their contribution to continence is not understood. Estrogen taken in pill form, or as a patch, clearly does not improve incontinence enough to warrant its use solely for this purpose. However, menopause seems to play a significant role in inducing the onset of leakage, which suggests that estrogen deficiency makes incontinence worse. The relationship remains under investigation. In addition, hormone replacement therapy in women must be carefully weighed against other risk factors, especially if you have a history of breast, uterine, or ovarian cancers.

Estrogen vaginal creams and suppositories, may help to boost the effects of other treatments. Through increasing the blood flow to the tissues, estrogen cream may beef up the cells of the urethra and help seal the tissues closed during coughing or laughing. Generally, estrogen cream alone will not cure the problem, but is it usually added to the treatment regimen of most postmenopausal women with stress incontinence.

Estrogen creams can be particularly helpful preoperatively in women who are preparing for surgery. If the vaginal tissues are dry and thin, cream applied nightly for a few weeks before an operation can increase the blood supply to the skin. Healing is improved and the infection rate may, theoretically, be reduced.

Duloxetine
The first medication that is being developed solely for the purpose of treating stress urinary incontinence is still awaiting FDA (Federal Drug Administration) approval. It is called **Duloxetine**. It is an SSRI (selective-seratonin reuptake inhibitor, like Prozac®, Zoloft®, and Paxil®). Duloxetine works at the level of the spinal cord and at the level of the pudendal nerve, the nerve that controls the urinary sphincter. The mechanism of action involves increasing the amount of the neurotransmitters, norephinephrine and serotonin, that bathe the nerves that help the urinary sphincter con-tract. The longer that these neurotransmitters are exposed to the nerves, the longer the nerve is stimulated to function. The longer the stimulation, the more durable the muscle contraction effected by the nerve. In this case, the pudendal nerve stimulates the contraction of the urinary sphincter for a longer period of time, resulting in better urinary control.

No other incontinence medication on the market works in the way that Duloxetine does. It is the only drug that has been developed solely for the treatment of stress incontinence. All of the other incontinence medications

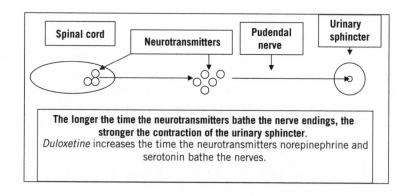

The longer the time the neurotransmitters bathe the nerve endings, the stronger the contraction of the urinary sphincter.
Duloxetine increases the time the neurotransmitters norepinephrine and serotonin bathe the nerves.

that are available treat urge incontinence. Although both problems are often present in the same patient, only the urge incontinence component can be treated with medication until Duloxetine is approved. We are eager to see how effective this new medication actually is in patients with stress incontinence.

Injection Therapy

Injection therapy is the next least invasive method of treatment for stress urinary incontinence. Different materials can be injected into or around the urinary sphincter to bulk up the tissue and improve its resistance to outflow. Using local anesthesia or a light sedative, the procedure can be done either in the office or in an outpatient surgical setting. Usually the agent is injected through a cystoscope, although some urologists will place the injecting needle next to the urethra and view the sphincter through a scope after the procedure is completed.

Only two agents have received FDA approval in the United States for use in the urethra. These agents are collagen and Durasphere®. Collagen is a protein that is found in the skin. The product that is used in the United States is called Contigen® and comes from pig skin, which has been denatured to eliminate the DNA, and irradiated to eliminate viruses and immunogenic materials. The collagen is highly purified, easily injected, and biocompatible (it is easily taken up by the tissues in which it is injected). The same material is used in plastic and reconstructive surgery to increase the volume of the lips and cheeks.

Approximately 3% of the population is allergic to collagen. One month prior to a urethral injection, every woman needs to be skin-tested. A tiny amount of collagen is injected under the skin of the forearm of the woman to be treated. If the area becomes red or swollen over the course of the ensuing weeks, then collagen cannot be used.

The problem with collagen products is that they are *too* compatible with the body. The tissues absorb the collagen over time so that the effect that the collagen creates is lost. It is a temporary solution to a chronic problem. The duration of the response varies from a few weeks to a few months. Most women will not become totally dry from collagen, but they may be considerably better. In nearly all cases, re-injection will be necessary.

I tell women that collagen is a temporary solution. If there is an event coming up in which you want to be dry but you are not ready to commit to surgery, collagen can be used for that purpose. Older women who are going on a cruise or who have a wedding to attend in the near future may want collagen to help them through the event without undergoing surgery.

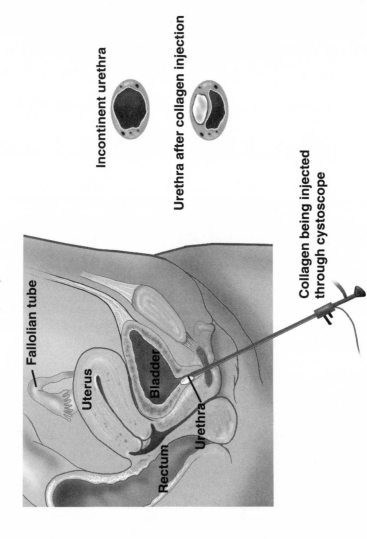

Incontinent urethra

Urethra after collagen injection

Collagen being injected
through cystoscope

Fallolian tube

Uterus

Bladder

Rectum

Urethra

FIGURE 3. *Collagen Injection.*

Collagen needs to be reinforced, however, and is by no means a permanent solution to your leakage problem.

In response to the temporary nature of collagen, a new agent was developed called Durasphere. The material is composed of carbon beads suspended in a gel matrix. These particles are not as easily incorporated into the tissues as collagen, so they remain in position for longer. Some physicians report improvement in symptoms for over two years in women who have been in injected with Durasphere.

The downside to Durasphere is twofold. The first problem is that although more durable than collagen, it is still a temporary solution. Even if it lasts for months or a year, most women will get recurrence of their leakage and will need re-treatment. The other problem is the difficulty of performing the injection. The beads can be sticky, requiring force to evacuate them from the syringe and into the patient's tissues. The new manufacturers are trying to address this problem by reducing the size of the beads. However, if the beads are too small, there is a risk of migration of the particles from the urethra to other parts of the body. This can be a problem. The jury is still out on Durasphere.

Surgery for Stress Urinary Incontinence

Surgery remains the mainstay of treatment for stress urinary incontinence. Although the other treatments mentioned previously will improve the condition, only surgery will cure it. The durability of the surgery and the best type of operation are debatable, but most urologists and urogynecologists would agree that surgery is the only definitive cure for this problem.

Over 200 different operations have been developed to treat stress incontinence. Conceptually, they are very similar. The idea of all stress incontinence surgeries is to replace the support of muscle on which the urethra sits. This support serves as a backboard against which the urethra compresses during activity. If there is no stable surface that the urethra can compress against, the two walls will not come together and urine will squirt out. The different operations are categorized by the area of the body through which the incision is made. The three types of surgeries are *abdominal operations* (in which an incision is made through the stomach muscles or through the bikini line), *laparoscopic surgery* (done through the abdomen but with multiple small incisions as opposed to one long incision), and *vaginal surgeries* (in which the incision is made from the vagina with the woman's legs elevated in stirrups during the surgery). Traditionally, all surgery on the bladder and the urethra was done through the abdomen. Therefore, the first operations that were developed to treat stress incontinence were done through large incisions through the abdominal wall muscles. Now, most surgery to treat stress incontinence is done vaginally.

Standard Abdominal Surgery

The classic Burch colpopexy became the standard surgery against which all others were compared. However, the hospital stay is long: from 5 to 10 days. The abdominal incision can be painful and the exposure of the intestines which results from an abdominal approach results in slow return to normal bowel movements in the early postoperative course. Once the intestines are touched or moved by an external source, peristalsis slows down or stops for a short time. The strong demand for less invasive surgery brought on the new methods of repair, whose results are still compared with the Burch.

Laparoscopic Surgery

Laparoscopic surgeries rely on the same principles as the abdominal surgeries without using a large incision. Carbon dioxide gas is infused into the space between the bladder and the pubic bone to create a cavity into which a camera and instruments can be passed. The surgery is then performed through these ports. Cystocele, rectocele, and enterocele repairs can be done simultaneously, as can hysterectomies.

The original laparoscopic methods were performed through the abdominal cavity, which involved immobilizing the intestines and other internal organs. The newer techniques allow access of the instruments below the vital organs in a space between the bladder and the pubic bone, called the retropubic space. Reinforcing materials can be inserted through the laparoscopic instruments to help secure whatever repair is done.

Laparoscopic surgery is based on sound principles and well-tested open techniques; however, it is not championed by many vaginal surgeons. My reservations regarding the application of laparoscopic technique to vaginal surgery are as follows:

- The defects that are being repaired are located vaginally, so a vaginal approach seems more sensible.
- It involves abdominal incisions, which, although small, some patients find unsightly.
- Instruments are placed near vital organs, such as the bladder and the bowel, which do not come into the surgical field if the vaginal route is taken.
- Finally, the technique is very difficult to learn. It would be comparable to learning to eat with chopsticks when you grew

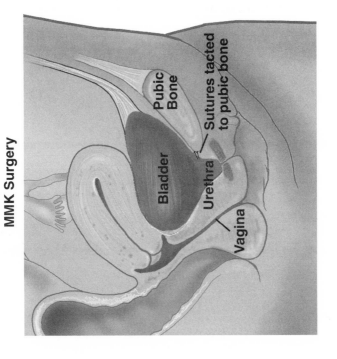

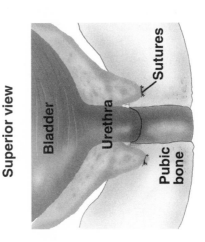

FIGURE 4. *MMK/Burch Surgery for Stress Incontinence.*

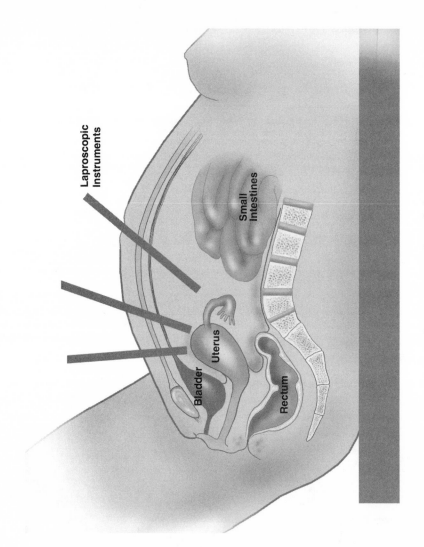

FIGURE 5. *Instruments go through these ports.*

up using a knife and fork. It can be learned, but because it does not offer an advantage over vaginal surgery (and may not even be as good), there is no reason to master the skills needed.

Laparoscopic surgery has many applications. However, in my opinion, it is not the optimal method for repairing urinary incontinence or pelvic floor prolapse. I feel that the vaginal approach is less invasive and offers the most durable repair because reinforcing materials can be placed at the site of greatest pressure, which is *under* the structures being supported. The vaginal approach accesses the structures in question from below. Of course, as with any surgery, the skill and comfort level of the surgeon is one of the most important determinants of the type of repair that should be done.

Vaginal-Approach Surgery

The vaginal approach is the most popular way in which stress incontinence surgeries are performed these days. Two main operations have been developed. They include needle suspensions and pubovaginal slings. The principles of the two techniques are similar in that they strengthen the backboard against which the urethra compresses. Needle suspensions use the native muscle to maintain support, whereas the pubovaginal sling involves applying a new backboard. Although many practitioners still do needle suspensions, the pubovaginal sling has become the mainstay of surgical treatment for stress urinary incontinence.

The pubovaginal sling is done through an incision in the vaginal wall. The vaginal covering is dissected off of the urethra and the muscle layer is exposed. A strip of material is then laid in place underneath the urethra and tacked into place. The vaginal skin is then closed over the material. There is tremendous variability in the type of material that is laid under the urethra and the location of the tacking stitches that hold the sling into place until it scars in naturally.

The type of material that the sling is made of is very important. The three main categories are native tissues, foreign tissues, and synthetic, or man-made, materials. The first slings were done using the patient's native tissues. A small piece of material is harvested from under the abdominal wall muscles before the vaginal incision is made. The strip of tissue is then inserted underneath the urethra and tied through the original incision above the pubic bone on the abdominal wall. The theory is that native tissue will create less of a reaction than foreign materials. Infections rates and rejection would not be a concern. The problem with using native tissues is

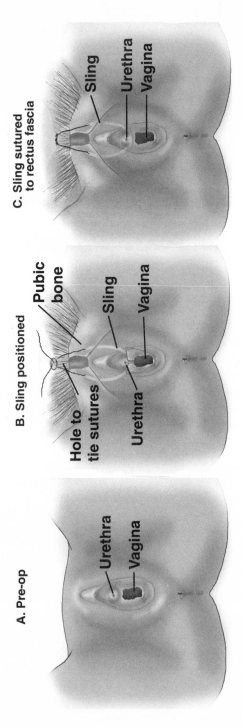

FIGURE 6. *Pubovaginal Sling.*

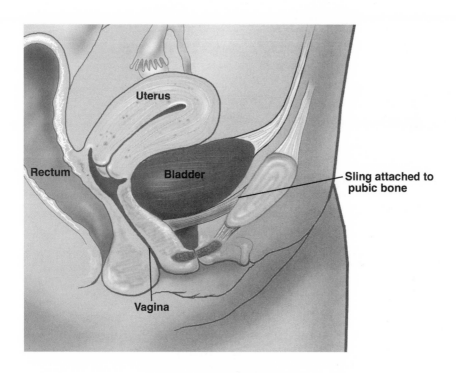

FIGURE 7. *Pubovaginal Sling.*

that they tend to have the same poor integrity as the muscles that failed, leading to the incontinence in the first place. Theoretically, the new strip of support will weaken and the problem will recur. The other criticism of using the harvested material is the extra incision that needs to be made in the abdominal wall. It can be uncomfortable during healing and leaves an unsightly scar that many women do not like.

PUBOVAGINAL SLING MATERIALS

Native tissues (autologous)
Foreign tissues (xenograft or allograft)
 Tissue from cadavers
 Tissues from animals
Synthetic (man-made) materials
 Nylon (polypropylene)
 Gortex(not used anymore)

These concerns led to the development of foreign tissues in the treatment of stress incontinence. When people donate their organs after death, part of their contribution goes into the preservation of tissue for grafts. Those grafts can be used in heart surgeries, joint surgeries, and incontinence surgeries. The material is harvested, frozen, and irradiated to remove all of the materials to which the recipient may react. The tissue is then stored in a bank from which it can be ordered by a hospital. Prior to surgery, the tissue is obtained from the bank and prepared for use in the operating room. Some hospitals will actually bank tissues on their own, although the more common source is private companies who prepare these tissues according to very strict guidelines. Because the harvesting and banking is so technical, these materials can be very expensive to use. The cost of the graft is included in the surgery and is not passed down to the patient.

The convenience of using a foreign graft appealed to surgeons, who did not want to make incisions abdominally. The problems with these cadaveric (coming from a cadaver, or dead person) materials, however, have made them less favorable over the newer materials that are now available. First of all, the theoretical risk of transmission of viral particles cannot be eliminated. I say theoretical risk because no one has actually reported any disease transmission through grafts used for incontinence. The materials are irradiated and chemically processed to eliminate all infectious agents, but there may be small prions that can survive. Prions are proteins that occur normally in harmless form, but by folding into aberrant shape can cause disease that is neither bacterial, viral, nor fungal. Secondly, the processing of the tissues is not uniform from source to source. Processing errors can lead to weakening of the material which jeopardizes the integrity of the surgery. Thirdly, the materials are expensive. A $\frac{1}{2}$-inch by 6-to-7-inch sheet runs a few hundred dollars. Because of these concerns, surgeons started turning to alternative materials.

Tissues from animals were being used with good results in orthopedic and cardiac surgeries. Heart valves from pigs and cows had proven extremely effective, so these same materials were developed for use in vaginal surgery. The durability of the tissues and their plentiful supply make them appealing. However, they do not solve any of the problems that the materials from humans presented. Disease transmission and cost, as well as questionable durability led us to search for alternative materials.

Synthetic mesh has been used in hernia repairs in the groin and the abdominal wall for decades. It is still the material of choice regardless of the method through which it is inserted—open surgery or laparoscopy. Fabricated materials for use in the repair of weakened muscle makes sense for many reasons. They are strong, durable, and inexpensive. Quality control is well-regulated because they are produced in factories through an entirely synthetic process. Their application to vaginal surgery is fairly new, and as with all new ideas, is open for debate.

The materials that have been used in incontinence surgery are all woven mesh, so they have small pores through which scar tissue can form. The size of the pores differs from material to material, but all are large enough to allow adequate healing. The criticism of some of the materials is that the pores are small enough for bacteria to pass through but not large enough for the white blood cells that chase the bacteria. No studies have compared the different synthetic materials with one another regarding infection rate, strength, or durability. All of them seem to have excellent characteristics. If they are inserted correctly, they should result in a good repair.

SYNTHETIC MATERIALS USED FOR PUBOVAGINAL SLINGS

Generic name	*Trade name*
Polypropylene	Marlex
	Proline
Polyethylene	Mersiline
Polytetrafluoroethylene	Gortex

A number of pharmaceutical and medical device companies have put together kits that surgeons can use to insert the sling. The kits come with a precut sling and the instruments that are needed to place the sling in proper position. The ease of using disposable instruments and a pre-fashioned sling has made these kits very popular. No study has shown that one kit is better than any other. All of them result in the placement of a piece of nylon mesh under the urethra. Each surgeon will have his preference. Many surgeons, including myself, do not use kits at all. We make our own slings and use reusable instruments.

SLING KITS

TVT: Transvaginal tape
SPARC
Obtape
TVT obturator
Monarch

The two main concerns with using synthetic mesh for repair of incontinence are infection and erosion of the mesh into neighboring tissues. The infection rate is very low—no numbers are available to even report on this occurrence. Erosions have been reported. Erosion means that the material pushes through tissues and winds up in a place in which it was not intended. In incontinence surgery, undesirable locations for synthetic mesh include the bladder, the urethra, and the vaginal wall.

If the mesh erodes into the bladder or the urethra, the results can be terrible. Nylon in the bladder will cause damage to the bladder wall, painful bleeding, and stone formation. It is very difficult to remove it once it scars into place. The same problems occur with mesh in the urethra. Proper placement of the mesh with careful inspection of the bladder through a cystoscope at the time of surgery will prevent this complication. If mesh is misplaced into the bladder, it can be removed and reinserted at the time of the original surgery with no problem. It is only if it is inadvertently placed and not immediately recognized and removed that serious problems can arise. Again, technique, good surgical skills, and experience will prevent these problems.

Erosions into the vaginal wall do occur, even with excellent technique. About 4% of women will reject the mesh for some unknown reason. No testing or history of allergies will determine which women will react to the mesh and which will not. When the mesh gets pushed through the vaginal wall, the patient will not feel pain or discomfort. She will complain of a pinkish, thick vaginal discharge. The incision will not heal completely, so the mesh can be identified by the doctor on physical examination.

Sometimes, the erosion will not occur for months or even years after surgery. Things are going well, when all of the sudden, a discharge is noted. An edge of the incision of the vaginal wall will be seen or felt by the examiner, and a bloody area is noted. In some cases, the rejected mesh can be cut out in the office using local anesthesia. In other cases, the procedure needs to be done with some heavier sedation in the operating room. The removal of this small area of mesh will not result in recurrence of the leakage. Although it is a nuisance for the woman affected, it is manageable with some simple revisions.

Besides the type of material that is used to create the new backboard for the urethra, the other variable in pubovaginal sling surgery is the location of the attachment of the sling. The sling can be secured to the abdominal wall muscles, the pubic bone, or through an anatomic hole in the pelvic bone called the obturator foramen. No studies have been done that prove the superiority of one location over another. They all have advantages and disadvantages. But, as I have said all along, the skill and experience of the surgeon will determine the outcome. If the surgeon performing the operation has a preference, then the patient is better off allowing him to do what he feels comfortable with. The location of the tacking sutures will not alter the success of the surgery nearly as much as the material from which the sling is made.

Complications of sling surgery need to be mentioned and discussed before any surgery is done. Generally, all of the complications that arise can be handled with a good outcome as long as they are recognized and managed expeditiously. At the time of surgery, bleeding can result from the dissection of the vaginal tissues and the muscle behind the pubic bone. A small space needs to be created to allow the sling to sit next to the urethra. If bleeding occurs during this process, it can be controlled at the time of surgery, or afterward, with pressure and packing the vaginal canal with gauze. If a large amount of bleeding occurs, you will need a transfusion until matters can be controlled. All surgery involves some risk of bleeding. In pubovaginal sling surgery, this risk is low. Although I have never had to transfuse a patient, it can happen.

COMPLICATIONS OF PUBOVAGINAL SLING SURGERY TO TREAT STRESS INCONTINENCE

Bleeding
Bladder injury
Urethra injury
Bowel injury
Urinary retention
New onset of urge incontinence

Injury to the bladder and the urethra can result because those organs lie immediately next to the area of dissection. Inadvertent injuries are easily repaired through the vaginal incision if they are recognized at the time of injury. Many surgeons inspect the bladder with a cystoscope after inserting the sling before closing the vaginal incision. This visual inspection will identify any injuries so that they can be repaired at the time. If an injury is made and repaired, a catheter will need to be left in the bladder for a few extra days to insure complete healing. This determination is made by the surgeon at the time of the repair.

If the hole that is made is large, some surgeons may opt to stop the operation, repair the injury, and close the incision. The sling would then be inserted after the bladder injury is healed. Each situation is dealt with individually. Discussion regarding the handling of this complication should take place when pre-surgical counseling is done. The way a surgeon handles her complications tells a patient a great deal about her skills, her experience, and her forethought.

Bowel injuries are rare in vaginal surgery for incontinence. The intestines lie high above the top of the vagina. Pubovaginal slings are inserted at the opening of the vagina, on the opposite end. Prolapse surgery is more likely to result in bowel problems than pubovaginal sling surgeries, but they can happen. Abdominal and laparoscopic approaches are more likely to result in injuries to the intestines because the intestines are exposed at the time of surgery. However, even in these cases, intestinal injuries are rarely.

Urinary retention, or the inability to urinate, after surgery is a fairly common outcome of pubovaginal sling surgery. It is nearly always temporary. Swelling around the urethra prevents normal urinary flow, which results in the inability to empty the bladder. It can be very unsettling to go from lack of control to no output at all. However, it nearly always resolves.

If you do not urinate immediately after surgery, a catheter will be inserted for a few days before another attempt is made to remove it and for you to urinate on your own. Some physicians will teach you to catheterize yourself to empty your bladder if you cannot urinate on your own. Self-catheterization is fairly simple to perform, but it can be very intimidating to learn. The advantage to self-catheterization is that the bladder will regain its normal function on its own. Before inserting the catheter to empty, you can try to empty on your own. In many cases, you will begin to go within a few days of surgery and not need to catheterize for very long. With an indwelling catheter, an attempt will be made at an arbitrary time, which may be longer than necessary. The only downside to this waiting is that you have to suffer with a catheter for longer than you really need to, and run the higher risk of infection.

If urination does not return to normal with self-catheterization, or removal of the indwelling catheter fails, then the sling may have been made too tight. Generally, physicians wait three months for the sling to loosen on its own and possibly result in normal urine flow. If that doesn't happen, the sling will either need to be cut or removed and a new one inserted. The decision to cut it or remove it is made on a case by case basis. It is determined by the type of material that the sling is made of and the philosophy of the surgeon. If you have normal urination prior to surgery, you will nearly always urinate after surgery. Permanent retention is extremely unusual and usually indicates some sort of underlying bladder disorder.

New onset of urge incontinence can occur after sling surgery. A woman with pure stress incontinence can develop urgency, frequency, and leakage related to the urge to urinate without having these symptoms pre-operatively. In many cases, you do not know that your leakage has changed; all you are aware of is that you still leak. This unfortunate outcome occurs in approximately 8% of women who undergo pubovaginal sling surgery. Often the symptoms will resolve spontaneously without any treatment. Occasionally, medications will need to be taken for the long term. Careful screening can usually predict if urge incontinence will result after surgery, but not always. Just be aware that communication with the surgeon postoperatively will help you manage whatever problems that you may be experiencing.

SUMMARY

To recap, stress urinary incontinence occurs when a woman leaks while coughing, laughing, sneezing, or lifting heavy items. Unlike urge inconti-

nence, stress incontinence results from a problem with the support structures of the urethra, not with the bladder itself. Weakness of the muscles on
which the urethra sits results in movement of the urethra with activity and
leakage. The treatment involves reinforcing or replacing that support,
usually through a surgical procedure. Medication, exercise therapy, and
injectable agents can be tried first, but as of now, the only real cure for stress
urinary incontinence is surgery. On the bright side, with the proper diagnosis, the management of stress incontinence is extremely successful.

CHAPTER 5

Urinary Urge Incontinence
Overactive Bladder Syndrome

Frequency **Urgency** **Getting up at night to urinate**	**Overactive bladder syndrome**
Leaks with urge to urinate **Key-in-the-door accidents**	**Urge incontinence**

Does this story sound familiar to you? R. mentioned to me that she is getting up often throughout the night. She has trouble falling asleep, and getting back to sleep after waking. Although sometimes her active thoughts keep her from falling back to sleep, the urge to go to the bathroom seems to be the cause of her awakening. She goes to the bathroom frequently during the day as well, but that does not bother her nearly as much as the nights. Recently, she has been feeling fatigued, which she attributes to lack of sleep.

For as long as she can remember, R. has gone to the bathroom often. Her family laughs about the fact that she cannot pass a bathroom without using it. At work, her desk is located fairly close to the ladies room, which is important since there are times when she has to go so badly that she is not so sure that she will make it. Indeed, she has had a few accidents in the last month. Those accidents compelled her to seek treatment.

The getting up at night, the frequency during the day, and the accidents have all started to get to her. She no longer enjoys going out to dinner or to the movies because she is self-conscious about needing to use the bathroom all the time. Shopping is a nightmare. She has to know where every bathroom in the neighborhood is before she can venture out.

It was funny at first. Now it is downright unbearable. At the age of 55, she is now wearing pads. In five years, just as she is about to retire, she will probably be in diapers.

The little reading that R. has done on the subject suggests that she should not be having these problems since she did not have any children. She has been healthy her entire life; the only operation she had was an appendectomy at the age of 25. Someone told her once that she should try to hold it longer and she would be able to stretch out her bladder. She must have a small bladder, or something, if it can only hold up to an hour's worth of fluid. If she drinks a cup of water, it will go right through her and she will be in the bathroom 15 minutes later. Of course she barely drinks at all during the day. Now R. is worried that she will become dehydrated because she is afraid to drink water.

She wants to go on a 10-day trip with friends to Europe, but the idea of being on a tour bus for hours every day absolutely terrifies her. At least on the airplane there is a bathroom. If she gets a seat on the aisle, she won't be so embarrassed every time she needs to go the bathroom. Of course, the fear of another accident has her totally preoccupied. The whole idea that her bladder has now taken over her life is very disturbing to R.

After listening to her problem and examining her, I reassured her that many women experience bladder problems as they go through menopause, and which, often, will continue after menopause. Usually, the problem begins with frequency of urination and waking up at night to go to the bathroom, and then it progresses to accidents both day and night. These bladder changes have nothing to do with childbirth. They are related to hormonal changes and age. Some women have worse problems than others, but most people of both sexes will notice some increase in frequency of urination as they get older.

If there was an operation to cure her problem, R. was willing to do it. But there is no operation for her kind of bladder problems. However, there are medications that she can take on a daily basis to control her urge to go and increase the volume of urine that her bladder will hold at one time.

Before she left the office, we discussed her goals of the treatment. I explained that the medication will help her get on with her life, but it will not perform miracles. If she can sleep for at least four hours at a time before waking up to use the bathroom, and hold it during the day for two to three hours at a clip, then the medication is working. It may cause dry mouth, so sips of fluid or sucking on ice or sugarless candy will soothe that side effect. All the side effects are reversible, so if she experiences anything terribly unpleasant, the pill should be stopped, and she should call the office.

R. began taking the medication the next morning. She improved within a week of starting the pills, has had no accidents in the past month, and she is sleeping much better. She is actually considering going with her friends on that trip to Europe, although she still wants that seat on the aisle!

Unlike stress urinary incontinence, urge incontinence occurs in women and men of all ages with varied histories and backgrounds. It is part of a spectrum of symptoms that starts with frequency of urination, urgency of urination, and, may ultimately progress to urinary incontinence. In general, urge incontinence occurs with age; as people get older they are more likely to develop urgency and urge incontinence. Unlike with stress incontinence, childbirth, delivery history, and surgical history do not necessarily contribute to the emergence of urge incontinence. Anyone is at risk for developing this problem. Likewise, everyone is in the position to have it treated.

This combination of frequency and urgency has recently been labeled overactive bladder. The incontinence is the extreme end of the spectrum of symptoms. That does not mean that if you have frequency and urgency you will necessarily end up with incontinence, but it does mean that you do not need to be incontinent to be bothered by your symptoms and want treatment. This newly named category of urinary problems was coined by the International Continence Society (yes, there is an actual organization) in 2002. The novelty of the name, "overactive bladder," suggests that it is only recently that these symptoms have become recognized by the medical community as important and, therefore, worthy of a name.

OVERACTIVE BLADDER

Frequency: urinates over 8 times in 24 hours
Urgency: strong, sudden urge to urinate, with or without leakage

Before we can understand overactive bladder as a syndrome, we first need to define the terminology, which, in and of itself, took decades to agree upon. Normal urinary behavior is defined by no more than eight trips to the bathroom to urinate in a 24-hour period, including awakening from sleep no more than twice at night. Anything more frequent than that is considered "overactive." As anyone who drinks a lot of water during the day can attest to, these criteria are rather loose. On any given day, a woman can go to the bathroom more than eight times and get up more than twice a night to urinate. The key is the degree to which you are bothered by the frequency and whether or not it interferes with your daily functioning. If the urge to go to the bathroom comes on suddenly, interrupting a phone call or a project, then perhaps you need treatment.

In my opinion, the leakage component is a clear indicator of problems requiring treatment. Under no circumstances should a woman wet her pants on a regular basis because she cannot get to the bathroom in time. Leakage due to the urge to urinate is not a normal state of affairs regardless of the degree of frequency. For this reason, I like to distinguish the frequency and urgency component from incontinence. Frequency and urgency is inconvenient; urge incontinence is debilitating.

Before the name "overactive bladder" came into vogue, other labels were given to these symptoms. Urethral syndrome, frequency/urgency syndrome, and urge syndrome were the more popular names.

Urge incontinence is very different from stress urinary incontinence in every way except that they both result in the loss of urine. Stress incontinence occurs mostly during the day, is caused by activity, and is treated with surgery or exercise therapy. Urge incontinence occurs both day and night, is not caused by any identifiable behavior, and is treated with medication and behavioral therapy. History alone can distinguish between the two types of leakage. Any remaining doubt is settled by physical examination. The real challenge lies in the fact that over half of you with stress incontinence also have urgency, frequency, and urge incontinence. Mixed incontinence, the presence of both stress and urge incontinence, can be difficult to tease apart and treat successfully. That is where referral to a specialist and sophisticated testing may come into play.

URGE INCONTINENCE	STRESS INCONTINENCE
Frequency	No frequency
Wakes at night to urinate	Does not awake to urinate
Urgency	No urgency
Leaks day and night	Leaks during the day
Leaks without activity	Leaks only with activity

HOW COMMON IS THIS CONDITION?

How many women in the country suffer from urge incontinence? We don't really know because so many variables are present in each person. First of all, the symptoms vary with fluid intake, physical activity, and the weather. So a questionnaire filled out one day may result in different data from one filled out on another day. Tremendous effort has been put into coming up with surveys that elicit reproducible results, but no foolproof method has been found. Secondly, the definitions are difficult to grasp. Awakening from sleep to urinate is different than getting up three or four times before falling asleep. Urgency with leakage may result because you live on the 22nd floor of an apartment building and you have to wait for the elevator before getting to your door and into the bathroom. Finally, people tend to minimize their symptoms. Denial is a coping mechanism for this embarrassing condition. Often women don't even realize how much they have altered their lives in order to adjust to the frequency and urgency. Therefore, recall bias can play into inaccurate statistics.

Now for some numbers that show that you are certainly not alone in your distress. The most recent information reveals that over 34 million Americans, or 16.5% of the adult population, suffer from urinary urge incontinence. Over 50% of women above the age of 66 have at least one symptom of overactive bladder. Most of these women have experienced at least one episode of leakage. One in three women has had multiple accidents and 14% report leakage on a daily basis. Two percent of women from the ages of 18 to 24 have frequency and urgency, with or without incontinence. The numbers steadily increase with increasing age. Men suffer from these problems nearly as often as women do, especially in the senior age group. Although leakage is less common in men, frequency and urgency occur in men as often as women at a rate of 16%.

Over $26 billion per year is spent on the diagnosis and management of urinary incontinence. This number includes $13 billion in hospital admissions for accidents related to injuries trying to get to bathroom at night, such as falls and fractures. Incontinent hospital patients remain institutionalized longer due to the leakage, which can cause urinary tract infections and rashes. Another $6 billion is spent on pads, diapers, catheters, medications, and outpatient office visits. Loss of income and home care costs round out the remainder of the expenses. This averages out to $3,565 per person per year over the age of 65 in the United States.

CAUSES OF URGE INCONTINENCE

So why do these symptoms happen? Women will say to me "I do everything I am supposed to do. I eat well. I exercise. I take really good care of myself. So how did this happen to me?" Like most chronic medical conditions, we don't really know why certain women develop frequency, urgency, and incontinence *when* they do. But, we do know that most women will eventually have some bladder symptoms. The older we get, the more likely we are to have health problems. Chronic medical conditions can contribute to the development of urge incontinence. Diabetes, Parkinson's disease, multiple sclerosis, dementia, Alzheimer's disease, and back problems predispose a woman to have urinary problems. The longer you suffer from any given illness, the worse your symptoms can become. Not every person with one of these diseases will necessarily have urological problems, but if you have one of these illnesses, your urological problem may be directly attributable to the disease.

An overall debilitated state will not help matters. If you are reliant on a wheelchair and get an urge to urinate, it may take you a while to make it to the bathroom. The delay may result in an accident that would not have occurred had the dynamics of your situation been different. Bed-bound people are more likely to have problems than ambulatory ones. On the other hand, if you are active, you may notice the frequency more than a woman who spends most of her time at home near the toilet.

A history of pregnancy and childbirth certainly predispose a woman to developing a problem. Actual pregnancy may play a role due to the hormonal changes to the pelvic organs and tissues. Vaginal deliveries increase the risk of getting a prolapse, which may lead to urinary problems. Although not proven, the low estrogen levels during menopause have been implicated in urgency and urge incontinence. Pelvic surgery, such as hysterectomy and colon resection, may lead to nerve damage, which alters the activity of the urinary bladder. Smoking, with the chronic coughing and nicotine damage to the nervous system, can increase bladder contractility, which can lead to spasms and leakage.

RISK FACTORS THAT CAN LEAD TO FREQUENCY, URGENCY, AND URGE INCONTINENCE

Older age
Chronic medical problems
History of pregnancy and childbirth

RISK FACTORS THAT CAN LEAD TO FREQUENCY, URGENCY, AND URGE INCONTINENCE—continued

---

Menopause
Pelvic surgery
Smoking
Immobility
Medications
Genetics?

Most women who suffer from frequency, urgency, and urge incontinence are healthy, active women over the age of 65 with no medical problems, or with medical problems that are well under control. Interestingly, the next largest affected group with this condition is younger women. It is true that many nursing home patients are incontinent, but the women who are driving the pharmaceutical industry to come up with treatments are the healthy, active, vibrant elderly who do not want to accept bladder problems as part of the aging process. Changes may occur in the bladder with age, but that does not mean that we have to live with those changes. We wear glasses to aid our failing vision and take medication to control our blood pressure. Bladder disorders should be treated no differently.

IMPACT ON QUALITY OF LIFE

In addition to being inconvenient, frequency, urgency and urge incontinence drastically alters the quality of the lives of those who suffer from it. Social, physical, and psychological functioning can become severely impaired as women take greater and greater pains to cope with their problem. Many women stop going out to movies and social events, exercise is curtailed, and depression sets in. Overall quality of life deteriorates as the preoccupation with bladder control gets worse. *Women with urge incontinence have a lower quality of life than women with heart disease, cancer, and depression.* The sense of shame is overwhelming. Women repeatedly lament to me "If I could only control myself," as if they are to blame for the humiliating accidents from which they suffer.

Physical deterioration is a real concern for the elderly woman who limits her activities as a result of the leakage. While on her way to the bathroom in the middle of the night in the dark, and barely awake, a woman can trip and fall, resulting in fractures and other injuries. Skin breakdown results from the acidic urine bathing the delicate skin of the genital region.

Urinary tract infections increase in frequency due to the moist environment created by the pads and wet undergarments. One of the most common reasons for nursing home admissions is the new onset of urinary incontinence. Families find this aspect of care one of the most daunting and unpleasant, prompting swift admission to a skilled environment.

Every woman who has a problem with frequency, urgency, or urge incontinence, whether she is 18 or 80 deserves to be recognized and treated. The recent recognition of this disorder by both the International Continence Society and the U.S. National Institutes of Health will provide more money for research into the cause and its treatment. At least now that bladder problems of this sort are characterized, and even given a name (overactive bladder), women will come forward and start enlisting their physicians to become more familiar with these disorders and treat them sooner.

THE SCIENCE BEHIND THE PROBLEM: WHAT IS GOING ON IN MY BODY THAT CREATES THESE SYMPTOMS?

Why does one woman develop frequency and another woman does not? The risk factors were mentioned above, but what if no risk factors differ between the two women? They are the same age, both have two children, neither has a prolapse, and both of their mothers passed away in their 70s with no urinary complaints. So, why does one woman have problems and the other does not? It is not clear why. If we can understand normal function, perhaps we will be able to grasp abnormal function and correct it with appropriate intervention. To understand the disease, we must first try to understand the normal activity.

Under normal circumstances, the bladder should not contract unless the conscious mind tells it to. Urine drains into the bladder from the kidneys as a passive process. We cannot "will" our bladders to fill. The bladder fills without increasing the pressure on the walls, sort of like a balloon filling with air. When the bladder reaches its capacity, about 400 cc or 13 ounces, the brain gets a signal that it is time to find a bathroom. The urinary sphincter (muscle) remains tightly closed until the brain signals that it is time to empty. The sphincter begins to open as the bladder contracts. All of this is done under semi-conscious control with very highly coordinated nerve signals between the brain and bladder that run through the spinal cord.

The nerves communicate with one another through chemicals called neurotransmitters. The neurotransmitters attach to receptors at the end of each nerve which sets off a series of signals that tells the organ what to do.

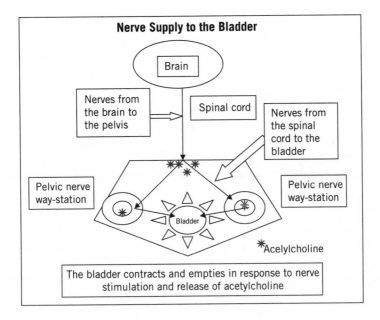

The body produces hundreds of neurotransmitters, each of which functions in a specific way. One neurotransmitter can affect the nerves of many different organs, which is why side effects can occur when medications interfere with the activity of a neurotransmitter. Let me explain.

The nerves between the brain, the spinal cord, and the bladder communicate through a neurotransmitter called *acetylcholine*. When acetylcholine is released by the brain, a signal is sent down the spinal cord, where more acetylcholine is released into the pelvic nerves. The message continues through the pelvic nerves into the bladder, which causes a bladder contraction and urine is evacuated. If the brain is taken out of the equation, the spinal cord and the pelvic nerves can set off a bladder contraction with the release of acetylcholine alone. The person in whom this happens will have no awareness that the activity is going on because the conscious brain has been left out. All of a sudden, a contraction will begin, the urge comes on, and leakage results. The first time that the brain is notified is when the bladder is already contracting. This is called *disinhibition*. The inhibition, or delay in urination, is absent. Inhibition is no longer present. But this explanation begs the question: why is the brain left out of the equation? What prompts the spinal cord to act on its own?

We get our answer from the list of risk factors that lead to the development of urgency and urge incontinence. Let's start with age. As we get older, our brain chemistry changes. Senility is the first sign of changes, and, ultimately, dementia is at the extreme end of the spectrum. But in the middle, subtle changes in the signaling can result in bladder impairment. Not everyone's brain deteriorates at the same rate or in the same areas, so perhaps this difference explains the variability in the presentation of the symptoms.

Chronic illnesses such as diabetes, multiple sclerosis, and degenerative disc disease affect the nerves in the spinal cord and the pelvis. The nerve damage can result in abnormal communication through the neurotransmitters. Pregnancy and childbirth can damage the pelvic nerves, as can hysterectomy and colon surgery. Any break in the communication among the three areas of control; the brain, the spinal cord, and the pelvis, can cause *disinhibition*, and result in urgency and urge incontinence.

Of course, this explanation is simplistic. Other neurotransmitters modulate the response of the bladder to acetylcholine. The effect that receptors play in all of this is also not clearly addressed here, mostly because it is not understood by scientists. The acetylcholine molecule attaches to a receptor which then affects the next nerve. If the receptor is altered in a certain way, it can affect the next nerve in a different way. For many illnesses, medications are available that alter the receptor and not the neurotransmitter itself.

Recent research has focused on the bladder control center in the brain. A number of areas in the brain are responsible for coordinating bladder activity. The cerebral cortex, which is the largest part of the brain in humans and controls thought and conscious behavior, clearly is involved in urinary function. However, the midbrain, which is the control center of the brain and is not under voluntary control, is also responsible for bladder control. A stroke that affects the cerebral cortex, but not the midbrain, will alter conscious control of the bladder, but not coordination. In other words, a stroke patient may urinate in her pants, but she will have an effective bladder contraction and empty completely. If the midbrain is affected, she may get urges with awareness, but not be able to empty, so her bladder will be full all the time.

FREQUENT URINATION AT NIGHT—NOCTURIA

The need to get up at night to go the bathroom is a whole other area of concern for many of you, but it is not included in this syndrome of frequency, urgency, and urge incontinence because it involves so many other factors that do not have to do with abnormal bladder function. An isolated symptom of awakening at night to urinate without frequency during the day is rare and often means that other problems are present as well. Awakening at night has to do with sleep disorders, fluid shifts at night, hormonal changes (not estrogen), and medical conditions. The urge to urinate at night is a different entity that may or may not be a part of the urgency and urge incontinence syndrome.

CAUSES OF NIGHTTIME URINATION

Bladder problem
Sleep problems
Fluid build-up in the legs
Changes in brain chemistry and hormones
Medical conditions
Medications

As people age, their sleep cycles change. Less sleep is needed and frequent awakening occurs. Everyone who awakens at night, regardless of the reason, will go to the bathroom. That seems to be a conditioned response to getting up at night. It is important to determine whether the awakenings are due to the urge to go to the bathroom or due to sleep changes. If this distinction is difficult to make, you can take a sleeping pill for a few nights to see how you do. If you sleep better and do not get up, then, most likely, you have a sleep disorder. If you sleep through the night, but are wet in the morning, then you clearly have a bladder problem in addition to your sleep disorder. If you wake up anyway, even with the sleeping pill, then you have a bladder problem.

Fluid shifts during the night play a role in getting up to urinate as well. During the day, fluid accumulates in the legs due to gravity. When the legs are elevated at night, the fluid enters the circulation and is eliminated by the kidneys. The bladder will fill more often, awakening you during the night. One solution to this problem is to elevate the legs earlier in the evening so that less fluid needs to be removed before bedtime.

Hormonal changes, as well, occur with age. Antidiuretic hormone is secreted by the brain in large volumes at night. Its function is to encourage the kidneys to reabsorb fluid and re-circulate it throughout the body so it does not enter the bladder and cause the urge to urinate. If this hormone is deficient, the kidneys will eliminate more fluid, resulting in bladder filling. Children produce large quantities of antidiuretic hormone at night, resulting in the ability to sleep for 10 or 12 hours at a time without awakening to urinate or wetting the bed. With age, the activity level of the hormone diminishes, resulting in bladder accumulation throughout the night.

Medical conditions also play a role in bladder function by causing inconsistent handling of fluids. Diabetes and heart disease are notorious for this problem. Medications also can wreak havoc on a good night's sleep. Diuretics, in particular, are problematic. Nowadays, many of the blood pressure medications have a small amount of diuretic mixed in with them. Some of you may not be aware of the presence of the diuretic in your particular blood pressure pill.

If nighttime urination is an isolated symptom, it may need to be addressed differently from urgency and urge incontinence. In my experience, most women with nighttime urination also have problems during the day. The problems at night may need to be handled slightly differently. Medications to treat the bladder can only do so much for the problems at night. Other treatments, such as sleeping pills and leg elevation, may need to be included to control that problem as well.

EVALUATION OF FREQUENCY, URGENCY, AND URGE INCONTINENCE

The evaluation of the woman who presents with urgency and urge incontinence is the same as with any other urological patient. A good history, followed by a thorough physical exam will usually determine most of the diagnosis. Some simple laboratory testing may help clinch it. Occasionally, invasive testing will be needed to define certain aspects of the problem to help direct treatment. *Under no circumstances should any instrumentation be done without you being told of what is to be done and for what reason.* In most cases, no instruments need to be inserted into your body to make a determination and initiate therapy.

The history is the information that the doctor obtains from you in your own words. Many women will say to me on the first visit, "You should have all of the information in my file," which may be true. But the information that I get is secondhand. Most doctors want to hear what you, yourself, have to say about your condition. The questions that you are asked include:

1. **Onset:** When did the problem begin? Was the onset sudden or gradual?
2. **Progression:** Has it gotten worse? Is it slowly progressive or quickly deteriorating?
3. **Severity:** How severe are the symptoms? Can you get on with your daily routine, or is it curtailed by the frequency and urgency?

4. **Duration:** How long have you been suffering with the symptoms?
5. **Response to treatment:** Have you tried any treatment? What was it and how helpful was it? Were there aspects of the treatment that were good and others that were not?

Unlike most medical conditions, incontinence is a problem whose treatment is dictated by the sufferer. It is true that underlying conditions can be present that manifest themselves with urinary leakage, but that is rare. Most cases of urinary frequency, urgency, and urge incontinence are not due to a life-threatening illness. But the condition is life-altering and needs to be treated, and you must be an active participant in the evaluation and treatment plan. You are there because of your symptoms, so helping you means understanding your symptoms and treating them to a degree to which you feel comfortable. You cannot be passive with this condition. You must be clear about your symptoms and your expectations so that an adequate plan can be devised.

Fluid intake and timing of the intake will be discussed as well. If large volumes of water are consumed during the day as part of a weight loss plan, this information must be conveyed. If coffee-drinking continues throughout the day or alcohol is enjoyed with dinner every evening, this information will play a part in managing lifestyle issues. Timing of medication may be important. If a diuretic is taken in the evening, then nighttime awakening may be managed with altering the time that the tablet is taken. It is helpful to have a list of the medications that you are taking and when you take them. It is also useful to have the names of the medications that may have already been tried for the urinary condition but did not work. Women come to me all of the time saying that they tried this or that drug but she cannot remember the name. It may save time and money if we can avoid reusing medications that were not effective.

EVALUATION OF FREQUENCY, URGENCY, AND URGE INCONTINENCE

History
Physical examination
Post-void residual urine determination
Urine analysis
    Urine culture
    Urine cytology

EVALUATION OF FREQUENCY, URGENCY, AND URGE INCONTINENCE—continued

---

Voiding diary
Urodynamics—optional

The questions about nighttime urinating are often very difficult for some women to answer. I want to know what awakens them from sleep. It is the urge to urinate? Is it noise, sirens, or the cat? Is it spontaneous, which indicates a sleep disorder? After awakening, I also want to know how quickly you are able to fall back to sleep. Difficulty falling back to sleep may indicate sleep problems as well, but it also means that the night is very disrupted by the awakenings. Is fluid consumed before going to bed? Are medications taken that require a glass of water? Is dinner eaten close to bedtime? Are sleep medications taken?

Another important question about the nighttime problems is the proximity of the bathroom to your bed. If you have problems with immobility, you may have leakage because it takes you so long to get out of bed and into the bathroom. A bedside commode may solve the problem.

Nighttime leakage usually does not occur in women with stress incontinence, but it does occur if you have urgency, frequency, and urge incontinence. Urge incontinence happens both during the day and while sleeping. This distinction is important but sometimes difficult to tease out. If you awaken from sleep with an urge to go to the bathroom, but you are dry until you get out of bed and walk to the bathroom, then you have stress incontinence. If you are wet when you wake up before moving, then you have urge incontinence. This information will help guide your doctor in recommending treatment.

MEDICAL CONDITIONS THAT CAUSE FREQUENCY, URGENCY, AND URGE INCONTINENCE

Delirium
Urinary tract infection
Postmenopausal changes to vagina
Medications: diuretics
Psychological problems: depression, anxiety
Immobility or walking with a cane
Severe constipation
Congestive heart failure and diabetes

Medical problems, past surgical history, and history of trauma and accidents will round out this aspect of the evaluation. As much information as possible should be provided to your doctor so that she can save time and minimize medication when treatment begins.

The physical examination will come next. A full exam includes a general evaluation of your overall health. Can you walk, or do you use a cane? A short memory test may be administered by the physician to test for changes in the brain. An abdominal exam reveals the presence of a scar suggesting a surgery that may have been missed during the history-taking. Lumps on the abdomen, suggesting tumors or fibroids, may be noted. The main part of the physical involves a pelvic exam. By examining the pelvis, the physician will notice the presence of a prolapse of the vaginal vault and any associated organs, stress incontinence, uterine fibroids, postmenopausal vaginal atrophy, and masses in the bladder. A neurological exam of the genital area can be done at this time as well. Anal sphincter tone is assessed through a rectal exam.

The *post-void residual* is the name given to the volume of urine that is left over in the bladder after you urinate. This measurement can be taken by the physician who inserts a catheter after you have urinated and drains the bladder of the leftover fluid. This method is invasive and can be avoided if the physician has an ultrasound machine in his office (see Chapter 12 and the Glossary). The amount is measured in cubic centimeters (cc), which is a metric measurement. Thirty cc equals one ounce. Normal post-void residual readings are generally considered to be under 100 cc or 3½ ounces. There is no absolute number that is abnormal. The lower the post-void residual, the better. That would make sense since the bladder should be as empty as possible after urinating. Readings taken in the doctor's office can be altered because you are anxious. Unfamiliar bathrooms, other waiting patients, and stress over the visit can all lead to abnormally high post-void residual readings. If the pelvic muscles are tense due to stress, the output will be reduced and emptying will be incomplete. If the post-void residual reading is low, then the bladder definitely empties. If the reading is high, it needs to be repeated at another visit before bladder pathology is considered. The abnormally high reading may be due to the circumstances more than anything else.

A urine specimen will be collected during the visit. Urine analysis helps eliminate causes of urgency, frequency, and incontinence that are unrelated to basic bladder problems. Blood in the urine can mean the presence of a stone, a tumor, or an infection (see Chapter 12 and the Glossary). It often does not mean anything, but it may be a sign of a serious condition and should be evaluated before it is dismissed. The urine can be sent for a cancer screening test, called a urinary cytology. This test will help in the determination of urinary cancer. It takes about one week to come back from the lab.

The presence of white blood cells in the urine indicates inflammation of the bladder wall. Again, it may have no significance, but proper evaluation by a specialist should be done to be sure that nothing serious is going on. Protein in the urine may indicate kidney problems. Bacteria in the urine suggest the presence of a urinary tract infection. If bacteria are suspected, the specimen should be sent to the laboratory for a culture. The definitive test for the presence of a urinary tract infection, the urine culture, may take three to five days to come back.

Some practitioners use a voiding diary to get a clear understanding of the pattern of urination and leakage described by the sufferer. For three days, you write down what you drink, what time you urinate, and how much you go each time. If leakage occurs, the time of the leakage and the presence of an urge at that time are recorded. The process is cumbersome because the urine has to be measured in a plastic container, which can be impractical at times. However, the information can be invaluable. If large volumes of urine are being voided throughout the day, perhaps an undiagnosed medical condition is present, such as diabetes. If large volumes of fluid are being consumed, then reducing fluid intake may solve the problem. If urgency occurs every six hours, then timed voiding will solve the problem. Instead of waiting for the urge, you can be instructed to attempt to empty your bladder every three or four hours. Not all practitioners use a voiding diary, but those who do rely heavily on the results.

Finally, urodynamic testing, or cystometrics, may be recommended. Urodynamic studies determine how the bladder functions as it fills and as it empties. Invasive testing, which urodynamics is, should be reserved for those of you with complicated situations, such as medical conditions that can be contributing to the problem, inadequate response to treatment, or mixed urge and stress incontinence. Straightforward presentations, in which no other medical conditions are involved, the physical examination is unremarkable, and the laboratory tests are normal, do not warrant urodynamic studies. Treatment can begin at the first visit.

WHEN TO SEE A SPECIALIST

Presence of pelvic floor prolapse
History of pelvic surgery
Elevated post-void residual

WHEN TO SEE A SPECIALIST—continued

Blood in the urine
Frequent urinary tract infections
Not responding to medication

Premenopausal women without pelvic floor prolapse or a history of pregnancy *do* get these symptoms with no other pathology present. However, the younger woman is not the usual patient that most of us see. I recommend that any young woman, that is, any woman under 50 (mean age for menopause is 52), should see a specialist. Neurological conditions, such as multiple sclerosis, can start with bladder problems. Although rare, I have diagnosed a few women with multiple sclerosis *because* of bladder symptoms. Interstitial cystitis (see Chapter 9), a painful bladder condition, may also start with frequency and urgency, but the symptoms are present for at least six months. Pelvic-floor spasms, which are treatable with exercise therapy, can have the same presentation.

I don't mean to be an alarmist, but I hate to see young women subjected to long-term medical therapy when a different diagnosis would cure their problem. Likewise, we don't want to miss a systemic problem that could have been caught earlier had the bladder symptoms been put into a different context.

TREATMENT OF FREQUENCY, URGENCY, AND URGE INCONTINENCE

There are five categories of treatment for urgency, frequency, and urge incontinence. Each treatment level builds on itself, so that behavior modification is recommended to those of you who go on to physical therapy and medication. The last two treatments are surgical and require exhaustive efforts to control the condition with nonsurgical methods first.

Because this problem is symptom-based, the success of the treatment is determined by the person suffering from the symptoms. It is not for the physician to tell you what is livable in terms of urinary symptoms. You can be told what is realistic to expect from treatment, but, success is decided together. One woman needs to be dry for nine holes of golf, and another may just want to get through a concert without interruption. A woman with daily frequency and nighttime awakening may be just as bothered by her symptoms as a woman who leaks and wears pads. Anyone with bothersome symptoms deserves to be heard and treated. It is collaborative between you and your doctor. Side effects need to be weighed against benefits. We have few objective ways of telling you that you are better; only *you* are the one to tell us when you are better.

TREATMENTS FOR URGENCY, FREQUENCY AND URGE INCONTINENCE

Behavior modification
Physical therapy
Medication
Botox
Surgery-neuromodulation

Reasonable goals include urinating no more than two hours during the day and getting up no more than twice in an eight-hour period at night. These time frames will allow you to carry on typical activities during the day, such as eating a meal and going to a movie, and also getting some sleep at night. Three or four hours of uninterrupted sleep should produce restfulness. However, not all women will agree that this result is acceptable. It is imperative that you discuss your needs with your physician so that both parties are working toward the same goals.

Behavioral therapy and medication aim to reduce the urgency, increasing the time interval between getting the desire to urinate and actually making it to the toilet. They also increase the capacity of the bladder, so that more urine can be collected before the urge sets in. Reduction in bladder contractions that are not under conscious control is an added benefit of the medications that are available. The ultimate outcome is less urgency, a larger-capacity bladder, and no accidents.

GOALS OF THERAPY

Day: Urinate every two hours
Night: Get up twice in eight
Carry on activities of daily living comfortably
No leakage

The ideal treatment provides rapid onset of effective relief. Side effects are minimal and do not interfere with other bodily functions. Few drug interactions would allow patients on multiple medications to use the drug. Finally, simple dosing would increase compliance. Because this condition is considered more of a lifestyle problem than a life-threatening one, most women will forgo treatment of bladder leakage if it means that their other medical conditions will not be adequately treated. For this reason, the available treatment has to fit into each one of your medical regimens without compromising other organ systems.

THE IDEAL TREATMENT

Efficacious
No side effects
Easily administered
No drug interactions
None exists!

Fortunately, there are a number of different treatment options, one or many of which can address each woman's concerns. Patience and attentiveness are important to coming up with a mutually acceptable regimen for both the patient and her doctor. If the first, or second, or even third effort is unsuccessful, try not to despair. The benefits and disadvantages of each option need to be investigated. Combination therapy may be effective if a single option is not working. The point is: come up with reasonable goals and work with your doctor to realize those goals. No one should be a prisoner to her bladder.

Behavioral Treatment
Behavioral therapy can be applied to nearly all bladder disorders, but is especially helpful in frequency, urgency, and urge incontinence. Even if medication is eventually instituted, modifications in lifestyle will maximize results. Fluid restriction is the first step. Many women drink six to eight glasses of water per day for health and diet-related reasons. Water is healthy, but not when it causes you to move into the bathroom. Nearly all of our foods contain water, as do fluids such as coffee, soda, and juice. Consumption of six glasses of water on top of drinks with meals, in addition to salad and fruit, may cause the borderline bladder to go off the deep end. Many women realize that decreasing their fluid intake will help, and they adjust

accordingly, while others are stubborn and don't want to "give into" the problem. Unfortunately, not everyone's bladder is created equal. Just because one person can drink like a fish does not mean that everyone can.

BEHAVIORAL THERAPY

Fluid restriction
Reduction in coffee, alcohol, soda
Bladder training
Timed voiding

As an experiment, try to decrease fluid intake for a few days to see if any of the symptoms change. It may take a few days for the body to get used to the reduction in water, so if thirst sets in, sip instead of gulp water. Over time, the urine will become more yellow, signaling that the kidneys have started to concentrate the urine and reabsorb water. That is one of their natural functions, which gets temporarily lost when they are flushed with too much fluid. The urine should be yellow, not clear. In many cases, the reduction in fluid will not cure the problem, but it may reduce the frequency and urgency to some degree, and perhaps eliminate the leakage entirely. An acceptable intake of fluid is four 8-ounce glasses per day.

Coffee, alcohol, and soda are all bladder irritants and diuretics. Bladder irritants will cause a fragile bladder to go into spasm, causing symptoms. A diuretic is a substance that pulls fluid out of the tissues and eliminates it through the kidneys. The body can become dehydrated.

Bladder training is the next step in behavioral therapy. Gradual increases in the time between the urge to urinate and the release of urine is meant to teach the bladder to delay emptying. The idea is to start slowly, with, say, counting to 10 before heading to the bathroom, then, increasing to 20, 40, and 60 seconds. Eventually, the bladder will "learn" not to contract with an impulse. Bladder training can be done under the guidance of a trained professional, or alone using diaries and voiding journals.

Bladder training is very difficult to do without instructions on how to hold off the urge without stimulating it. There are methods of contracting the pelvic floor muscles in such a way that the urge is suppressed while holding in the urine. Specialty trained physical therapists and biofeedback technicians can work with you to master these skills. I think it is very difficult to produce effective results without, at least, some instruction. In conjunction with fluid restriction, bladder training is especially effective in young, motivated women with intact pelvic floor muscles. Women with weak muscles, and especially those with prolapse, generally do not do well with these interventions alone.

Timed voiding can be very helpful in the elderly woman who has lost some of her bladder sensation. With age, the urge to urinate may not be particularly strong. The first signal that she needs to empty her bladder is the wetness that she feels from the leakage. If prompted to try to empty before the urge sets in, she may avoid accidents. This technique is particularly effective in women in nursing homes, those with cognitive impairment, and neurologically impaired women.

Medical Treatment

Most (but not all) of the medications on this list work mainly through interfering with the activity of acetylcholine. Because they work against the effect of acetylcholine, they are called *anticholinergics*. The method of interference differs from drug to drug, but the effect on the bladder is the same. Urination does not stop completely. Only involuntary bladder contractions are reduced or eliminated. The reason that the bladder doesn't become paralyzed is that acetylcholine is constantly being released by the nerve endings.

Medications Available to Treat Frequency, Urgency, and Urge Incontinence

Medical name	Trade name	Dosage
Oxybutynin, short acting	Ditropan	5 mg up to 4x/day
Oxybutynin, extended release	Ditropan XL	5–15 mg 1x/day
Oxybutynin, extended release patch	Oxytrol	1 patch 2x/week
Tolterodine	Detrol	2 mg 2x/day
Tolterodine, long acting	Detrol LA	2 or 4 mg 1x/day
Darifenacin	Enablex	7.5 or 15 mg 1x/day
Solifenacin	Vesicare	5 or 10 mg 1x/day
Trospium	Sanctura	10 mg 2x/day
Propantheline	Pro-Banthine	15–30 mg up to 4x/day
Hyocyamine	Levsin/Cystospaz	0.325 mg up to 3x/day
Dicyclomine	Bentyl	20 mg 3x/day
Flavoxate	Urispas	100–200 mg 3–4x/day
Imipramine	Tofranil	10–75 mg 1x/night
Vasopressin	DDAVP	0.2–0.6 µg 1x/night
Botulinum toxin	Botox	500 units injected in bladder

The side effects of the medications are due to the presence of acetyl-choline in other organs as well, such as the eyes, the intestines, and the salivary glands. The drug will interfere with the effect that the neurotransmitter has on those organs as well. The newer bladder medications attempt to target the bladder more than the other organs by acting on the bladder receptor, the area on the nerve to which the acetylcholine molecule attaches. The receptors in the eyes, the intestines, the brain, the salivary glands, and the bladder are subtly different. By working at the receptor level, it may be possible to reduce, or even eliminate, the side effects. That is what the term "organ-specific effect" refers to. Therefore, differences among the many medications lie mostly in the side effects and the ability to tolerate the medication.

All of these medications aim to increase the volume of urine that the bladder will hold before it contracts. The bladder contractions, both voluntary and involuntary, are reduced in their strength. The idea is that if the contraction is weaker, the muscles of the urinary sphincter will be able to squeeze closed and hold off an accident. Very strong bladder contractions will force open the sphincter and leakage will result. A larger capacity bladder will solve the problem of frequency. If the bladder can hold more, then less frequent emptying is necessary.

Although the body is able to hold more water while taking these medication, there is no retention of fluid in the tissues. The kidneys will continue to flush fluids as necessary, but the bladder will hold more of that fluid before there is a need to evacuate it. So, if you are on a diuretic, you will not be interfering with the diuretic effect by taking bladder medications. The diuretic will still pull excess fluid out of the body and filter it rapidly through the kidneys, while the bladder medication will allow the bladder to expand and hold more water before it becomes full. The result is still going to be elimination of fluid and more frequent urination than without the diuretic. However, there should be more control, less frequency, and no leakage.

Short-acting medications, such as oxybutynin and tolterodine require more frequent dosing throughout the day. The long-acting medications (Detrol LA, Ditropan XL, Vesicare, and Enablex) will allow you to take one pill a day with effects that last the entire 24 hours. The patch requires even less frequent application: only twice per week. Although they cost more, long-acting formulations are not necessarily better than the short-acting options. Short-acting medications permit more flexible dosing, so you can take one dose in the morning and a different dose at night. The peak level in the bloodstream of the active ingredient is not as consistent with the short-acting medications as with the long-acting ones. The fluctuations in the tissue levels may result in periods where no active ingredient is in the bloodstream. The symptoms may come back during these periods during the day. Generally, long-acting drugs are preferable, but the short-acting option may be better for certain patients or may be used to supplement the effects of the long-acting choices.

Short-Acting versus Long-Acting Medications

	Short	Long
Frequency of dosing	More than 1x/day	1x/day
Side effects	Worse	Better
Cost	Low	High
Effectiveness	Good	Good

Besides the length of time during which the medication is active, the available treatments differ in the method through which the body breaks them down, the combined effects some of the medications offer, the different dosing options, and the route through which they are administered in the body. We will go through each of the options, discussing how they work, and what benefits and drawbacks each one offers.

Oxybutynin
The first medication to become available for the treatment of urinary urge incontinence was oxybutynin. Containing both anticholinergic properties and antispasmodic properties, this medication relaxes the bladder, effectively treating the incontinence component as well as the frequency and urgency. With a half-life of approximately 6 hours, that is, its potency or effectiveness decreases by one-half every 6 hours, it needs to be taken multiple times throughout a 24-hour period. The tablets come in 5-mg doses and can be taken up to four times per day. It is metabolized by the liver, as are most pharmaceutical drugs. Once it is broken down, it releases an active metabolite, which is a part of the drug that is activated by the liver, and contributes to the increased side effects without really helping the bladder symptoms. This metabolite is one of the reasons that the side effects are so bad for this medication. Up to 60 percent of you will suffer from dry mouth while taking oxybutynin. Constipation and blurry vision can also result. Because it crosses the blood–brain barrier, it can also lead to dizziness, headaches, and lethargy. None of the positive or negative effects are permanent, which is why the medication has to be taken regularly to work.

Ditropan XL (Extended Release)

In response to the frequent dosing and high incidence of side effects from oxybutynin, the longer acting Ditropan XL came into being. The active ingredient is still oxybutynin but the casing around the tablet has been chemically altered to release the medication slowly over a 24-hour period. The metabolism is the same as with oxybutynin but less medication needs to be administered to get the same effect. Therefore, fewer side effects result, and they are better tolerated. The tablets come in 5-, 10-, and 15-mg doses. The usual dose is 10 mg, but the physician has the flexibility to increase or decrease the amount as needed. There is no generic choice for the extended release oxybutynin. It is considerably more expensive than the short-acting choice.

Oxytrol Patch

In response to the poor side-effect profile but good response of oxybutynin, a patch became available. The patch is applied to the skin overlying the abdomen twice per week. You can shower, swim, and exercise with the patch affixed in place. The patch is impregnated with oxybutynin, which slowly seeps through the skin and directly enters the bloodstream. Immediately active on the bladder, the medication does not go through the liver before it becomes effective. The side-effect profile is much better than either the short-acting or long-acting formulations because no active metabolites are produced. The problem with the patch is that it comes in only one dose, which is often too low to produce effective results. The company that produces the patch is looking to offer higher doses. It can also cause local skin irritation at the site where the patch is affixed.

Tolterodine (Detrol and Detrol LA)

Tolerodine acts at the level of the receptor. It does not actually inhibit the release of acetylcholine; it mitigates the effect that the acetylcholine has on the receptors. The bladder has receptors that are different than the receptors on the salivary glands, the eyes, and the intestines, even though all of these organs respond to acetylcholine. The idea is that the medication will only affect the bladder, without altering the interaction of acetylcholine in those other organs. Originally available in twice per day dosing, the newer long-acting Tolterodine is taken once per day. Both formulations are metabolized through the liver with active metabolites.

The tolerodine molecule is larger than the oxybutynin molecule so it does not cross the blood–brain barrier, and thus should not cause problems with mental function. The result is fewer side effects such as dizziness,

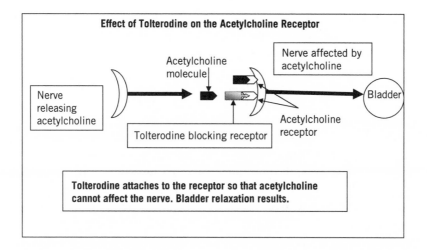

headaches, and fatigue. However, the side effects involving other organs are still present. Blurry vision, constipation, and dry mouth are the most common. The longer-acting medication has fewer side effects than the twice per day choice. As with oxybutynin, Tolterodine leaves the system, so none of the effects, both good and bad, are permanent. In order to maintain the benefits, the medication must be taken regularly.

Newer Agents: Enablex, Vesicare, and Sanctura

Darafenacin (Enablex), solifenacin (Vesicare), and trospium (Sanctura) all became available in early 2005. They were developed to reduce the side effects seen in the other two medications more than to increase the efficacy. All three work on blocking the receptor. The types of receptors that they interfere with are supposed to be more bladder-specific than tolterodine. Enablex and Vesicare are taken once per day, while Sanctura is taken twice a day. They are all costly, but work well. With better understanding of the bladder receptor, more specific medications will become available.

How to Choose the Right Medication

With all of the medications mentioned so far, the benefits are seen within about a week of taking the pills. Immediate results are unrealistic. Because it takes a few days for the effects to set in, they cannot be taken as needed. For long car trips or special occasions, a single pill will not give the user the advantages that she is looking for. The short-acting oxybutynin and tolerodine may work for some women. I recommend using the short-acting formulations for specific instances as opposed to the longer-acting choices. The reason is that a large boost of drug given by the short acting medications that enters the bloodstream quickly will also affect the bladder quickly. The slower onset of the 24-hour pills will not give the targeted benefit that is needed.

The daily pills should be taken every day. The time of the day is not important as long as the medication is taken at the same time every day. If it is taken in the morning one day and the evening the next day, 36 hours will have passed and the dosing will be off, with noticeable changes in bladder symptoms. If other medications are also being taken, any of these drugs can be taken with those other pills. There is little drug interaction with any of these medications. The body will sort out all of the various pills that are being taken, with each pill doing what it is supposed to even though everything is bombarding the system at one time.

Over-the-counter medications, such as antacids, Tylenol, aspirin, and laxatives will not alter the effect of these medications. If a reaction occurs that you find disagreeable, just stop taking the bladder pill immediately. No tapering of the dose is necessary for either the long- or the short-acting formulations. They can also be taken in combination. If a long-acting pill is helpful during the day, but the nights are still interrupted with awakening to urinate, a short-acting drug can be added to extend the effects. Theoretically, the two different medications should work together. Playing with the combinations and the doses is perfectly safe and may result in excellent bladder control.

Other Medications

The older medications that are seldom used now include propantheline, hyocyamine, dicyclomine, and flavoxate. Propantheline was one of the first agents to be used to treat urge incontinence. It needs to be taken every 4 to 6 hours on an empty stomach. A non–organ-specific receptor blocker, propantheline's (Pro-Banthine) side effects are much more severe than those seen in the short-acting oxybutynin. Hyocyamine (Levsin or Cystospaz) is also a receptor blocker that works similarly to propantheline. It is still used by some physicians for bowel disorders. Dicyclomine and Flavoxate are each taken up to three times per day. They also have limited efficacy in regard to reducing urgency and urge incontinence. These agents are rarely used anymore in the United States because the newer agents are better.

Imipramine is an antidepressant that was found to have bladder relaxation effects when taken in low doses. The antidepressant effect occurs at doses of 150 mg or higher, whereas the bladder effects can be seen with as little as 10 to 25 mg per day. The main problem with imiprimine is that it sedates the user, so it cannot be taken during the day. The effect of the medication lasts for about 6 hours, so it can be highly effective in women who have nighttime urinary problems. The bladder will not only relax, but the sedative effects will help with the sleep disturbances. It does cross the blood–brain barrier, so it can cause mental status changes, such as lethargy and confusion in the older woman. If this side effect is noted, the medication should either be reduced in strength or eliminated all together. It clears the bloodstream in a matter of hours, so no permanent changes will result. In spite of this one side effect, imiprimine is an effective treatment and is still used often. It can be combined with the other medications, such as oxybutynin and tolterodine, to maximize treatment at night.

DDAVP is an artificial hormone that mimics the activity of vasopressin (antidiuretic hormone), the native hormone that induces the kidneys to reabsorb water. Because the kidneys release less water, the bladder will not fill up as quickly, resulting in fewer trips to the bathroom. With age, natural vasopressin levels are reduced, and they lose their circadian release. Children have surges of vasopressin at night, which allows them to sleep for 10 to 12 hours without awakening to go to the bathroom. These surges diminish with age. The kidneys function in excreting fluid during the night the same way they do during the day. The result is frequency of urination during the night that mirrors the day. DDAVP can be taken in tablet form before bedtime. Blood work needs to be done every few months for women who take DDAVP because it can lower the sodium levels in the blood. Like all of the other medications mentioned, it can be taken in combination with other treatments.

Botulinum toxin can be injected into the lining of the bladder through a cystoscope, either in the office or in an outpatient hospital setting. It is indicated for use in women who have failed to improve with traditional medical therapies. The toxin paralyzes the bladder, preventing involuntary bladder contractions. It reduces leakage, as well as the symptoms of frequency and urgency. Very few centers offer this treatment because it is expensive and difficult to perform. The poison is fragile and not easy to handle. Each vial costs a few hundred dollars. Usually one to two vials are injected at one time. The results last for approximately 6 to 8 months before another instillation is required.

Side Effects of Medications
All of the anticholinergic medications have the same potential side effects. The reason that I say *potential* side effects is that no woman will experience all of them. You may not have any negative reaction to the medication. The lists of side effects that are written in the package inserts include all of the

adverse events that were experienced by the participants in the clinical trials. I tell people not to read the side effect profile until you experience something that you do not like. At that time, you can look at the list and see if your reaction is mentioned. If it is, then you know that what you have is coming from the medication, and you can either stop the drug or continue it with the side effect. If it is not listed, then your problem is not coming from the medication. **None of the side effects is permanent. Stopping the medication will alleviate the adverse reaction in every case with these medications.**

POTENTIAL SIDE EFFECTS OF ANTICHOLINERGIC MEDICATION

Dry mouth
Constipation
Blurry vision
Urinary retention
Headaches
Confusion

The most common problem is dry mouth. Sometimes it is mild, at other times it is intolerable. Sucking on a sugarless candy, chewing gum, or sipping water may help lubricate your mouth. With time, the dryness gets a little better. The dry mouth comes from the medication interfering with the salivary gland secretions. You are not dehydrated; you are just not secreting saliva. Excessive water drinking is not necessary.

Constipation is a short-term side effect that occurs in anywhere from 2–30% of people tested on these medications. It usually goes way after about a month of continual use of any of these drugs. Increasing fiber in your diet and, perhaps, using a laxative for a short time will help with bowel movements until this resolves.

Blurry vision and urinary retention are rare problems seen with these medicines. Again, both will go away with discontinuation of the pills. Narrow-angle glaucoma is an absolute contraindication to taking any one of these medications because they will cause irreversible exacerbation of the condition. Less than 10 percent of glaucoma sufferers have the narrow-angle variety. Check with your ophthalmologist before starting one of these medicines if you have glaucoma.

Confusion, dizziness, and headaches rarely occur. Many of the neurological side effects that are listed are very suggestive: if you know that you may experience that symptom, you probably will. Therefore, I suggest, once again, don't read them unless you feel something that you think is coming from the medication.

Symptom relief from urge incontinence is a balance between the side effects and the efficacy of the medication that you and your doctor have selected. The likelihood that you will have a problem with the medicine is related to the dose: the higher the dose, the more likely you are to experience an adverse reaction. If the drug works, you are more likely to tolerate the bad points of taking it. If you cannot tolerate one medication, you may tolerate another. It's all about balance through trial and error.

Surgery
Finally, neuromodulation can be offered to those of you who do not respond to any other treatments. Neuromodulation refers to the insertion of a pacemaker into the nerves in the spinal cord that supply the bladder. Wires are surgically inserted into the spinal canal and attached to a pacemaker that sits under the skin of the lower back or buttocks. The pacemaker fires low-voltage, low-amplitude electrical stimuli into the wires that transmit that energy into the nerves. The nerves go into overdrive from the constant stimulation, and eventually, they fatigue. The bladder then stops the involuntary contractions. The system works very much like a pacemaker for the heart, and is even made by a company that produces cardiac pacemakers (Medtronic). Very little is understood about the scientific effect of this treatment, but experience has shown that it can work very well in the woman who does not respond to medication.

A test stimulation can be done before the final pacemaker is inserted. The test stimulation is done in the office using local anesthesia. The wire is inserted into the spinal canal and attached to an external pacer. The pacer determines the intensity and the frequency of the stimulation. The external pacer is worn on a belt, like a beeper, and can be adjusted by the user depending on the results and the level of discomfort. The test stimulation can last for three or four days, which will give you ample time to see if the system will work. If it is effective, then the permanent pacemaker can be inserted in the operating room in an ambulatory setting. X-rays are used to help position the wires correctly. The pacer is set using a magnet over the skin where the battery pack is sitting. The batteries are changed every five years.

Some practitioners will insert the permanent pacemaker at the outset. They feel that since the procedure is simple enough, it warrants permanent placement at the outset. Whether a test stimulation is done or not can be decided by you and your doctor. Experienced practitioners are available throughout the country.

Neuromodulation is an effective treatment in the correct patient. All other options for relief must be exhausted before this option is considered. It sounds drastic, but it is not at dangerous as it sounds and is worth trying if you have not found any relief with other treatments. The test stimulation, at least, should be considered.

SUMMARY

The most effective treatment for frequency, urgency, and urge incontinence is a combined approach using both behavior modification and medication. Reduction in fluids, pelvic muscle exercises, and combination medication should work in nearly every woman with this condition. Often, trial and error is needed to get the right dose and the right mix of treatments to balance the relief of the symptoms with reduced side effects. It is important to be patient and communicative with your physician. If something is not working or creates too many problems, let the doctor know so that he can change the strength or the class of the drug. Women are often embarrassed that they are not getting better, or they think it is their fault. They think they "just can't control themselves." That is by no means the case. This is a physical condition that should be treated that way. Your doctor is there to help you get better. Be honest, and be persistent.

CHAPTER 6

- -

The Golden Years
Incontinence in the Elderly

R. remembers her 80th birthday party vividly, even though it was over two years ago. She was surprised at how many of her friends had reached 80 or over and still live active lives. J. teaches aerobics at the senior center two mornings a week. S. still sings in the church choir and organizes fund raising events once or twice a year for the youth group. R., herself, still drives and volunteers to help her friends and neighbors with groceries and doctor's visits. R.'s mother lived to be 78, and her father 75, but they seemed so old compared with R. and her friends.

One morning, R. was in her yard doing some work, when she tripped and fell over a rock sticking out of the ground. X-rays at the hospital revealed a broken hip. She was admitted and scheduled for surgery. Her son and daughter-in-law arrived in time to see her in the recovery room. The doctor told them that the repair went well, but R. would need about 6 weeks of intensive physical therapy in a rehabilitation hospital before she could go home and resume her busy life. He reassured both R. and her family that she would be able to function as well as she did before, including driving around town, even if it took a few months to return to normal mobility. He said patience and hard work would get her back on her feet, literally, in no time.

The rehabilitation facility that R. was transferred to was more like a nursing home than a short-term unit for patients like her, people who would return to their active lives "in no time." She was put into a room with a woman who was completely disoriented. She screamed out in what sounded like fear and confusion all day and all night. R. could get no peace and quiet. Between all of the noise and the pain in her hip, she barely slept the first night. When the doctor came to see her in the morning to evaluate her, she reported her concerns and frustrations

131

regarding her roommate. She was worried that she would never improve without rest. The doctor listened with empathy. He prescribed a sleeping pill and an antidepressant to help R. cope with her situation. He would try to get her room changed, but he couldn't promise anything.

The following week R.'s son visited his mother. When he walked into the room, he found her lying in bed at lunchtime, lethargic and slightly disoriented. He called the nurse who told him that she cannot get out of bed because of her confusion. She has not started physical therapy because she cannot get out of bed. She is wearing a diaper due to incontinence that began shortly after she arrived at the facility. She pretty much sleeps all day, and eats only when she is fed. She has even lost a few pounds. R.'s son was rightfully upset. The orthopedist assured them that she would be better "in no time," and here he is staring at a woman who is confused, incontinent, and cannot feed herself. How will she ever return to a life where she lives independently, let alone drives.

R.'s son called the doctor immediately who met him at the bedside. He reviewed her chart and began to make some changes. He stopped her sleeping pills and antidepressants, both of which were contributing to her lethargy and incontinence. He examined her, finding that her bladder was distended and full. A catheter was put in and 300 cc of foul-smelling urine was drained. After removing the catheter, he started her on antibiotics to treat a urinary tract infection. She was also placed on stool softeners to keep her bowels regular. The last thing he did was transfer her to another room. Her noisy roommate was put into a single room so no other patients would be subjected to her disconcerting outbursts.

Within two days R. was awake and alert. Although she had some urgency of urination with a few accidents, she was able to make it the toilet or into the bedpan 90% of the time. Her physical therapy began the following week. Within six weeks, she was discharged home with home therapy and the use of cane. She resumed driving three months after the surgery.

Incontinence in an elderly woman like R. is often considered an unavoidable aspect of aging. Fortunately, many of the causes of urinary leakage in older people are treatable. " Elderly" is defined as anyone over the age of 65. Of course, these days, elderly people live longer, healthier, more active lives than they did 20, or even 10 years ago. People over 65 years old do not need to live with incontinence any more than people under the age of 65 do.

Most elderly people are continent. In other words, most of you do not leak urine and do not wear diapers. However, many of you do, often because you do not want to see a doctor for yet another ailment, or to take yet another medication. Although the prevalence of incontinence increases with age, uncontrolled urinary leakage is not a *natural* part of the aging process. It is common among the elderly, but not *normal*. Incontinence is an unacceptable aspect of aging that can be treated effectively in nearly every person over the age of 65.

Despite our ability to manage urinary problems in the elderly, nearly 50% of the nursing home population sits around in diapers and leaks uncontrollably. Over $1 billion per year is spent just on managing incontinence in nursing home inhabitants. Management includes diapers, catheters, ointments to treat skin conditions, treatment of bed sores from sitting in wet clothing, and dealing with fractures from falls at night from struggling to get to the bathroom. If we include those of you who live in the community, we spend $26 billion per year, overall, on the management and treatment of urinary incontinence.

As we age, we become increasingly different from one another. It is difficult to make general statements regarding the health of the elderly versus the health of infants. Elderly people have multiple medical and surgical issues, take medications, and have histories of childbirths, all of which will affect this condition, Therefore, if one of your friends has a problem that sounds similar to your problem, it may, in fact, be treated totally differently because of your different make-up history. After all, we are dealing with 65 years worth of living in the body that we are treating.

Factors outside of the urinary tract can affect the functioning *within* the urinary tact. The ability to control one's urine is affected by medications, mobility, dexterity, social appropriateness, and fluid balance. Like R. experienced, medications can cause problems with urinary emptying, which can lead to infections and leakage. Medical conditions, such as diabetes and heart disease, can affect urinary behavior. Very simple changes in the toileting behavior of the woman may improve matters without actually changing anything major in her medical program. Moving the chair closer to the toilet, providing a commode next to the bed, or bringing her to the bathroom every 2 to 3 hours to try to empty, may get her out of diapers. Older people with senility may need to be reminded to use the bathroom. They may have lost their inhibitions, emptying their bladders wherever they are. Suggestive voiding may be enough to keep them dry. Fluid intake is one of the most common mistakes that people make. We are told to drink at least eight glasses of water per day. However, older people do not concentrate the urine as effectively as children. The fluid, literally, goes right through them. Decreasing your intake to four glasses per day may make a huge difference in your problem.

Incontinence in the elderly population is multifactorial, but eminently treatable. Each patient needs to be managed individually because so many aspects of one's health and history can be contributing to the problem. Patients and their families need to report incontinence to their doctors so that changes in medication can be made and treatments begun.

THE AGING BLADDER: NORMAL CHANGES TO THE LOWER URINARY TRACT THAT OCCUR WITH AGING

The bladder and the urethra undergo changes with age just as other organs of the body do, such as the bones and the eyes. There are natural changes that predispose us to developing incontinence as we age. Illness and medications often exacerbate the underlying changes and throw us over the edge, resulting in leakage. Certain baseline changes that occur in the elderly urinary tract involve the muscles of the pelvic floor, the length of the urethra, and the capacity and functioning of the bladder.

Changes to the Urethra

In women, the urethra is already a short organ. As the supply of estrogen to that organ diminishes, it shortens even more as we age. The neck of the bladder, where the urethra attaches, becomes weak as well. This area is called the bladder outlet. Weakening of the bladder outlet is caused by childbirth, low estrogen, muscle weakness, and previous surgery. In addition, the urinary sphincter, which is a muscle that surrounds the urethra, begins to shrink and thin with age. Weakening of the outlet coupled with a shortened tube and loss of the muscle fibers in the urinary sphincter allows urine to squirt out more easily during activity. These defects evolve out of changes that are natural to the aging urethra, and lead to stress incontinence (see Chapter 4).

Changes to the Bladder

Changes to the bladder that occur with aging are more complex. The bladder must carry out two tasks in order to do its job effectively. It must store urine during periods of filling, and empty completely during periods of voiding. The aging process can affect both the ability of the bladder to

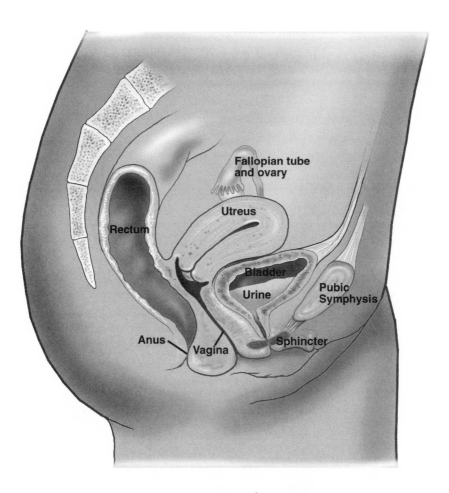

FIGURE 1. *Normal Anatomy.*

fill adequately and to empty efficiently. Most elderly people will show some diminished function in both the storage and the emptying phases of urination, even if they are continent of urine and highly functional. However, it is easy to throw this fragile balance off kilter, leading to urinary leakage.

- **Cannot Fill Bladder**
  - **Involuntary bladder contractions**
  - **Reduced bladder capacity**
  - **Poor compliance**
  - **Poor urinary sphincter tone**
- **Cannot Empty Bladder**
  - **Blockage**
  - **Poor bladder muscle contractions**

Failure to Fill the Bladder

Involuntary bladder contractions occur when the bladder muscle begins to contract and evacuate urine before the brain tells it to. There will be a sudden urge to go to the bathroom, which may result in the loss of a *few drops* of urine or loss of an *entire bladderful* of urine. With the sudden urge, some women will make it to the bathroom without leaking. Caused by an uncontrolled bladder contraction, the natural response to the sudden urge is to squeeze the pelvic muscles as hard as possible. With the squeezing, the urge may go away by itself. At times, leakage will result in urge incontinence (see Chapter 5).

Uncontrollable bladder contractions are common among elderly people. Nearly two-thirds of you will describe symptoms of urgency, frequency, and waking up at night with a strong desire to urinate. Over half of incontinent elderly women will have involuntary bladder contractions. In other words, bladder spasms are common in those of you with incontinence and need to be addressed as part of the treatment of the incontinent elderly woman.

Reduced bladder capacity also occurs with age. The bladder capacity of a normal healthy adult woman is between 300 and 400 cc or 10 to 13 ounces of fluid. The capacity decreases by about one-third in women over age 65. The reason for the reduced capacity is probably due to loss of the elasticity of the bladder muscle and the increased incidence of bladder spasms. Because the bladder is stiffer as it fills, the pressure exerted on the walls can be transmitted to the kidneys. Involuntary bladder spasms cause emptying of the bladder, relief of the pressure on the walls, and thus, preservation of the kidneys. In many older women, the urge to void kicks in before the pressures get too high, thus preserving the kidneys. In this way, loss of elasticity, reduced capacity, and bladder spasms go hand in hand in the aging bladder.

If the muscles below the bladder begin to weaken due to estrogen depletion, muscle weakness, prior surgery, or childbirth, leakage will result. This type of leakage is called **stress incontinence.** The bladder is able to hold water, but it seeps out because the outlet is not closed tightly enough. Women who suffer from stress incontinence will leak with activity. In contrast while sitting or lying down, the urine is contained within the body of the bladder and will not seep out. If the seeping out of the urine occurs in high volumes, the bladder may never be able to fill.

Failure to Empty the Bladder

The failure of the bladder to empty occurs for two reasons. One is that there is a blockage that prevents the urine from exiting, and the second is that the bladder does not contract effectively enough to squeeze out the urine. **Blockage to the flow of urine** in women is caused by either prolapse or prior surgery. Women do not have any organs between the bladder and the urethra that can block urine flow. Of course, in men, the most common cause of urinary blockage is prostate disease. Women do not have prostates.

Pelvic-floor prolapse is described in detail in Chapter 7. Briefly, if the bladder or the uterus falls into the vaginal canal, they can block the flow of urine. The urethral canal becomes kinked, making it very difficult for the bladder muscle to exert enough force to overcome the resistance of the blocked urethra. The result is incomplete bladder emptying. Women will walk around with residual volumes (the volume of urine left in the bladder after urinating) in their bladders from 100 to over 1000 cc. If the residual volume is high enough, the kidneys can become blocked as well. The system works just like the plumbing in a house. If a drain gets clogged, it will result in stagnant water that will continue to build up as long as the faucet is running. Eventually, the clogged drain will result in a backup and a flood will result. In a patient, the backup of fluid in the bladder will extend into the kidneys, which will eventually become permanently damaged. This is very rare. Usually women are well aware of the prolapse before then and will seek treatment.

Poor bladder muscle contractions are a common and difficult problem that we see in elderly women. The bladder muscle must be able to mount a contraction in order for the urine to exit the organ. As women age, the force of that contraction diminishes, but it is still adequate enough to empty effectively, especially since the outlet is weak as well. Therefore, some degree of impaired muscle contraction is expected, but if it gets bad enough, the bladder will never empty. Incomplete contractions result in increased residual urine volumes. That means that there is still urine in the bladder even after you urinate. If the residual urine volume is high, over 200 cc or 6 ounces, then you are at risk for developing urinary tract infections. Stagnant urine harbors bacteria that will multiply and create problems.

As women age, the bladder undergoes changes that we expect to see. The ability to store urine and the ability to empty urine are not as efficient as they were in the earlier years. However, the bladder should be able to function well enough for us to do our daily activities, even if that means that we urinate more often than usual or get up once or twice each night. When urinary leakage results, the degree of impairment becomes unacceptable and a gynecologist or urologist should be consulted. Many factors may play into why the fragile balance in the bladder is off. Each aspect of your history, physical exam, medications, and illnesses must be evaluated to determine if any confounding factors can be found. Correction of the problem or treatment of the defect can ensue, thereby restoring continence and allowing you to function at your fullest capacity.

TYPES OF INCONTINENCE SEEN IN THE ELDERLY

TYPES OF INCONTINENCE

Stress
Urge
Overflow
Functional

Stress incontinence is the involuntary loss of urine during activity. It is called stress incontinence because it is caused by mechanical stress or pressure on the intra-abdominal muscles, which is transmitted to the bladder. Urine is, effectively, squeezed out of the bladder, resulting in leakage. It is caused by weakness of the bladder outlet, which is the point at which the urethra meets the bladder. The causes of weakness in this area include poor muscular support from below these structures or weakness within the

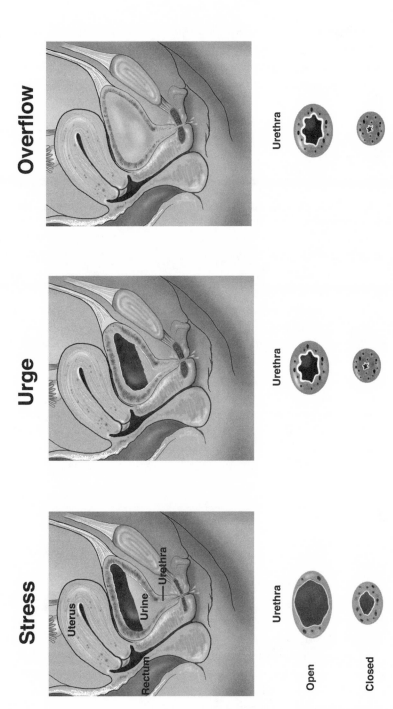

FIGURE 2. *Incontinence.*

urethra. The urinary sphincter is a muscle that surrounds the urethra. When you are not urinating, it is usually tightly closed, preventing the passage of urine through the urethra. During urination, it opens. After childbirth, trauma, or with aging, the fibers of the sphincter will weaken. The seal is not so strong, and urine can leak if you laugh, cough, or sneeze. If stress incontinence is mild, it does not need to be treated.

STRESS INCONTINENCE

Cause: **Urethra cannot seal shut with increases in pressure on the bladder**
Amount of leakage: **Usually small**

Urge incontinence occurs with a sudden and uncontrollable urge to go to the bathroom. This is the "key in the lock" type of incontinence. As soon as the key is in the door, the wave comes on and your parts are wet. Sometimes, the leakage is small, but usually, when this comes on, it comes on in full force. Urge incontinence is caused by bladder contractions that are not under the control of the brain. These uncontrolled contractions occur more often in the elderly, but also occur in younger women. They can be caused by treatable problems, such as cystitis, bladder stones or polyps, urethral irritation, and infected urethral cysts. They can also be caused by neurological disorders such as a stroke, Parkinson's disease, spinal cord problems, or dementia. The presence of urge incontinence does not mean that a woman has a neurological condition. These spasms are seen in women who have no neurological disorders at all.

URGE INCONTINENCE

Cause: **Uncontrolled bladder contractions**
Amount: **Usually large volume, but not always**

Overflow incontinence results from leakage of urine with an overly distended bladder. The bladder literally overflows with urine. If you have this, you will have a constant, slow leak that occurs both day and night. No urge or activity is associated with the drip. Most commonly seen in men with prostate disorders, overflow incontinence is rare in women.

OVERFLOW INCONTINENCE

Causes:
Blockage of urine flow
Poor muscle tone in bladder
Amount: **Usually slow drip**

It is caused by either the blockage of the outflow of urine or by the inability of the bladder to contract and empty. Blockage in women results from pelvic floor prolapse or from prior surgery that prevents urine from exiting. One of the problems that can result from incontinence surgery is the inability to urinate due to blockage. Usually, if a woman cannot urinate after surgery, she will be very uncomfortable. In women with prolapse that blocks outflow, the process is slow-growing enough that she can build up urine over years. She does not sense that the bladder is not emptying, and ultimately, she will come to the urologist with overflow incontinence.

The inability of the bladder to contract at all can occur with aging alone, or as a result of an underlying disorder. If it results with aging, nothing can be done to rejuvenate the muscle and get it to contract. If an underlying condition is causing the problem, correcting the problem may help the muscle to repair itself. Diabetes mellitus is one of the more common causes of overflow incontinence. In diabetes, you loose sensation in the bladder, just like you can loose sensation in the feet and the hands. With loss of bladder sensation, you cannot respond appropriately to the urge to urinate. The bladder fills more and more with urine before the sensation of fullness hits. Eventually, the bladder muscle gets overstretched and cannot contract. The result is overflow incontinence.

Functional incontinence is when a person leaks because of factors not related to the bladder at all, but to circumstances. For example, a woman with Altcheimer's or Pick's disease cannot tell that she is not on the toilet, and may evacuate directly into a diaper. If a woman is physically impaired, such as after hip surgery, she may not be able to get out of bed to get to the toilet before she empties. Women with functional incontinence have normal urinary tracts with no abnormalities in function. Testing will not reveal any correctable disorders within the bladder or the urethra. The problems are all external. Some of the causes of functional incontinence are depression, severe dementia, anger and hostility, and immobility, such as a hip fracture. Treatment of functional incontinence involves timed toileting, where the women is brought to the toilet on a regular basis, or placement of a commode at the bedside. Good supportive care will often correct this problem with little other intervention.

FUNCTIONAL INCONTINENCE

Causes: Immobility, depression, dementia, anger
Amount: Whole bladder volume

Not all cases of incontinence in the elderly are clear-cut. A woman may have a combination of problems that may be resulting in uncontrolled urination. The impulse is to add another medication to the armamentarium already being prescribed. However, it is often more productive to take the time to evaluate each aspect of the incontinent woman's care. Perhaps decreasing or stopping certain medications in combination with available toileting will maintain an adequate dryness.

TYPES AND INCIDENCE OF URINARY INCONTINENCE

Urge incontinence:	
With good bladder function	31%
With poor bladder function	30%
Stress incontinence	21%
Overflow	8%
Outlet obstruction	4%
Mixed stress incontinence/urge incontinence	6%

CAUSES OF URINARY INCONTINENCE

The causes of urinary incontinence can be divided into those that cause *short-term, or transient or reversible, incontinence* and those that cause *long-term, or persistent, incontinence.* Short-term incontinence can be treated by treating the underlying condition. Long-term incontinence persists even if all of the underlying conditions have been adequately addressed. A woman may present with a baseline level of incontinence that is manageable for her or her caregivers, but worsens when something in her life changes. Correcting the exacerbating factor will bring her back to her baseline. In managing elderly women in whom multiple medical problems treated by multiple different medications all coexist, a careful and thoughtful approach to addressing changes in urinary behavior is essential.

Disorders that may predispose a woman to developing urinary incontinence include urological and gynecological problems, neurological problems, impaired physical and/or cognitive functioning, environmental obstructions, and problems caused by medical treatment, such as surgery or medication. Irreversible conditions such as dementia can *predispose* elderly patients to incontinence but do not *cause* incontinence. Women with poor brain function can forget where they are and urinate into their clothing, or they forget where the bathroom is, so they can't make it in time to empty.

If incontinence comes on or worsens suddenly, it is usually caused by an underlying condition that can be treated. The eight reversible causes of incontinence account for up to one-third of the cases of urinary leakage in the community-dwelling elderly population, and up to one-half of the cases of leakage in hospitalized and nursing home women. Gradual onset of leakage, or leakage that persists in spite of treatment of all the possible underlying conditions, is called *persistent* or *long-term* incontinence. The types of persistent incontinence include the types of incontinence that were described above: stress incontinence, urge incontinence, overflow incontinence, and functional incontinence. Persistent incontinence is diagnosed when all reversible causes are eliminated. Once it is determined that persistent incontinence is the cause of the problem, the type of incontinence is diagnosed and treated.

Reversible Causes of Incontinence

TREATABLE CONDITIONS THAT CAN CAUSE INCONTINENCE

D	Delirium/confusion
I	Infection: urinary tract
A	Atrophic vaginitis
P	Pharmaceuticals (medications)
P	Psychological (depression)
E	Excessive urine output
R	Restricted mobility
S	Stool impaction

Delirium is a dramatic change in a person's behavior that is marked by confusion, fluctuations in attentiveness, and disorientation. These changes can be alarming, but when the underlying condition is treated, baseline cognitive abilities often return. Delirium can be caused by medications and illnesses, such as infection, heart disease, pain, and uncontrolled diabetes. Simple urinary tract infections that can be treated with a few doses of antibiotics can present with confusion in elderly people. Small illnesses can present with big changes in personality in the fragile elderly woman. If the cause of the delirium is not recognized or treated, it can progress to serious illness and even death. Women with delirium *and* incontinence must be evaluated for the *cause* of the delirium and the incontinence, not just be treated. These two conditions can be symptoms of a more ominous problem that must be addressed swiftly, like in the case of R.

Infections, specifically urinary tract infections, can present exclusively with leakage. Some of you experience burning, frequency, and urgency, the classic symptoms of an infection, but many of you may not. The rapid onset of urinary incontinence can be the only indication that an infection is present. Treatment of the infection will cure the leakage if the infection is the cause. Treating the incontinence and leaving the infection untreated may result in progression of the infection to kidney involvement and possible sepsis, which is a life-threatening condition. A urine analysis and culture are essential components to the evaluation of sudden onset of urinary incontinence.

There is no need to treat bacteria that are found in the bladder when no symptoms of infection, including incontinence, are found on a routine physical exam in an elderly woman. The presence of bacteria in the bladder with no symptoms of infection is called *asymptomatic bacteriuria*. This condition is not treated because the bacteria will not cause any harm to you. If harm is being done, signs or symptoms will occur, such as incontinence. The antibiotics used to treat these bacteria will result in more problems than these organisms. Therefore, asymptomatic bacteriuria goes untreated, but leakage of urine in the presence of bacteria in the bladder *should* be treated. If the leakage persists despite a clear bladder, another cause of the leakage needs to be found.

Atrophic vaginitis results when women stop producing estrogen naturally. The tissues of the vagina and the urethra become thin and dry. They lose their elasticity and tend to bleed easily. Women experience itching, discomfort, and dryness during sexual intercourse. Oral estrogen will not usually treat this problem effectively, although vaginal creams, rings, and suppositories do. The dry, thinned tissues of the vagina and the urethra predispose elderly women to infections and incontinence. Generally, atrophic vaginitis itself will not cause leakage, but it contributes. Vaginal estrogen will often supplement treatment of other conditions that are causing the leakage.

Pharmaceuticals, also known as medications, used to treat potentially life-threatening conditions in the elderly population can contribute to incontinence. The average person over 65 is on five medications or more on a regular basis.

In older people, medications can take longer to digest. Over days, the level of the medication in the bloodstream can build up without you or the doctor realizing it. Sleeping pills, sedatives, and antianxiety medications are examples of drugs that can remain in the system longer in the elderly. A woman, like R. discussed previously, may wind up lethargic and confused after one or two days on a low-dose sleeping pill. This lethargy may lead to incontinence because she cannot get out of bed or doesn't realize that she is not in the bathroom. Stopping the medication for a few days, and then restarting it on a different schedule or discontinuing it altogether, may solve the confusion and leakage problem. Sedatives, antianxiety medications, and sleeping pills in the elderly may be very effective and useful. However, they need to be dosed properly with careful monitoring.

Medications That May Affect Incontinence

Type of Medication	Examples	Effect on Incontinence
Diuretic (water pills)	Lasix®, hydochlorothiazide	Frequency, urgency, leakage
Anticholinergics	Antihistamines, dicyclomine	Urinary retention, overflow incontinence, delirium, stool impaction
Antipsychotics	Haldol®, thorazine	Retention, sedation, immobility, delirium, impaction
Antidepressants	Elavil®, Amiltryptiline	Retention, sedation, overflow, impaction
Anti-Parkinson's	L-dopa, Sinemet®	Retention, sedation, overflow, impaction
Sedatives/hypnotics	Valium®, Ativan®	Sedation, delirium, immobility
Narcotics/pain killers	Morphine, codeine	Retention, sedation, overflow, impaction
Alpha-adrenergic agonists	Cardura®, hytrin®	Urethral relation may lead to stress incontinence

Medications That May Affect Incontinence—continued

Type of Medication	Examples	Effect on Incontinence
Calcium channel blockers (blood pressure medication)	Nifedipine	Retention
Alcohol		Frequency, urgency sedation, immobility
ACE inhibitors (blood pressure medication)	Captopril, enalopril	Cough may cause stress incontinence
Chemotherapy	Vincristrine	Retention

Many medications have different characteristics that can contribute to the onset of leakage. For example, antipsychotics, antidepressants. antihistamines, antiparkinson's, antispasmodics, antiarrhythmics for the heart, and opiate painkillers all have anticholinergic properties. Anticholinergic medications affect the nerves of the parasympathetic nervous system, which helps balance the sympathetic nervous system. The sympathetic nervous system modulates the fight-or-flight response. It causes the heart beat to increase, the blood pressure to go up, and the body to move into action during danger. The parasympathetic nervous system is involved in digestion, salivation, and urination; the functions we need for daily living. The main chemical that helps deliver messages between the brain and the target organ of the parasympathetic nervous system is called acetylcholine. Medications that interfere with the function of acetylcholine are called *anticholinergics* (see Chapter 5 for more detail).

One of the remarkable aspects of these medications is that pharmacologists have been able to isolate the specific activity of acetylcholine on nearly every organ. So, an anticholinergic medication may only block the affect of acetylcholine on one organ and not on the others, like the bladder or the eye or the brain. The more specific the medication is, the less effect it will have on other organs. Specificity of effect is considered good in most cases. However, many physicians want to cut down on the number of drugs that an individual is taking, so a medication that will help two or three problems may be desirable. A balance between medications and side effects has to be made on an individual basis. Always bring a list of your medications to the physician's office when you go for an initial consultation. If any of your medications change, alert all or your physicians of the change to be sure that no interactions or side effects will bring on other problems. Generally, physicians will communicate with one another. If each physician has a list of your other doctors, each will notify the other of changes to protect you from problems.

Sometimes, we have no choice and must prescribe something that will cause an undesirable side effect. Incontinence is a terribly debilitating and embarrassing problem, but compared with the risk of heart failure or a stroke, it pales by comparison. For example, if you must take a diuretic to maintain fluid balance in the heart and lungs, but you urinate six times in the morning before you can leave the house, or you are up all night going to the bathroom, then we have to work within the framework of you taking the diuretic. Some suggestions would be to restrict fluids (which should be done on diuretics anyway), take the medication in the morning and stay near the bathroom, and elevate the legs for an hour or two before bed after a full day of walking or standing. Although these are hardly radical steps, they may help make the situation more bearable.

There are occasions where the urologist will have to treat the incontinence even though it is being caused by a medication. Usually in these cases, the problem is multifactorial. You have an underlying predisposition to incontinence that is being made worse by the medication. If the medication cannot be stopped, then we will deal with it. Just because a medication is contributing to the problem does not mean that the problem cannot be solved. It is important for women with heart disease, vascular disease, depression, diabetes, and every other condition to be active. If the medications are causing a problem that precludes exercise and an active lifestyle, the condition is not being adequately managed. Part of effective treatment is treating the condition to allow for an active, healthy, fulfilling quality of life, Incontinence will interfere with that. It must be addressed to get you out of the house to enjoy those golden years!

Rarely, **psychological problems** can lead to urinary incontinence in the elderly woman. Depression is the most common psychiatric disorder seen in older people. In the most extreme cases, the depression itself may be the source of the leakage. Many elderly people are depressed *and* incontinent, but they are not causally related. In other words, treating the depression will not cure the incontinence. The fact that many depressed elderly women also suffer from incontinence has led researchers to study the relationship between the two disorders. There is some speculation that the areas in the brain that control mood and continence are near one another. Elderly people suffer loss of brain tissue secondary to age and mini-strokes, which are caused by microscopic blood clots. The blood clots get stuck in the smallest blood vessels in the brain, killing off the nerves that are supplied by those blood vessels. These events are called microinfarcts. You do not feel these tiny strokes as they are occurring. Over time, the cumulative effect of all of these blockages can result in noticeable changes in brain function. The theory of microinfarction has not been proven because our imaging studies do not pick up blood flow in these tiny vessels. As technology improves, investigators will be able to study smaller and smaller changes within the brain that occur with aging. Microinfarcts and loss of brain tissue to the area of the brain that control depression and continence can result in both conditions presenting at around the same time.

Excessive urine output can result from untreated metabolic abnormalities, such as high blood sugar, congestive heart failure, and high blood calcium. In these conditions, the excessive urination is caused by overproduction of urine by excessive fluid in the body. The bladder is responding appropriately to the increase in volume by signaling that it is time to empty because it is full. The problem is that it is filling too rapidly, precipitating the urge to urinate, which may come on quickly before you can make it to the toilet. An aged bladder that is stressed by high volumes of urine may not be able to handle the fluid as efficiently as it needs to. The result is frequency, urgency, and urinary leakage. Although treatment of the underlying problem is the most sensible solution, it is not always possible. *Every effort should be made to control the original derangement before the bladder is treated.*

High blood sugar signifies diabetes mellitus. Excessive thirst drives diabetics to drink fluids, which produces urine and precipitates the urge to urinate. The woman with uncontrolled diabetes, who drinks water, produces high volumes of urine, so the urge to urinate is justified. The bladder is actually full of water and needs to be emptied. The signals are not crossed, and the problem is not with the bladder. Many diabetics have reduced bladder capacities because of age, but increasing their bladder capacity with medication will not improve the problem. Treating the diabetes is of paramount importance, plus it will reduce the frequency of urination and the leakage.

Congestive heart failure is caused by a weak heart. Women with weak hearts cannot pump blood quickly enough to the rest of the body, so they get a backup of fluid. The backed up blood will pool in the lungs and the body tissues. The treatment is twofold: (1) reduce the work that the heart has to do with medication and (2) reduce the excess fluid in the body with diuretics, also called water pills. Water pills eliminate fluid from the body through the kidneys. Therefore, diuretics cause us to urinate frequently. The excess fluid circulates through the kidneys and collects in the bladder until it is evacuated. The frequency brought on by diuretics is a normal reaction of the bladder to being filled rapidly and fully. Many people drink water to keep up with the frequent evacuation of fluid, but this behavior only perpetuates the problem. The point of the diuretic is to *eliminate* water, so drinking and replacing it is counterproductive. If the bladder fills too much, too often, you will have urgency and incontinence in addition to the frequency. In this case, water restriction is a must in order to help manage the problem while the diuretics are still on board.

Management of the incontinence that results from congestive heart failure can be tricky, but it is doable. Fluid restriction is the hallmark of therapy. Reduction of fluids that increase urination, such as caffeinated beverages and alcohol, is part of fluid restriction. Eliminating or replacing medications that cause pooling of fluid in the legs is also helpful. These medications include antiinflammatory agents, such as ibuprofen (Motrin®, Advil®, Aleve®, Vioxx®, Celebrex®, and Bextra®). Calcium channel blockers, such as Verapamil® and Nifedipine®, increase urination at night through mobilization of fluids in the resting position. Elevation of the legs in the late afternoon and early evening will evacuate fluid that has pooled in the legs during the day. If this fluid is eliminated before bedtime, it will help decrease the need to awaken from sleep and get to the bathroom before leakage sets in.

Although less common a problem among the elderly than diabetes and congestive heart failure, high blood calcium, called hypercalcemia, can also lead to excessive urine output and incontinence. Medications can cause elevated blood calcium, which should be checked in any elderly, incontinent woman.

Restricted mobility, which is the inability to move around easily, prevents you from getting to the bathroom when the urge comes upon you. The result is obvious: you wet the bed. Immobility can be caused by acute illness, injury, restraints, impaired vision, low blood pressure, weakness of the legs, arthritis, poor circulation, spinal cord problems, bad shoes, and imbalance or fear of falling. Many of these conditions are treatable. If the underlying problem can be solved, then, obviously, it should be so that you can move around. If the underlying problem cannot be solved, then some changes need to be made to allow you to empty your bladder without soiling the bed. One solution is to place a commode next to the bed which is readily available to you, especially at night. If that is not effective, medications, surgery, or catheterization may need to be started.

Stool impaction causes incontinence. This is one of the most common causes of urinary problems in the elderly population. Some investigators gauge that about 10% of geriatric incontinence is caused by stool impaction. Although clearly evident, the relationship between constipation and urinary problems is not understood. Two theories can explain the association: one is that the buildup of stool mechanically blocks the outflow of urine. The second is that the bladder responds through crossed nerve impulses that result in reflex bladder contractions when the rectum is distended. Whatever the reason for the leakage, treating constipation should be a part of the program in the elderly incontinent woman. Screening colonoscopy should be done every five years in the low-risk patient (no family or personal history of colon cancer). If no problems are found, such as polyps, tumors, or diverticuli, then the constipation can be treated with fiber products, stool softeners, and diet.

The reversible causes of incontinence can be completely responsible for the leakage in many incontinent elderly women. If they are the not the sole cause, they will surely factor in to some degree. The combination of an aging bladder with a reversible problem will result in intolerable incontinence. Correction of the underlying problem may allow you to function adequately. In some cases, correction of both the underlying problem and the bladder or muscular defect will maintain dryness. Without correction of the underlying problem, however, total continence usually cannot be restored. Recognition of a reversible cause of incontinence is the most prudent first step in the approach to managing your condition if you are an elderly woman.

Persistent or Long-Term Causes of Incontinence
The long-term causes of incontinence are those conditions that have altered the function of the bladder in a way that causes permanent damage. Incontinence due to irreversible causes can still be treated, and often cured. It is just that the underlying condition cannot be altered. These causes of incontinence included poor bladder function, pelvic floor prolapse, and muscle weakness leading to stress incontinence. We distinguish between reversible and irreversible causes of incontinence in elderly women because we want to treat any underlying condition before we treat the incontinence itself.

EVALUATION OF THE INCONTINENT ELDERLY WOMAN

The initial evaluation can be done by a general internist or gynecologist, or you can go to a urologist. Many internists feel more comfortable having the urologist treat incontinence in older people because the condition can be complicated. If you see a urologist, it does not indicate a serious problem. It just means that the internist is being especially careful. No matter who sees you and begins treatment, the evaluation should be similar in its thoroughness.

KEY POINTS THAT NEED TO BE COVERED IN THE INCONTINENT WOMAN'S HISTORY

1. Nature of leakage: Day vs. night, urge vs. no urge, with movement
2. Patient's feelings about leakage: interference with daily living
3. Fluid intake
4. Past urological history
5. Other symptoms: Neurological problems, bowel problems, leg swelling, history of radiation, heart problems, diabetes
6. Vaginal deliveries
7. Gynecological surgery
8. Environmental factors: Location of bathroom
9. Medical conditions
10. Medications

All medical evaluations begin with a thorough history, which includes your own complaints, as well as reports from your family and direct caregivers, and other physicians. Confused women or women with poor short-term memory may need some help in defining the problem. Many elderly people with dementia don't realize that they leak. A phone call to a reliable source who knows you well will prevent confusion. If the most direct caregiver is present at the initial consultation, it will help expedite the evaluation. A list of your medical problems and medications is essential to bring to the appointment. Previous surgeries will also be discussed. All aspects of your past and present medical history need to be mentioned to the physician. A good history will point to the correct diagnosis in most people. Of all the aspects to the evaluation of the incontinent person, the history is the most important (see Chapter 5 for the types of questions that you should be prepared to answer).

Following the history-taking, the physician will examine you. The physical exam includes an abdominal exam to locate scars and assess for bloating, suggesting intestinal problems. A gynecological exam must be done to evaluate for atrophic vaginits and pelvic-floor prolaspe, such as a cystocele, rectocele, or uterine prolapse. A rectal exam is done to check for sensation around the anal opening, anal sphincter tone, and stool impaction in the rectal vault.

A urinalysis and urine culture will be sent from a specimen that you will provide in the office. Catheterized specimens are not necessary unless you can't empty your bladder. The urine studies will evaluate for infection, inflammation, and suggestions of a urological disease. If blood is found in the urine with no evidence of infection, then a full examination of the urinary tract should ensue to look for causes of the microscopic blood. This includes a urine cytology (a urine test sent from the doctor's office that looks for cancer cells in the sample), a kidney ultrasound or CT scan, and a cystoscopy. These last three studies do not need to be done for incontinence unless red blood cells are seen on a urine analysis.

EVALUATION OF URINARY INCONTINENCE IN THE ELDERLY WOMAN

History
Physical examination
Urine analysis and culture
Post-void residual measurement
Optional: Voiding diary
Pad test
Urodynamic studies

Sugar in the urine is also tested in the urinalysis. Occasionally, someone with no prior history of diabetes will see a urologist with frequency, urgency of urination, and incontinence, and will be found to have sugar in the urine. If a woman without diabetes has sugar in the urine on analysis, she should be tested for diabetes with a blood test. Elevated blood sugar levels suggest a diagnosis of diabetes. If you have a known history of diabetes and you are spilling sugar into the urine, then this elevated sugar in the urine may indicate that the diabetes is not being well controlled. It is possible that getting the blood sugar under control will help with the urinary leakage. Certainly, anyone with sugar in the urine on analysis who does not have a diagnosis of diabetes should be sent to an internist for evaluation.

The ability of your bladder to empty is evaluated on this first visit as well. Most urologists have an ultrasound (same as sonogram) machine in the office. Through a probe placed on your abdomen, an image appears on a screen. The amount of fluid in the bladder can be seen easily and no catheters have to be used. The physician can see how much urine is left in the bladder after you urinate. This reading is called the *post-void residual*. A post-void residual over about 200 cc, or $6\frac{1}{2}$ ounces, suggests that your bladder does not empty well. Further testing may be warranted in this situation. Usually, an ultrasound of the kidneys is performed to be sure that the increase in urine sitting in the bladder is not blocking the kidneys. If the blockage extends up to the kidneys, then a catheter will need to be inserted to drain the bladder, and further testing is warranted. In this case, the incontinence becomes a symptom of a more serious urological problem. Although this is rare, a careful evaluation will pick up all of these abnormalities.

If the history, physical exam, and urine tests are normal, most women can be treated directly for one of the four causes of urinary incontinence not related to reversible incontinence. These causes include urge incontinence, stress incontinence, overflow incontinence, and functional incontinence. **Urge incontinence, caused by bladder spasms, is the most common cause of purely urological incontinence in the elderly woman.** Treatment without invasive testing is safe and generally effective. If the medication fails, then further testing can be done.

If the medication does not work or if you are found to have a large volume of urine left in your bladder after urinating, then a urodynamic test should be performed to determine the ability of the bladder to hold urine and its ability to empty (see Chapter 12). Through this testing, the problem can be identified and treatment can be directed. The choice to go ahead with the study or try medications first is up to you and your doctor.

The voiding diary is a helpful adjunct to diagnosis and treatment. The voiding diary is a three-day record of the frequency of urination and the amount that is emptied each time. You record the time of your urge to urinate, the time you actually get the bathroom, the amount you urinate, and the whether or not leakage has occurred, all over a three-day period. Preferably, you choose one day at work, one day at home, and one day out socially. The activity that you are doing and the proximity you have to the bathroom may play a role in your urinary behavior. Important information comes out of the voiding diary. If you are emptying large volumes of urine all throughout the day, perhaps a problem with your metabolism is present, such as diabetes or high calcium in the bloodstream. If you go frequently at home or at work, but infrequently when you are out shopping, then behavior plays a role in your frequency.

After treatment has been instituted, a second three-day voiding diary can be used to measure the degree of improvement. Some women like to measure improvement by the reduction in the number of pads they wear. Some want to see a reduction in the number of times they go the bathroom during the day and during the night. The diary can be a nuisance, but it is a helpful addition to the evaluation of the degree of leakage.

Some physicians also use a pad test to determine the amount of leakage a woman has. The pad test is another objective way of determining how bad your incontinence really is. You collect your pads for an entire day in a zip-lock baggie and bring them into the doctor's office. You need to bring a dry pad in a separate bag. The doctor will weigh the dry pad first, and then weigh the wet pads. The amount of leakage is determined when the dry weight of the pads is subtracted from wet weight. This value will give you the amount of urine that you leaked that day in grams. This test can be repeated after treatment to see how effective the intervention is.

If you seek help for incontinence from a urologist or urogynecologist, a long, painful, invasive evaluation will not be recommended. Fearful from past experiences at the urologist's office, many women are afraid of what will happen to them if they seek treatment. Even if urodynamic tests or catheterization is necessary, it is not painful or unpleasant if done gently and with care. No invasive testing should be initiated without you and your family's or caregiver's full understanding of what is to be done and how that information will be used to help you with your problem.

TREATMENT OF URINARY INCONTINENCE

Two thirds of elderly patients with urinary incontinence can be cured and the other one third can be dramatically improved. No nursing-home- or community-dwelling woman should be suffering from debilitating urinary leakage. The treatments range from alterations in your daily routine to provide for frequent toileting to dramatic surgeries and catheterization. The physician, the patient, and the caregiver need to make some decisions regarding the risks and benefits of whatever treatment is being offered. In general, if a careful evaluation is done, treatment can be both effective and minimally traumatic for every woman.

Treat the Reversible Causes of Incontinence
The first order of business is to eliminate one of the eight reversible causes of incontinence that were discussed above. If your incontinence is being caused by a correctable problem, then the problem should be taken care of

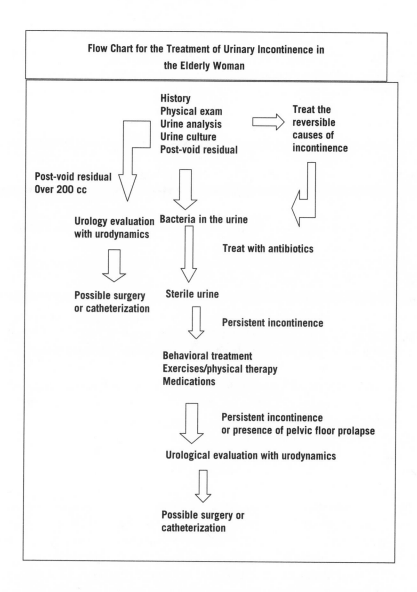

Flow Chart for the Treatment of Urinary Incontinence in
the Elderly Woman

History
Physical exam
Urine analysis
Urine culture
Post-void residual

Treat the
reversible
causes of
incontinence

Post-void residual
Over 200 cc

Urology evaluation
with urodynamics

Bacteria in the urine

Treat with antibiotics

Possible surgery
or catheterization

Sterile urine

Persistent incontinence

Behavioral treatment
Exercises/physical therapy
Medications

Persistent incontinence
or presence of pelvic floor prolapse

Urological evaluation with urodynamics

Possible surgery or
catheterization

first. Although that seems obvious, it is not always done. Demented women are the ones who get cheated the most in terms of trying to find a workable program of dryness. Surprisingly enough, these women do just as well as every other woman with incontinence if they are managed within the framework of their abilities. Access to a bathroom, reminders to urinate, and reducing fluid intake will often be all that is needed to maintain some level of urinary control.

Small improvements in many areas of an elderly woman's life will ultimately result in changes for the better with urinary behavior. Increased mobility, improved attention, motivation to stay dry, and improvements in manual dexterity through physical and occupational therapy all play important roles. Adjusting fluids and toileting schedules, especially in nursing homes, may get an elderly woman out of diapers. Many people force themselves to drink eight glasses of water each day, only to get the urge every hour during the day and awaken six times a night. Reducing the amount of fluid taken in may help the problem and reduce the urgency by 50%. That fluid is obviously not going to good use because it is being evacuated as quickly as it is being consumed. What a logical intervention for a problem that throws people into major depression!

Bacteria in the Urine
Once the reversible causes of incontinence have been identified and treated, persistence of the problem will warrant continued investigation. It is not unusual to have some residual problems with leakage even though all other medical issues have been addressed.

Bacteria in the urine is a tricky subject. If you have symptoms of an infection, such as burning with urination, frequency, and leakage, with a finding of bacteria in the urine, then we say that you have a *urinary tract infection*. If you do not have any symptoms even though bacteria have been found in the urine, we say that you have *asymptomatic bacteriuria*. Young women usually have symptoms when the bladder becomes colonized with bacteria. Older women will often have bacteria in the urine with none of the usual symptoms of an infection. You may feel fine even though the bladder is loaded with bacteria.

Whether or not to treat these bacteria is dependent on what else is going on. If you have urinary incontinence or frequency, and bacteria are found in your bladder, then you should be treated with a course of antibiotics. Posttreatment cultures should be done to document that the bladder is clear of bacteria. If the incontinence persists in spite of sterile urine, then the leakage was not due to the bacteria and other causes need to be investigated. If the leakage goes away, then incontinence becomes a sign of an infection in your system, and you need to be treated for a urinary tract infection when the leakage recurs. Symptoms of a bladder infection are not always so straightforward. Urinary leakage may be the only sign of one in an elderly woman.

Incomplete Bladder Emptying

If no bacteria are found in the urine or the incontinence persists in spite of an adequately treated infection, then interventions to treat the incontinence, specifically, can begin. If incomplete bladder emptying is noted on the post-void residual ultrasound test, then you are not emptying your bladder completely. You need to see a urologist to evaluate why this is happening. Urodynamic testing in the urologist's office will determine whether the incomplete emptying is due to the blockage of outflow or poor bladder muscle function.

TREATMENT OF INCOMPLETE BLADDER EMPTYING

Cause	*Treatment*
Obstruction	Surgery/pessary
Bladder muscle weakness	Catherization
	Self-catheterization
	Chronic indwelling
	Urethral
	Suprapubic
	Neuromodulation

Blockage of Outflow

Incomplete emptying may be due to blockage of the outflow of urine. Causes of outflow obstruction in women include urethral masses and pelvic-floor prolapse. The most common urethral masses are **urethral prolapse** and urethral caruncles. Even though the names are the same, prolapse of the inner lining of the urethra is unrelated to pelvic-floor prolapse. With excessive bearing down, as one would do to make a bowel movement, the lining of the urethra can protrude through the opening. It looks like a beefy, red mass at the top of the vagina. It may be sore and painful to the touch, and occasionally it can bleed, often producing clots. They are treated with the direct application of estrogen cream, or surgical excision if the bleeding is profuse. A **caruncle**, on the urethra, is analogous to a hemorrhoid, which is on the anus. It is a blood vessel that gets clogged with a blood clot. It looks like a small grape-like lesion on the tip of the urethra. They are usually not painful, although, on occasion, they can bleed. Rarely, they are removed surgically. Urethral tumors are extremely uncommon. They present with bleeding and a firm mass in the urethra. They need to be removed surgically. Urethral prolapse, caruncles, and tumors seldom cause blockage of urine.

Pelvic-floor prolapse is discussed in detail in the next chapter. In some cases, a pessary can be inserted to alleviate the blockage. In other cases, surgery may need to be performed to fix the prolapse and preserve urinary tract function, in addition to treating the incontinence. Surgery in older women can be a delicate proposition, but it should be entertained if the prolapse is causing serious quality-of-life issues. With proper preoperative evaluation and optimization, most women can undergo a surgical procedure that will correct a problem that, if untreated, could result in disastrous consequences.

Loss of Bladder Muscle Function
One of the more unfortunate outcomes of the aging bladder is the loss of muscle contractions within the bladder muscle itself. If outflow obstruction is not the cause of the incomplete bladder emptying, then loss of muscle function is. If this diagnosis is being entertained, urodynamic studies will show if the bladder muscle has lost its ability to squeeze urine out of the bladder. There is no way to regain the bladder muscle's ability to function once it is lost.

INDICATIONS FOR CATHETERIZATION

Overflow incontinence
Kidney impairment due to bladder fullness
Skin breakdown due to incontinence
Pressure ulcers that cannot heal due to wetness
Patient/caregiver preference

Incomplete bladder emptying can only be treated with catheterization or, in select women, neuromodulation. The bottom line is that a woman with a bladder muscle that does not work will need to mechanically empty her bladder by herself or by wearing a catheter all the time. Catheters in the elderly woman can be very useful and very liberating. If the choice is either being homebound with leakage or being active with a catheter, most people would rather have a catheter. Good catheter management is essential to the success of this form of treatment.

Intermittent self-catheterization remains the best option from a medical standpoint for a woman in whom catheterization becomes necessary. With intermittent self-catheterization, you or your caregiver inserts a small catheter into your bladder through the urethra and drains the urine into the toilet. You then remove the catheter until the next time. It is done when you feel the urge to urinate or arbitrarily, such as every four to six hours. If you have lost the sensation of needing to void, then you will have to empty at regular intervals so that the bladder does not overfill and you begin to leak. You can be taught the technique in the doctor's office using a mirror. Eventually, insertion of the catheter becomes second nature and you can catheterize yourself in public places as easily as you do at home. Of course, when presented for the first time, most women gasp in horror at the idea of catheterizing themselves. I tell them that it is just like putting contact lenses in your eyes. One never thinks that she can touch her eyeballs, but after a few attempts, it becomes easy.

The advantages to self-catheterization are enormous. The bladder continues to function as it would if you were urinating normally. It fills to its capacity and drains completely. The risk of infection is low because the bladder is continuously being drained and flushed of bacteria. No stagnant urine is sitting around waiting to become infected. Sterile catheters do not need to be used. You just wash off the catheter before use and insert it. It is kept in a baggie until the next use. The same catheter gets used over and over, until it begins to look dirty. Even though it is not a natural way to empty the bladder, it is the best option for the woman with incomplete emptying and a high post-void residual in whom no bladder function is seen on urodynamics.

The downside to self-catheterization is obvious. In women, the urethra is not as accessible as we would like it to be for this maneuver. In order to find the hole a women needs to bend over and look down into the genital area. Many older patients with osteoarthritis and spinal problems are not so agile. With practice, it is done by feel. The next best option is for a caregiver to insert the catheter when needed. This alternative is not as great as it sounds because a caregiver may not be around 24 hours a day. Also, when another person catheterizes a woman, she needs to be lying on her back so that the other person can see where the catheter is going. This limits activities because a bed must be available every couple of hours for bladder emptying. Usually, if a woman is unable to catheterize herself, then one of the other catheter choices may have be selected.

If intermittent self-catheterization cannot be done, then an **indwelling foley catheter** will need to be inserted. A foley catheter is a long rubber tube with two ports at one end and a balloon at the other end. The tube is hollow so urine can drain through it from inside the bladder, out though one of

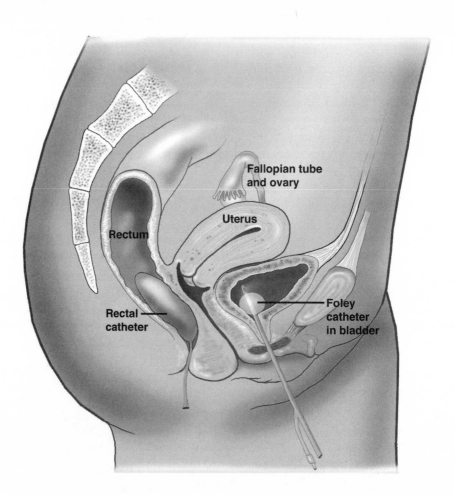

F I G U R E 3 . *Urethral Foley Catheter.*

the ports. When inflated, the balloon holds the catheter inside the bladder. The diameter of the balloon is larger than the outlet from the bladder into the urethra. The other port allows water to be injected into the balloon for inflation and deflation. In its simplicity and function, the foley catheter is one of the most ingenious inventions in medicine. It was invented by a third-year medical student who revolutionized urinary drainage and changed our management of urological patients dramatically.

SIDE-EFFECTS OF CHRONIC INDWELLING CATHETERS

1. **Chronic bacteria in the bladder**
2. **Bladder stones**
3. **Abscesses around the urethra**
4. **Bladder cancer (very rare)**

A foley catheter can be inserted into the bladder and attached to a bag that is secured to your leg under your clothes. With the bladder deflated, the urine drains continuously from the bladder into the leg bag. The leg bag is emptied when it gets full. Because no odor is identified and the bag is hidden under your clothes, other people will not know that you have a foley catheter. You never have to think about going to the bathroom except to empty your bowels. The catheter gets changed every month or six weeks, either by a doctor or a visiting nurse.

In some cases, the catheter irritates the bladder wall as the balloon bounces around inside the body. You may leak urine as a result of the bladder wall contracting around the balloon. In women with absolutely no bladder function, this problem never becomes an issue because the muscle is not responsive. In women with some function of the muscle, it may create an annoying problem with leakage, and sometimes, it may cause pain. These spasms can be treated effectively with medication. Just be sure that the doctor is aware of the problem.

Besides spasms, the catheter can be irritating between your legs while you sit. Because the catheter is inserted into the urethra, which lies under the pubic bone, women, especially those in wheelchairs, may wind up sitting on the catheter all day. This pressure can be painful and result in ulcers around the urethra. The walls of the urethra can break down causing a horrible problem with leakage and fistulas (see Glossary). A solution to the pain associated with urethral catheterization is to put the catheter into the body through a hole on the abdominal wall just above the pubic bone. This location is called *suprapubic* (above the pubic bone). In women, **suprapubic tubes** are exceptionally easy to manage for you, your caregiver and the doctor. Not painful, it can be cleaned easily with water in the shower. A small piece of gauze will cover the site to keep your clothes dry. In this location, the tube can even be plugged and taped to your belly. The bladder will fill normally and the tube drained into a container or the toilet when you have the urge to urinate. No bags are necessary, so you will have maximal mobility throughout the day. During the night, the tube can be attached to a large bedside bag for continuous drainage. You will then be able to sleep through the night without awakening to urinate.

Indwelling catheters must be changed on a regular basis. Usually, once a month or every six weeks is enough to keep you comfortable and dry. Catheter changes can be done by visiting nurses, caregivers, or physicians at the office. Occasionally, the catheter can clog with debris. If you are prone to catheter clogging, irrigations can be done at home on a daily basis to keep the tube open. Cystoscopy, a visual inspection of the bladder performed by a urologist, should be done every year in the catheterized person. The irritation of the bladder wall by the catheter and the balloon can induce cellular changes that need to be watched. Some of the more serious complications of chronic catheterization include bladder stones, abscesses around the urethra, and bladder cancer. All of these are unusual and easily managed if they are found early and you are surveyed regularly.

Infections in the catheterized patient are always a source of concern for women and their families. All catheterized women will have *colonization* of bacteria, that is, the bladder will always have bacteria sitting there. Most of the time, the bacteria are not dangerous. They will live in the bladder symbiotically with you, minding their own business, not causing trouble. Sometimes, the bacteria will get out of hand, multiply, and cause trouble. Trouble includes new onset of leakage, urgency, pain, fever, nausea, lethargy, or loss of appetite. If a catheterized woman manifests any of these symptoms, a urine sample should be obtained and a culture grown. Treatment can begin and the catheter changed. Upon completion of treatment with antibiotics, the symptoms should have resolved. If they have not, another source of the symptoms needs to be identified or you will need to see a urologist. Routine urine cultures are not necessary in the catheterized women. These cultures will invariably be positive for bacteria and unnecessary treatment will result. Nursing home residents, in particular, should be spared from unnecessary courses of antibiotics because resistance to antibiotics is very high in this patient population.

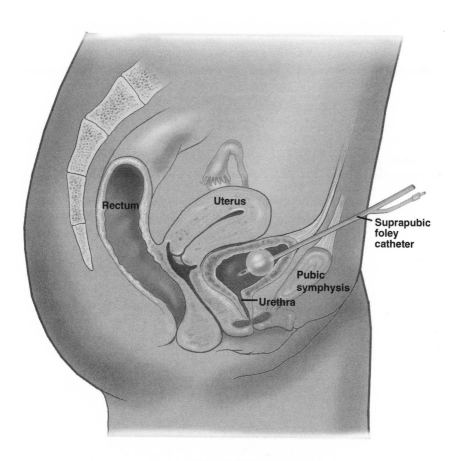

FIGURE 4. *Suprapubic Foley Catheter.*

As with all problems, risks and benefits have to be weighed. The humiliation, discomfort, and inconvenience of urinary leakage mixed with the risk of kidney deterioration needs to be weighed against the unpleasantness of catheterization. Neither option is great, but one will allow you to be mobile, active, and social. The other keeps you isolated and depressed. Encouragement and a positive outlook on the part of your caregivers and doctors will help you accept some of these less appealing options.

Persistent Incontinence: Urge Incontinence and Stress Incontinence
If overflow incontinence is not the problem because the post-void residual urine measurement is below 200 cc, then you are experiencing either urge incontinence or stress incontinence. These conditions are managed the same way in older women as they are in younger women (see Chapters 4 and 5.) Surgery will not correct urge incontinence and medication will not correct stress incontinence. However, many of you have components of both types of incontinence, which is addressed in those previous chapters.

TREATMENT OF URGE, STRESS, AND FUNCTIONAL INCONTINENCE IN THE ELDERLY WOMAN

Behavioral Intervention
  Fluid restriction
  Prompted voiding
Exercise/Physical therapy
Medication
Surgery
Catheterization

Behavioral Therapy
Behavioral therapy is the first line of treatment with any type of leakage. Reduction of fluid intake will alleviate the work of the bladder. The kidneys lose their ability to concentrate urine as they age. The hormones that control the reabsorption of water by the collecting ducts of the kidneys become less effective with age. They also lose their circadian rhythm of secretion. In children, the activity of antidiuretic hormone increases at night, reabsorbing water back into the bloodstream. Less fluid enters the bladder with each pass of blood through the kidneys. The result is that children can sleep for 12 hours without waking up to use the bathroom. With age, the amount and timing of the release of these hormones changes, resulting in the need to

awaken at night to urinate. Reducing the amount the fluids consumed, especially at bedtime will help reduce the volume of fluid that makes it into the bladder.

Many people register concern when I tell then to reduce their fluids. Four glasses of water per day, or 32 ounces, is enough to maintain hydration. In some cases, the extra fluid is consumed to help with bowel activity. However, eight glasses of water per day is not necessary to make a bowel movement. Fruit, vegetables, and grains in combination with the four glasses of water will provide enough fluid and enough roughage to maintain a balanced system in most people.

Prompted voiding works well in elderly women, especially if they are slightly confused or have problems sensing fullness of the bladder. In prompted voiding, the woman is asked if she has to urinate every two hours or so during the day, and every four hours at night. A commode is placed within reasonable proximity to her bed. If she has to climb stairs in order to reach the bathroom, she may have a problem making it in time. Many nursing home inhabitants do well with the combination of fluid restriction and prompted voiding. The lack of sensation to urinate is a common problem among elderly women. Diabetes and pelvic-floor prolapse predispose us to the lack of sensation for the urge to urinate. Some women will leak with a sudden urge to urinate. In these patients, prompted voiding is particularly successful. If she is reminded to go to the bathroom before the sudden urge comes on, a woman will likely be able to make it to the toilet before she leaks.

Exercise and Physical Therapy

In motivated women, exercise therapy and biofeedback can produce wonderful results. *Kegel exercises* help to strengthen the pelvic-floor muscles. When you get an urge to urinate, you contract those muscles, giving you a few extra seconds to get to the toilet. Kegel exercises are easy to teach (see Glossary). If you are having trouble identifying the muscles that you need to work, then you can see a specialist in biofeedback and pelvic-floor physical therapy.

Physical therapy for incontinence is more involved that is biofeedback. Physical therapists are experts in the activity and repair of damaged muscles. An area within physical therapy is emerging, in which practitioners work on pelvic-floor muscle disorders. Incontinence can be improved in certain women. Motivation is the most important component of a good outcome. Like any muscle exercise, you have to be cooperative and willing to continue with the program after the completion of the most intensive training.

Confused women are not candidates for this. Not all physical therapists work in this area, so some effort may be needed to find a therapist interested in pelvic-floor disorders. Older women can do very well with these interventions as long as they are willing to put in the effort.

Besides Kegel exercises and biofeedback, physical therapists will use massage therapy, stretching, vaginal weights, and electrical stimulation to work with their patients.

CAUSES AND TREATMENTS OF PERSISTENT INCONTINENCE IN THE ELDERLY WOMAN

Cause	*Treatment*
Urge incontinence	Medication
	Nerve stimulator implant
	Botox
Stress incontinence	Injection of bulking agent
	Surgical insertion of pubovaginal sling
Pelvic floor prolapse	Surgical repair of the prolapse
	Catheterization
Urethral masses (RARE)	Surgical removal

- *Massage therapy* helps release tension in the pelvic floor so that the muscles can be worked.
- *Stretching* also opens up the area for easier identification of the muscles.
- *Vaginal weights* are used to tense certain muscle groups. Different size weights are inserted into the vagina and you have to hold them in position. As you get stronger, you can hold heavier weights.
- *Electrical stimulation* is a passive method through which muscles can be exercised. A low-voltage electrical current is directed into a muscle, which will twitch in response. The twitch is a contraction that increases the tone of the muscle being worked.

Although these methods seem a bit barbaric when they are described, they are actually painless. This part of the female anatomy is neglected in so many ways. Education about the mechanics and increasing the tone of these muscles can do wonders for issues of incontinence.

Improvements usually result after behavioral therapy, exercise therapy, and physical therapy have been implemented. Many of you will be better just because you are out of bed and moving around more. Some of you will still be wet. The next step in treatment depends on the type of incontinence from which you suffer. If you have urge incontinence, medications can be offered. If you have stress incontinence, surgery will be discussed. In that case, either medication or surgery will need to be discussed.

Medication

Medication is available to treat urge incontinence only. The options that are available to older women are the same as the choices for younger women. Some of them affect older people differently, but they are all effective. Tolerance to a medication is specific to each individual. You and you doctor can discuss the pros and cons of the different formulation and come up with a choice to start with. The most important thing to keep in mind is that any of them can be stopped immediately without any bad outcome. If you suspect a problem, stop the medicine right away. The list of medications and the way they work are discussed in Chapter 5 in detail.

If all efforts at treatment have not yielded an improvement or if you have stress incontinence or prolapse, then invasive measures have to be taken. Now it is time to see a urologist who either specializes in incontinence or a urogynecologist. Surgery or catheterization may be indicated, but neither should be considered without some information about the bladder function. Urodynamic testing will give the physician the informations he needs to recommend either surgery or long term catheterization.

Urge Incontinence

Urge incontinence that does not respond to medication may respond to a bladder pacemaker or botulinum toxin (Botox) injections into the bladder wall. The bladder pacemaker (Intersim® made by Medtronic) is a relatively new development in the urological armamentarium. A wire is inserted into your sacral spine where the nerves that supply the bladder come out of the spinal cord. The wire is attached to a device that is inserted under the skin of the buttock. The device is adjusted with a magnet that raises and lowers the voltage that is delivered through the wire into the spinal nerves. This nerve stimulator overrides the native impulses from your spinal nerves, resulting in relaxation of the pelvic and bladder muscles. The science behind these nerve stimulators is not clear, but there can be dramatic results in those of you who suffer from urge incontinence not responsive to medication.

The beauty of this device is that it can be tested before a permanent implant is done. A test stimulation is done in the physician's office and you will go home for three days with an external pacing device. The external voltage control can be increased or decreased by you depending on the amount of leakage weighed against the discomfort of the electricity. If the method works, a permanent implant will be done in the hospital. The device lasts for about five years before it needs to be replaced. Nerve stimulators are being tested for urinary retention and pelvic pain syndromes as well.

Botulinum toxin injections into the bladder paralyze the muscle, preventing it from going into spasm. A relatively new procedure, Botox injections are reserved for patients with urge incontinence that does not respond to any other interventions. The injections can be done in the physician's office or in a surgical center under light sedation. Like Botox injections elsewhere in the body, the effect wears off in about six months. Research is ongoing in this area.

Stress Incontinence

If the persistent leakage is due to stress incontinence, then surgery is going to be the next option that is offered. Stress incontinence results from an open urethra. Unfortunately, medications to treat stress incontinence are not available. A few companies have drugs in the pipeline, but none is ready for prime time yet. The options for the treatment of stress incontinence include injections of bulking agents into the urethra or surgery to support the urethra in the way that the pelvic floor muscles no longer can (see Chapter 4).

Elderly women can be excellent candidates for surgery, as long as proper precautions are taken preoperatively. The risk of anesthesia is much lower than it has ever been before. With a healthy heart and lungs, people of any age can undergo successful operations. If the quality of life is severely impaired by the incontinence and surgery is the only option to control the problem, then it should be done. In good hands, a successful outcome will not only enhance your lifestyle, but it will prolong your life. The resolution of the leakage will encourage you to be more active, more social, and, ultimately, healthier. The details of anesthesia and the postoperative course are outlined in Chapter 11.

Pelvic-Floor Prolapse

If a prolapse (the bladder, uterus small intestine or rectum has descended into the vaginal canal) is found on physical exam, intervention does not have to be done immediately to correct the prolapse. In many cases, correcting the prolapse will not necessarily improve the incontinence. Before surgery is done to reduce the prolapse, testing is warranted to correlate the prolapse with the incontinence. These are two separate issues that may *or may not* impact on one another. The presence of an anatomical abnormality does not in and of itself mean that it is causing the symptoms.

If pelvic-floor prolapse is identified and noted to be causing the urinary problems on urodynamic testing, then either a repair will need to be done, or a pessary inserted (see Chapter 7). A pessary is a rubber ring that, when inserted into the vagina, supports the prolapse. The prolapse is pushed back into the vagina, but leakage, frequency, urgency, and nighttime waking to urinate may persist. Urinary problems due to pelvic-floor prolapse may not be helped by inserting a pessary. But the bladder may empty better, which would allow medications to work for the urinary symptoms. A trial with a pessary can be attempted. No harm is done by trying it before surgery is done.

When done correctly and for the right reasons, pelvic-floor prolapse surgery can be very effective in older women. Urodynamics must be done first to correlate the prolapse with the incontinence. Just because a prolapse exists in the same patient who has incontinence, does not mean that one causes the other. Once the relationship is determined, then surgery should be done. Elderly women can do exceptionally well with prolapse repairs. If the repair is done vaginally, you will have minimal side effects from the operation.

A few words on the surgery for prolapse: either spinal or general anesthesia is required. You come into the hospital the day of surgery on an empty stomach. The surgery will take anywhere from one to three hours depending on what needs to be done. Sometimes just the bladder and the urethra need to be lifted, sometimes the uterus has to be supported or removed, and sometimes the rectum needs to be tacked out of the way. After the surgery, you will go to the recovery room for two or three hours to come out of the anesthesia. While you are there, your vital signs and urine output are monitored. Once you are stable, you are sent to a room on a regular floor to convalesce for the next day or two. Depending on your overall health, some doctors will allow you to leave the hospital within one to two days after the surgery.

Once at home, most women will have discomfort without much pain. The biggest concerns postoperatively are bowel movements and urination, especially in the older woman. Usually, a urinary catheter is left for a few days to allow for all of the swelling to go down in the area. Once the tube is removed, normal urination will return within a few days. Some physicians

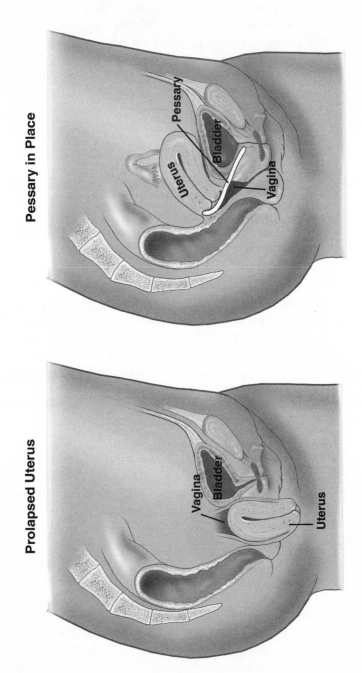

Pessary in Place

Pessary

Bladder

Uterus

Vagina

Prolapsed Uterus

Vagina

Bladder

Uterus

FIGURE 5. *Pessary for Uterine Prolapse Label*

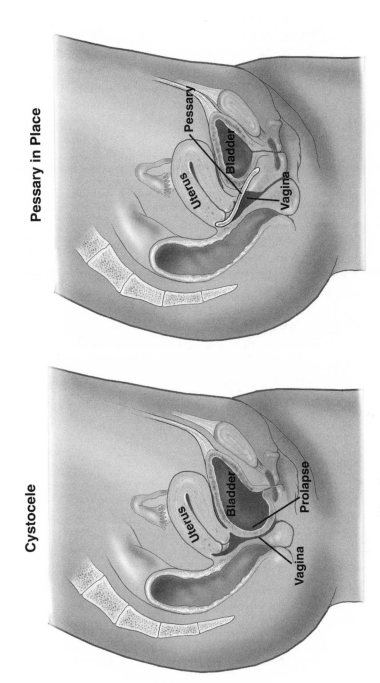

FIGURE 6. *Pessary for Cystocele label.*

will leave a tube that does not come out of the urethra, but comes out through a small puncture immediately above the pubic bone. This is called a *suprapubic tube*. This tube gets capped and taped to the belly. You go home with the tube. When you get the urge to urinate, you try to go naturally. Once you have gone as much as you can, you can then uncap the tube and drain out the left over urine, or the residual. When the residual is less than 50 cc, the tube is removed in the office. This method of catheter management prevents the tube from being removed too early, which can cause retention of urine. In any case, urination ultimately will return to normal and you will be much better off after surgery than before.

Bowel function after surgery also becomes a preoccupation. Elderly women have bowel problems to begin with. Surgery only exacerbates the problem in the short term. Stool softeners and bulking agents help until everything ultimately returns to normal. It always does.

Prolapse surgeries are very successful in women in their 70s and 80s who need them. Correction of the defects allows you to be mobile and active. In this age group, remaining active is essential for survival. Incontinence and prolapse can interfere with overall lifespan in older women. I always tell families that fret over correcting this problem in women in their 80s and 90s, "What is the point of getting to this age if you can't live your life comfortably?" With proper preoperative evaluation and optimization, and careful correlation of symptoms to the physical exam, successful surgery will result and you can be dry and happy.

If All Else Fails . . .

If you have untreatable incontinence and cannot have any surgical or procedural intervention at all, catheterization may be the only choice. A chronic indwelling catheter can be left to drain in a woman who has terrible leakage, especially if she is wheelchair bound. The catheter will keep the bladder drained, so spasms will not occur and you are not running to the bathroom all day and all night. The bag can be secured to the leg under the clothing so no one will see it. If spasms occur around the catheter, medications can be added to quiet the bladder down. The catheter will need to be changed every month and flushed on a daily or weekly basis with water. Overall, catheter care is simple and clean. Although it seems horrible conceptually, this option may be the best chance in getting you both dry and active.

Occasionally infections will result from the catheter, but these are rare. Most of the time, the infection rate is much lower with the catheter in than with the constant wetness that you have without the catheter. Skin breakdown, pressure ulcers, and urinary tract infections will all improve from a chronic indwelling catheter.

An alternative to an indwelling urethral catheter, is an indwelling suprapubic catheter. This tube is inserted into the bladder through a small puncture above the pubic bone. The first time the tube is inserted, it is done under sedation, usually in a surgical setting. The urologist inserts it the first time. Then it can be changed by a caregiver or a visiting nurse every six to eight weeks. The catheter can be plugged during the day while you are out and about. When you get the urge to urinate, you go into the bathroom and unplug the tube, draining the urine into the toilet. The tube is then replugged until the next urge occurs. With this method, no bag is needed.

SUMMARY

Urinary incontinence is common in the elderly woman, but not acceptable. With effective treatments available for nearly every situation, women and their families need to inform their physicians of this depressing, debilitating, and embarrassing problem. Urinary leakage in the elderly can cause terrible problems that go beyond the inconvenience of soiled clothes and bed sheets. Infections, pressure sores, limitations to physical activity, and falls that result as you try to get to the bathroom in time to prevent an accident will all lead to an early demise. Careful evaluation and thoughtful treatment can save you and your caregivers from the difficult and painful consequences of urinary incontinence. Medication and surgery are not the only options out there. Many less-invasive interventions can be attempted, many of which will cure you without any painful testing or expensive procedures. Communication between you and your doctor will ensure that good results are achieved. A little persistence and a lot of patience will produce effective results for almost all elderly women with incontinence.

PART THREE

DROPPED ORGANS: PELVIC-FLOOR PROLAPSE

CHAPTER 7

Pelvic-Floor Prolapse

A. came to see me after her gynecologist told her that her bladder had descended into her vaginal canal. She had no idea what that meant, but it sure sounded like something that needed to be attended to sooner rather than later.

Upon questioning, A. told me that she feels pressure and pulling in her lower body as the day progresses. In the mornings when she wakes, she feels fine, but by the late afternoon, she just wants to take a break and put her feet up for 20 minutes or so to relieve the pressure. Recently, she noticed a ball in her vagina when she wiped herself after urinating and defecating. That ball has been present for a few years and never really bothered her. It hasn't gotten any bigger, nor has it ever come out and not gone back into her vagina.

In terms of her urination, she reported getting up once or twice per night and going every few hours during the day. Frequency is not a problem, but sometimes, she gets the urge to empty her bladder, but nothing will come out. She may wait a few minutes, but the urge nearly always passes. Occasionally, she will try to urinate and an intermittent stream will result. Not feeling empty, she will go back a few minutes later and drain the rest. She has had a few accidents where she gets the urge to urinate and will lose a few drops of urine on the way to the bathroom. She does not wear pads on a daily basis.

A. has had two children through natural childbirth, a fact that she is proud to report. She had a hysterectomy for irregular bleeding over 20 years ago. Otherwise, her past medical and surgical histories are not remarkable. She works every day and exercises two to three times a week at a gym.

Examination of her pelvis reveals a round ball in her vagina which, I explained to her, is her bladder, covered with vaginal skin, sitting in the canal. The urethra sits on top of the vagina. A small red blood vessel is pushing out of the urethra. This is called a urethral caruncle and appears in women who push to evacuate the bladder. When the ball in the vagina is pulled out of the way with a speculum, the vaginal canal is noted to be long and well supported. There are no other organs falling into the canal besides the bladder. The urine analysis revealed some red blood cells, some white blood cells, and was cloudy in color. The volume of urine found in the bladder on ultrasound after A. urinated was 250 cc, or 6 ounces. She felt empty.

Her two vaginal deliveries and hysterectomy put A. at risk for developing pelvic floor prolapse. The fact that she has minimal urinary symptoms means that either the bladder has not been affected very much at all or it is so badly affected that it barely functions. This distinction will be made with further testing. The physical examination reveals a grade 2 to 3 out of 4 bladder prolapse, called a cystocele. The grading system helps physicians communicate with one other regarding the degree of the descent. The worst prolapse is a grade 4; the least, a grade 1. The fact that she has no other organs falling into her vagina, such as a small intestinal prolapse, a rectal prolapse, simplifies the problem. She had a hysterectomy, so her uterus is not involved.

The urine analysis suggests that A. has a urinary tract infection, which may be due to the incomplete emptying. The residual urine acts as a stagnant pool of fluid in which bacteria can replicate. Prevention of infections will only occur if the bladder can be drained.

I offered A. a number of approaches to tackling her problem. The simplest intervention would be to insert a pessary into her vagina. A pessary is a rubber ring that slips into the vagina, like a diaphragm, only it is stiffer. It sits against the pubic bone and the back wall of the vagina, supporting the bladder. The bladder sits in the middle of the ring. The pessary can be left in place for three months at a time, at which point it is removed and cleaned. Many women prefer to have a physician take care of the pessary, while others will remove, clean, and reinsert it themselves. A pessary will not cure the problem, but it will manage it safely.

The more permanent option would be surgery. Surgery will fix the prolapse once and for all. Before surgery is done, urodynamic tests or cystometrics should be performed to evaluate her bladder function. Urinary problems that may surface after surgery can be identified on this office procedure. Kidney tests to evaluate for stones and fluid buildup is required by some physicians, as is cystoscopy.

Because A. did not have the time right away to devote to healing from an operation, she decided to try the pessary first while she did all of her preoperative work and scheduled the surgery. In the office, the pessary was inserted into her vagina without any pain or discomfort. She walked around for a few minutes and urinated before leaving with the pessary neatly tucked away under her bladder.

Unfortunately, later that night, it fell into the toilet while she was making a bowel movement. So much for the pessary. Needless to say, the pessary remained out until she came back to the office. We tried to insert a larger pessary, but it was uncomfortable. The following month, she came for urodynamic testing. The test revealed that she would do well with surgery; her bladder function was excellent. The kidney ultrasound showed that she has two healthy kidneys with no stones or blockages. Now that she knew what the plan was, A. could not get the surgery out of her mind. She cancelled her plans and scheduled the surgery for the following month.

On the morning of the operation, she met the anesthesiologist who reviewed her chart and discussed the options with her. She could either go to sleep or have the surgery done under a spinal anesthetic. She chose the spinal in an effort to reduce postoperative nausea and disorientation. The operation took a little over an hour and involved supporting the bladder and the urethra with a nylon netting. Her legs came back to life about two hours after getting to the recovery room, after which she was transferred to her room for dinner. She was hungry and tired, but, aside from some pressure in her bladder, she felt remarkably well.

The following morning, a long gauze packing was removed from A.'s vagina and a catheter was removed from her bladder. She ate breakfast, urinated in fits and spurts and was discharged home. Aside from feeling like she was hit by a truck, A. did not feel as badly as she thought she would. She slept for most of the next few days and ate in small quantities. The urine flow improved daily until it returned to nearly normal about two weeks after the operation. She was able to return to her activities of daily living gradually. On her two-week postoperative visit, her bladder was well supported, it was emptying well, and she had no leakage. She was actually going to the bathroom less often, and even sleeping through the night, on occasion.

Six months after surgery, A. is thrilled that she committed to getting the prolapse fixed. She has no sensation of fullness in her vagina, nor *does she have the pulling and pressure that would plague her as the day wore on. She has no leakage or bladder problems either. On the contrary, her bladder function has improved since the surgery.*

Pelvic-floor prolapse, which sounds like a construction or civil engineering problem, is a common condition among women that has remained a virtually unknown entity among most people because it is such an embarrassing problem. Women who discuss their health issues among their friends will often hide the fact that they have a prolapse. Erectile dysfunction and urinary incontinence seem to be less stigmatized than pelvic floor prolapse. When women come to see me, I will often suggest that they look at their vagina with a mirror to see the problem. Invariably, the response is "Ugh, I don't want to look at that mess. It is so ugly." To which I reply, "It is not ugly at all. It is part of your body that happens to be a little out of position." Since so many women avoid addressing the problem, the exact statistics regarding the prevalence of prolpase are not known. Some of the numbers that we have available are reviewed in Chapter 13, but they vastly underestimate the true prevalence of the condition.

DEFINITION

Pelvic-floor prolapse describes the decent of the pelvic organs into the vaginal canal. Prolapse is another word for hernia, which is a defect in a supporting muscle, sort of like a hammock that gets too loose. Pelvic prolapse is a hernia of the muscles that lie under the pelvic organs. Weakness of the muscles under these structures results in the collapse of their support. The vaginal canal is an empty space that fills with these displaced organs. Men cannot have a pelvic floor prolapse because they lack a vagina, which is the space into which the surrounding organs can fall. The uterus is one of the most important support structures of the female pelvic floor, whose ligaments lose their integrity with time and pregnancy. Men don't get pregnant and they don't have uteruses. Men have a prostate, which sits under the bladder and pushes against it, preventing it from shifting in any direction. All and all, men cannot get pelvic-floor prolapse.

The organs that can be seen falling into the vagina include the bladder, the uterus, the small intestine, and the rectum. The woman with this problem cannot tell what organ or organs have prolapsed. All she knows is that a ball is falling into and maybe even out of her vagina. The doctor can tell which organ has prolapsed based on the origin of the ball. If you are

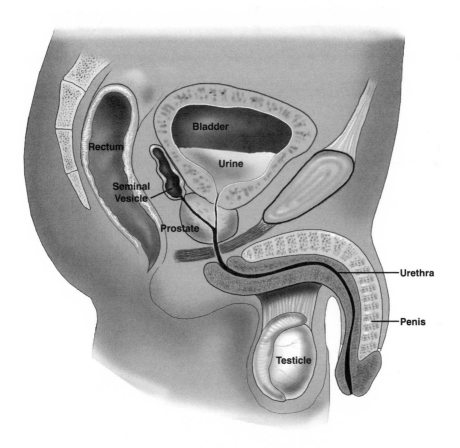

FIGURE 1. *Normal Male Anatomy—Side View.*

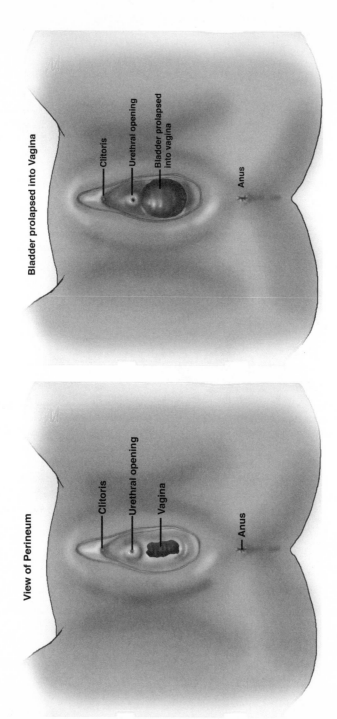

FIGURE 2. *Female Pelvic Floor—View in Stirrups.*

lying on your back with your legs up in stirrups, the ball can fall from the top of the vagina, it can slide down the entire length of the vagina, or it can push up from the bottom of the vagina. A ball falling in from the top will include the bladder. A ball sliding down the length of the vagina will include the cervix if you have not had a hysterectomy. If you have had your uterus surgically removed, the ball sliding down the length of the vagina may include the small intestines. A ball pushing up from the back wall will include the rectum.

Pelvic-floor prolapse is a general term that refers to the descent of any of the four pelvic organs into the vagina. It does not describe which organs have fallen. We have terms to refer to each of the four organs that can fall into the canal. If the ball falling down contains the bladder under the vaginal tissue, it is called a cystocele. *Cyst* in Latin means bladder, and *cele* refers to a weakness resulting in a protrusion. If a woman has a cystocele, then, by definition, she has pelvic-floor prolapse, but, specifically, of the bladder. If the uterus has fallen, the term is called uterine prolapse, no other fancy term is used. If the small intestine has fallen through the top of the vaginal canal, the problem is called an enterocele. If the rectal wall is pushing up into the vaginal canal, we call it a rectocele. Once the area of weakness is determined, physicians tend to use the more specific terminology to describe the problem because it helps in understanding the symptoms, the risks that may occur as a result of leaving the prolapse alone, and the treatment.

TYPES OF PELVIC-FLOOR PROLAPSE

Name	Organ out of position
Cystocele	Bladder
Uterine prolapse	Uterus
Enterocele	Small intestine
Rectocele	Rectum

CAUSES

Once the diagnosis is made on a simple exam, most women want to know how this problem could have happened. The answer is not as simple as we would like it to be, especially to the daughters of the woman who present with this problem. A number of risk factors have been identified, although no single event will definitely lead to its occurrence. Vaginal delivery, in which the pelvic muscles are pulled apart as the baby descends through the birth canal, remains the most popularly identified risk factor. However, not every woman who has had a vaginal delivery will develop pelvic floor prolapse. As a matter of fact, *most* women who deliver their children vaginally will not develop a prolapse problem. At least they will not have enough of a problem to seek medical treatment. The issue is not only *who* will develop prolapse, but who will develop prolapse that leads to symptoms requiring medical intervention. Most women who deliver their children vaginally will never develop symptomatic pelvic-floor prolapse. They may have some weakness of the vaginal muscles, but a problem requiring treatment will not result.

CAUSES OF PELVIC-FLOOR PROLAPSE

Vaginal delivery
Menopause
Genetic factors
Hysterectomy
Constipation

This begs the question: What else could predispose a woman to developing a prolapse? If we analyze the profile of the woman who presents with this problem, she is most commonly in her late 60s or early 70s. Menopause, specifically estrogen depletion, seems to play a significant role. Exactly how estrogen affects the muscles and organs of the pelvis is not known, but clearly, some relationship is present since most urinary tract disorders that women suffer from (incontinence and prolapse specifically) occur in women who are menopausal (see Chapter 10). Younger women in their 30s and 40s can suffer from the symptoms of pelvic floor descent, but most commonly, it is seen in older women. A mild prolapse may progress to a symptomatic one as the years of estrogen depletion weaken the tissues. The loss of elasticity that hormones provide leads to worsening of the problem.

Genetic factors play a role as well. Women whose mothers had a problem are more likely to have similar issues. Because these matters were not discussed openly in previous generations, many women do not know exactly what was wrong with their mothers. The degree of descent and the treatment administered may not be known by the family, but many women will know that their mother had some sort of bladder problem. In addition, people did not live as long in the past as they do now. Many mothers did not live long enough or active enough lives to even address their bladder issues. However, upon questioning, many of my patients will vaguely remember that their mother or aunt, or even grandmother, had some sort of bladder condition.

The other epidemiological observation that points to genetics as a risk factor is the predominance of Caucasian and Hispanic women with this problem. African-American and Asian women do not suffer from prolapse nearly as often as the other two groups. The collagen composition in the skin of the various races differs. Women with pale, fragile skin and light hair tend to be at the greatest risk for developing a bothersome prolapse.

Hysterectomy, or any pelvic surgery that violates the pelvic floor muscles, can produce pelvic muscle problems. The uterus and cervix buttress the vaginal tissues. If the uterus is removed, this disruption in the ligamentous support can lead to prolapse. Most hysterectomies do not lead to further pelvic-floor problems, but on occasion, usually many years later, pelvic organ descent can be identified.

Constipation, which involves straining or bearing down, rarely, but occasionally, can cause problems with the muscles of the pelvis. The constant pressure involved in pushing out bowel movements will strain the muscles that support the pelvic organs. The degree to which constipation contributes to this problem is unclear, but there certainly seems to be a theoretical relationship between the two conditions.

Picking out a single risk factor and blaming that as the cause of a prolapse is incorrect. Many factors in a woman's medical history will each contribute to the development of the problem. Family history, constipation, vaginal delivery, and a hysterectomy may all be part of any woman's history. To pinpoint the vaginal delivery or the hysterectomy, for example, as the reason for this to have happened would be faulty reasoning. When young women or the daughters of my patients ask me what to do to prevent this problem from happening to them, I tell them to live their lives; whatever will be, will be. Many conditions may afflict us, but we cannot go around worrying about what will befall us. If we were to conduct our lives that way, every woman would be counseled to have a mastectomy to prevent breast cancer, a cholecystectomy to prevent gallbladder attacks, and an appendectomy to prevent appendicitis. Performing a C-section in an attempt to avoid pelvic floor prolapse will not ensure that this condition will not eventually develop anyway. Prevention would be nice, but it is not guaranteed.

SYMPTOMS

The symptoms of pelvic-floor prolapse fall into two categories: symptoms specific to the prolapse and symptoms specific to the organs that have descended. These two sets of symptoms may be present at the same time, or there may only be symptoms specific to one problem. Let me explain.

Symptoms of the prolapse itself include pressure in the vagina, a mass protruding from the entrance of the vagina, pulling in the pelvis or the back, or difficulty walking because of a mass falling out of the vaginal canal. The woman who has this problem will not be able to tell which organ or organs specifically are protruding. All she will see is a ball at the opening, or she may feel a ball when she wipes after going to the bathroom. Some women describe pressure and pulling in the groin area, especially by the end of the day, or after standing for a long period of time. There are women who push the ball back inside their vaginas after urinating or defecating.

SYMPTOMS OF PELVIC-FLOOR PROLAPSE IN GENERAL
  Pressure
  Pulling
  Ball in the vagina
SYMPTOMS RELATED TO A PROLAPSED BLADDER
  Frequency/urgency/ incomplete emptying
  Stress incontinence/urge incontinence
SYMPTOMS RELATED TO A PROLAPSED UTERUS
  Same as pelvic floor prolapse
SYMPTOMS RELATED TO A PROLAPSED SMALL INTESTINE
  Same as pelvic floor prolapse symptoms
SYMPTOMS RELATED TO A PROLAPSED RECTUM
  Constipation
  Mucous discharge

Symptoms related to the organs that have prolapsed are described differently, depending upon which organ has fallen through the muscle defect. If the bladder has fallen, which is the most common organ to fall, you may only have symptoms related to your bladder, and not to the actual protrusion of tissue. If your bladder is hanging down, the urine must be forced up and out by the bladder muscle in order to be evacuated. In this common condition, you will experience frequent urination, a sense of incomplete

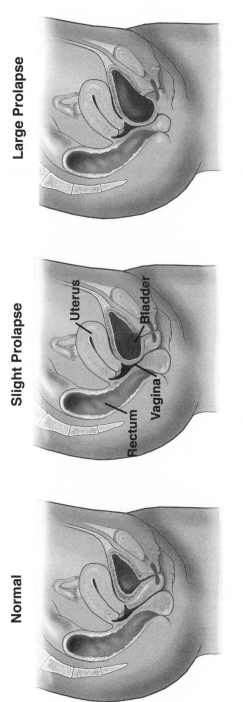

FIGURE 3. *Bladder Prolapse.*

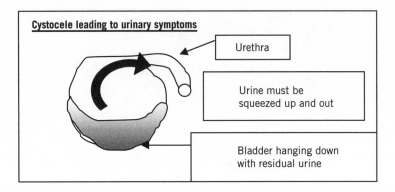

emptying, difficulty getting the stream started, and urgency. You may have recurrent bladder infections due to the incomplete emptying and the presence of stagnant urine.

Many of you may suffer from stress incontinence, which is leakage of urine when coughing, laughing, or sneezing. The general weakness in the muscles of that area affects the urethra as well as the bladder. This weakness is manifested by stress incontinence. Not all women with a cystocele will have stress incontinence. If the bladder is hanging out of the vagina and the urethra is fixed in its normal position, the urethra will be kinked. The symptoms will reflect an obstruction from the kinking more than they will leakage from weak muscles.

URINARY SYMPTOMS THAT MAY BE PRESENT IN WOMEN WITH BLADDER PROLAPSE

Stress incontinence
Frequent urination
Urgent onset of need to urinate
Urination at night
Urge incontinence
Sense of incomplete emptying
Difficulty initiating stream
Weak or intermittent flow

To complicate matters, a woman with a cystocele may develop urgency, frequency, and urge incontinence. These symptoms do not come from the descent itself as much as from changes within the bladder that are caused by the abnormal position. Over time, the effort that the bladder has to make to empty will take a toll on the organ. It will begin to go into spasm from the increasing effort to empty. These spasms present as frequent urges to urinate, the sudden onset of the need to empty, and even uncontrolled leakage.

The bottom line is that if you complain from either urinary problems or the feeling of a mass falling into your vagina, it is the responsibility of the doctor to determine if a prolapse is present, and if it is contributing to the symptoms. Either set of symptoms can bring you to the doctor. The treatment strategy is determined by the findings on exam and the symptoms that you report.

Uterine prolapse does not present with symptoms other than those involving a mass in the vaginal canal. However, uterine prolapse does not usually occur on its own. As the ligaments of the uterus weaken and allow the organ to slide into the vagina, the bladder and the rectum often get pulled into the canal as well.

Like uterine prolapse, an enterocele is usually silent and occurs in the presence of descent of other pelvic organs. The entire top of the vagina falls down, bringing the small intestine, the bladder, and the rectum with it. Vaginal depth is lost in the process. In many cases, an enterocele is not recognized because the bladder protrudes so far out that it blocks the bowel component. Radiographic studies can identify bowel prolapse, or it may be recognized during surgery to correct a cystocele and rectocele.

Rectocele can present with just a ball of tissue falling out of the vagina or with symptoms specific to defecation. Some woman will describe the sensation of a ball of stool sitting in a pocket that just won't seem to empty, which is exactly what is happening. No matter how hard they push, they cannot evacuate completely. In some cases, women experience fecal soiling on their clothes or pads. Other women will insert a finger into the vagina to complete a bowel movement.

The degree of prolapse does not always correspond to the symptoms that a woman presents with. The level of activity will certainly contribute to the bother that any one person will experience. The symptoms should be regarded as an independent variable in the assessment of the severity of the condition. In other words, if you are very bothered by your problem, but the prolapse is noted to be small on exam, it should not be disregarded. The two aspects of your condition, symptoms and physical presentation, need to be weighed equally.

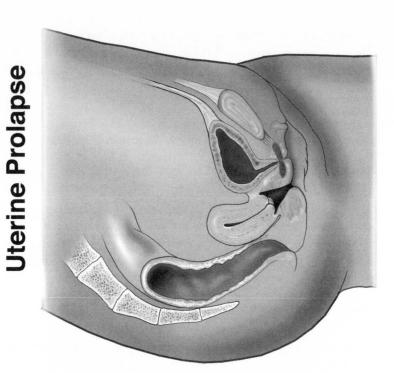

Uterine Prolapse

Normal Anatomy

Uterus

Bladder

Vaginal
Canal

FIGURE 4.

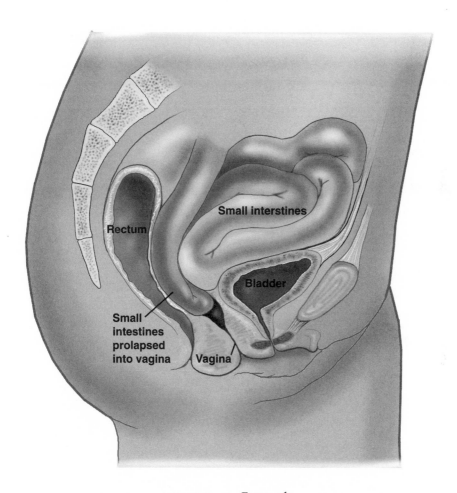

FIGURE 5. *Enterocele.*

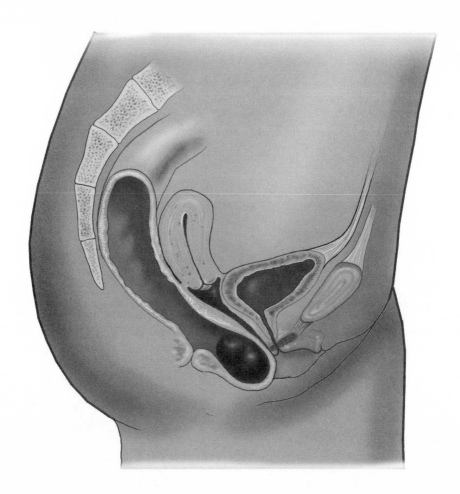

FIGURE 6. *Rectocele.*

EVALUATION

After presenting her symptoms, a woman with prolapse needs to be examined. The examination may include any number of tests, which should be described to you before they are performed. You will be asked questions regarding your symptoms during the history-taking part of the visit. The areas of questioning that you should be prepared to answer are covered in detail in Chapter 5. Bring a list of all of your medications. All consultations precede to a thorough physical exam. The pelvic exam is the most important aspect of the physical exam, because a prolapse is seen vaginally.

EVALUATION

Physical examination
Urine analysis
Urine culture
Urine cytology—optional
Post-void residual urine measurement
Cystoscopy—optional
Radiographs—optional
Urodynamics

Physical Examination

With the legs in stirrups, the vaginal opening in inspected for color, lubrication, and size. Postmenopausal women who do not use vaginal estrogen can have a pale, dry vagina. If a rash is present, it may indicate irritation from leakage or pads. The distance between the anal opening and the back wall of the vagina indicates a defect in the deep muscles of the pelvis.

A speculum may be inserted to pull the back wall away and open the canal. Defects deep inside will become more evident. In many cases, a prolapse will retract while you are lying down. You may need to stand up and be examined in order to find the defect. Coughing or bearing down as if to make a bowel movement may also bring out a prolapse. There may be leakage of urine at this part of the exam. It is important that the examiner try to elicit all aspects of the prolapse and it is associated symptoms. There is no reason to be embarrassed or to hold back. Now is the time to let it all out so that all of the symptoms that were described earlier can be observed objectively.

Once an organ is seen descending, the speculum can be used to move it out of the way and look for something else coming through further back. The actual organ is not seen protruding into the canal. Rather, it is the imprint of that organ on the vaginal tissues. The pink ball that descends is the bladder, the small intestine, or the rectal wall covered in the pink tissue of the vagina. If the cervix falls down, that is not covered.

GRADING OF PELVIC-FLOOR PROLAPSE

Grade 1: Ball is only seen with bearing down
Grade 2: Ball is seen in the vaginal canal
Grade 3: Ball comes to the vaginal opening
Grade 4: Ball is hanging out of the vagina

Grading of Prolapse
The degree of prolapse is graded by the examiner as a way of documenting the findings that are seen. Complicated descriptive tables have been devised to help in communicating various defects to other clinicians, but these systems are not practical for most of us to use when we want to relay information from one clinician to another. The simplest and most widely used system includes four grades of prolapse. The same grade is used no matter what organ is falling into the vaginal canal. All the grading system does is describe how far out the ball of tissue extends.

Grade 1 prolapse means that the vaginal canal looks normal when the woman is lying down. If she coughs, the descent is visualized. Grade 4 prolapse, which is at the other extreme, refers to a ball of tissue that is actually hanging out of the vagina. Grades 2 and 3 fall in the middle. Grade 3 refers to a ball of tissue that sits just at the opening of the vagina, but does not actually dangle outside of the body. Grade 2 prolapse refers to prolapse that is seen on exam while you are lying down, but it does not necessarily hang far down through the vaginal opening.

Grade 4 prolapse is usually symptomatic. Women who have a ball of tissue hanging outside of their vaginas are aware of its presence, unless they are bedbound or mentally deficient. The other grades of prolapse are not always noticeable to women. Sometimes grade 2 or 3 prolapse will present as pulling and pressure in the groin and pelvis.

Urine Studies
After the physical exam is completed, urine studies will be done to be sure that no concurrent urological problems are present, such as blood in the urine or an infection. If blood is present, it needs to be evaluated first and foremost. Testing of blood in urine includes cystoscopy, kidney x-rays, and cytology, a cancer screeing test done on the urine sample that you provided

in the office. If an infection in present, it needs to be treated to see if the symptoms resolve with eradication of the infection. If antibiotics treat all of your complaints, you may not need to manage the prolapse unless it is determined that the prolapse in some way caused the infection.

Bladder-Emptying Studies
Most physicians will want to check the bladder for its emptying ability. This can be done in a number of ways. After you urinate, a catheter can be gently inserted into the urethral opening and advanced into the bladder. If any urine is left over in the bladder, it will be drained into a measuring container. The other method that is gaining in popularity is performed using an ultrasound (same as a sonogram) machine. Either a handheld device or a large, freestanding machine will project an image on a monitor while a probe is rubbed over the pelvic area by a technician. No invasive instrumentation is necessary, which appeals to most of us. The volume of urine sitting in the bladder is calculated automatically by the machine.

The volume of urine left over after urination has been completed is called the *post-void residual.* No absolute number reveals abnormal bladder function. Generally, if the amount of urine left in the bladder after urination is less than 100 cc, or 3 ounces, the bladder is emptying efficiently. If the post-void residual is higher, a number of concerns may arise. First, the residual may be elevated due to the circumstances of the visit. Strange bathrooms, urinating on demand, and rushing to finish going to the bathroom can all lead to incomplete emptying. Visits to the doctor can induce anxiety that will lead to an elevated residual. If any of these concerns affect you, your residual volume will be elevated, but your bladder function is not impaired. This abnormality is purely situational. Second, the residual may be elevated due to the prolapse blocking the outflow of urine. One of the hallmarks of obstruction is an elevated post-void residual. Third, the residual may be elevated because the bladder is not contracting effectively to eject the urine. Poor bladder function may be related to a prolapse, age, or neurological problems.

CAUSES OF AN ELEVATED RESIDUAL WHEN PROLAPSE IS PRESENT

Anxiety/circumstances
Blockage of outflow due to the prolapse
Poor bladder muscle function

Once the post-void residual is determined on that initial visit, the meaning of the number that is recorded needs to be interpreted in the context of the entire history and physical exam. If you report that you feel empty most of the time but noted that you did not empty well on that visit, your residual is not a cause for concern. On the other hand, if you report that you feel perfectly empty, but your residual is 10 ounces, further evaluation needs to be undertaken. Each aspect of the evaluation is put into the context of the big picture. In general, any abnormal test should be repeated. If an elevated post-void residual is found on the next visit, the consistent findings may warrant further testing.

Cystoscopy

Many physicians like to do cystoscopy to look at the inside of the urethra and the bladder before any determinations are made regarding treatment. Cystoscopy is an office-based procedure in which a scope is inserted through the urethral opening and into the bladder (see Chapter 12). The lining of the urinary tract can be viewed for polyps or tumors. Characteristic findings can suggest long-standing obstruction, which may play into your treatment choices. If blood is found in the urine on any urine analysis, cystoscopy should be done. Separate from the prolapse issue, microscopic or obvious blood in the urine should be assessed with cystoscopy to eliminate the possibility of bladder cancer. Aside from this indication, I do not routinely perform cystoscopy in the evaluation of pelvic floor prolapse, but many clinicians do.

X-rays

Radiographic testing is also recommended by some physicians for various reasons. I like women to get kidney ultrasounds, especially if surgery is being considered in the treatment plan. Kidney tumors, stones, and anatomical abnormalities will be seen on this noninvasive, non–radiation-dependent test, which will help avoid problems during and after surgery. If the prolapse is high grade (grade 3 or 4), the kidneys can be blocked as the ureters are pulled into the vaginal canal and kinked. This blockage will be seen on ultrasound (as well as CT scan) and will indicate that immediate treatment is necessary.

Some physicians recommend obtaining a standing MRI to evaluate the prolapse itself. If the test is done with you standing up and bearing down for the 20 seconds it takes to run the scan, the prolapsed organs can be identified. In large prolapses, it is sometimes difficult to tell which organs are falling through the defects. Enteroceles, high rectoceles, and cystoceles can get confused with one another. These distinctions can be made on standing MRI. I do not recommend MRI routinely because I will find whatever defects are present at the time of surgery. Some physicians want the information before surgery.

Although VCUGs and IVPs can be performed in the assessment of pelvic floor prolapse, they will not provide nearly as much information as an MRI and they both involve either catheterization or contrast injection, neither of which is required for an MRI (see explanation of all tests in Chapter 12). If a physician orders one of these tests, be sure to ask him what information he is looking for, and if the same information can be obtained another, less-nvasive way.

CT scans are sometimes performed to look at the ovaries and the uterus for surgical planning. Large fibroids can be difficult to remove vaginally if a hysterectomy is being considered as part of the treatment. A pelvic ultrasound will provide the same information without radiation exposure or the injection of contrast media. If the ultrasound reveals an abnormality that needs to be characterized further, a CT can be ordered. In general, most women with prolapse will not need a CT as part of a routine evaluation.

Urodynamic Testing
Urodynamics, on the other hand, are generally included in the routine evaluation of a woman with pelvic-floor prolapse. As described in Chapter 12 and the Glossary, urodynamic testing looks at the function of the bladder, while cystoscopy looks at the anatomy of the bladder. Urodynamics, also called cystometrics, tests the two main bladder functions: filling and emptying. Problems with bladder filling result in frequent urination, urgency of urination, and leakage. Problems with emptying result in elevated post-void residual volumes and slow urinary flow. If only it was as simple as matching the symptoms with the defect, we would not need to subject patients to this 45-minute test that includes catheterization of both the urethra and the rectum.

Urodynamics helps in many aspects of the evaluation of a woman with pelvic-floor prolapse. Most cases of prolapse involve the bladder, so bladder function plays into both the presenting symptoms of the condition and the long-term effects that the prolapse will have on the body. If you have bladder symptoms in addition to your symptoms of prolapse (in other words if you have frequency, urgency, and leakage as well as a sense of pressure and pulling in your pelvis), then urodynamics can help relate the bladder symptoms to the prolapse. The two sets of symptoms may be independent of one another or they may be cause and effect. If they are cause and effect, the prolapse is causing the bladder symptoms, so fixing the prolapse will cure the bladder symptoms. On the other hand, fixing the prolapse will not help the bladder symptoms. If surgery is performed, you may still need treatment for the frequency, urgency, and leakage. Large prolapses can cause bladder deterioration that is not always noticeable to you because the changes occur over years. If the prolapse is repaired, the bladder problems may be revealed postoperatively.

Urodynamics helps in both scenarios. Obstruction caused by prolapse will be found. Abnormal bladder function can be seen. Postoperative bladder difficulties can be anticipated. I think that cystometrics are essential in the evaluation of any woman with a pelvic-floor prolapse who has either bladder symptoms, bowel problems, or feels her organs falling out.

Some clinicians use x-rays to augment their findings during urodynamics. The radiographic data are optional because they will not change the results on the test. What they will do is document the prolapse and show film images of the findings. The information is helpful, but whether or not it is worth the radiation exposure is a personal matter. My feeling is that you should listen to your physician. If she does the test with x-rays, then that is fine; if she does not, that is okay as well. The radiographs are not essential to the test and they do not involve imaging of the kidneys, so the kidney studies will need to be done as well.

TREATMENT

Now, the problem is out in the open and the testing has been done. What is the next step? Before we even get to the treatment options, the question always comes up: who should be taking care of this, my gynecologist or a urologist (see Chapter 3)? Many general gynecologists and urologists do not feel comfortable treating pelvic-floor prolapse. It is an extremely complicated and specialized area of women's medicine which is evolving quickly as our surgical techniques and medical treatments improve. Most medical communities have a few physicians who specialize in this field. These physicians may be urologists or gynecologists, usually with extra training or experience in prolapse surgery and incontinence treatments. It doesn't matter which area of medicine the specialist comes from as long as she is comfortable, interested, and experienced in treating women with these problems. Internists, gynecologists, and urologists will know who the appropriate person in their community is and will refer accordingly. It is always helpful at ask around and see if other physicians, health-care personnel, and patients point you to the same few practitioners.

Once the proper physician has been identified and the problems have been elucidated, treatment options can be offered. The treatment may include a number of different choices as well as a combination of these options. As I have mentioned previously, some of the presenting symptoms may be related to the prolapse itself which needs to be treated, while other symptoms may be related to the organ that has prolapsed. All of the options should be laid out and discussed before any decisions are made. Most importantly, nonsurgical treatment choices should be exhausted before surgery is discussed.

PROLAPSE TREATMENT

Bladder symptoms:	
NO	YES
Pessary +	Medication
Surgery +	Medication

Pessary

Prolapse can be treated in two ways: pessary or surgery. A pessary is a rubber ring that resembles a diaphragm used for birth control. The ring is made of silicone, which is a flexible, rubbery material. The pessary is inserted vaginally and remains in place for up to three months at a time, after which point it is removed, cleaned, and reinserted. Differently shaped pessaries are made to accommodate differently shaped vaginas and different defects. The clinician fits you with the appropriate pessary which should hold up the tissues without exerting undue pressure that could cause ulcerations and bleeding. If properly fit, you do not feel the pessary at all. Some women can be taught to remove, clean, and reinsert the device on their own. Most women need to see the doctor every two to three months to have it done.

Although every woman with a prolapse is a candidate for a pessary, active, sexually active women often find them cumbersome. They tend to fall out because women with large prolapses have wide open vaginal vaults. An open vaginal vault makes it difficult to hold the pessary in position. The vagina tends to produce a discharge in response to the silicone. Some women find the discharge offensive. It rarely causes infections, but some women interpret the presence of the discharge as evidence of infection.

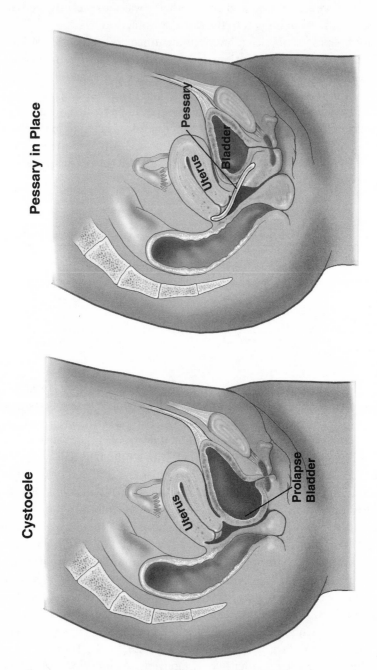

FIGURE 7. *Pessary for Cystocele.*

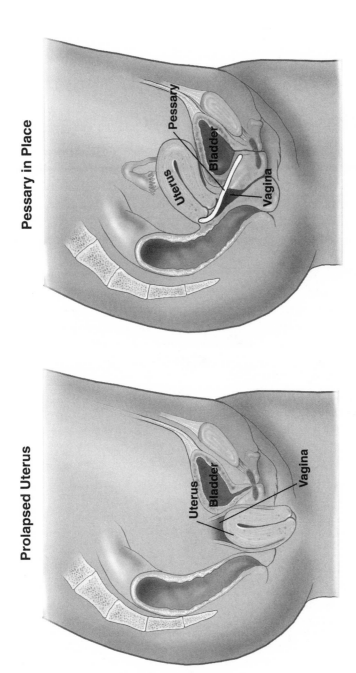

FIGURE 8. *Pessary for Uterine Prolapse.*

Usually estrogen creams need to be applied to lubricate the vaginal tissues and prevent rubbing of the pressary against the skin.

Ideal patients for use of a pessary are elderly women who are not highly active. Poor surgical candidates would also do well with a pessary. There is no reason why any elderly women with a prolapse would not try a pessary, even for a short time. I do not recommend pessaries in younger women because it is a temporizing measure, not a cure. A woman who is active, healthy, and sexual will need a treatment that will allow her to continue with that lifestyle well into her old age. If she delays definitive treatment, she may require surgical intervention when she can least afford it medically.

Once the pessary is inserted and the bladder is shifted back where it belongs, bladder symptoms may begin. Stress incontinence (leakage with coughing, laughing, or sneezing) sometimes becomes problematic because the obstruction between the bladder and the urethra is eliminated. Weakness under the urethra is present for the same reason that weakness occurred under the bladder. The result is stress incontinence. No medical therapy is available for stress incontinence yet, so, either you live with it, you elect for surgery to repair everything, or the pessary is removed and you live with the symptoms of the prolapse. Kegel exercises usually do not work when this degree of muscle weakness is present. Treatment of stress urinary incontinence after a pessary is inserted is one of the more difficult problems.

More commonly, women with pessaries will have frequent urination day and night and leakage of urine with an urge to urinate. This symptom complex reflects the aging bladder, which can be treated quite effectively with medication (see Chapter 5). The first plan of treatment in an elderly woman who is a poor surgical candidate is a pessary combined with medication. If a comfortable pessary cannot be found, then surgery will be your only option.

Who Should Be Repaired Surgically?
Having just said that, should every woman with a prolapse who is a surgical candidate have it repaired? The answer is no. Prolapse repairs should be done in women with symptomatic prolapse or in women who have urinary or bowel symptoms that cannot be corrected without correcting the prolapse. Urodynamic studies as well as the rest of the evaluation discussed earlier will determine this. I do not believe in preventive surgery. Surgery is only done for a condition that is bothersome now, today, at this moment. If a woman reports to me that her quality of life is affected by her bladder or bowel condition, or by her prolapse, I will recommend that surgery be

done if our testing confirms that it will solve her problem. If the bladder or bowel symptoms can be treated without repairing an asymptomatic prolapse, then I do not recommend surgery. If the prolapse becomes symptomatic or if the bladder or bowel problems stop responding to our treatment, then surgery may become necessary. All of these conditions can be dealt with as they arise. The relationship between the specialist and the patient is ongoing.

Surgery

Symptomatic prolapse in an active woman is ultimately going to be treated with surgery. A number of different operative techniques have evolved over the years because the surgery has traditionally been regarded as complicated and unsuccessful. Newer instruments, intraoperative medications, and reinforcing materials have transformed the surgical results into one of the most satisfying areas of treatment for both patients and their surgeons.

Traditional surgical technique to treat prolapse involves access to the area of interest through an incision that is made on the abdominal wall. The bladder is reached after the intestines and other neighboring structures are identified and tucked away from the operative field. The vaginal canal is nearly impossible to get to from this angle, but the ligaments above the vagina can be pulled up and tacked to the sacral bones or the nearby muscles. Modern techniques have dispensed with large abdominal incisions and manipulation of the bowel, which has reduced the complication rate of the surgery and improved on the results.

Vaginal surgery to correct prolapse makes the most sense because the problem is vaginal, therefore the solution will be found vaginally. The tissues *under* the bladder and the other prolapsed organs are the problem, so why not only work *under* those organs, through the vagina. Trying to pull tissues together or place material under organs is difficult if the approach is from above. However, there are still many surgeons who perform prolapse surgery through the abdominal cavity. If the surgeon is comfortable with this approach, has good results, and can manage the complications, then it is reasonable to undergo the surgery using this technique. Although rare, there are instances in which the abdominal approach is preferable. These few indications can be discussed if the surgeon can justify his choice of abdominal over vaginal surgery.

All prolapse surgery must be performed under anesthesia (see Chapter 11). Either a spinal/epidural or general anesthesia will allow the surgeon to operate without movement, pain, or anxiety on the part of the patient. You are placed on the operating table with your legs high up in stirrups in order to allow the vaginal opening to be widened for adequate exposure. The position, in and of itself, requires heavy enough sedation to warrant anesthesia. No matter what organs have prolapsed into the vaginal cavity, all repairs can be done this way. Intravenous antibiotics are routinely administered before the first incisions are made. Prevention of infection is of the utmost importance, especially since we are dealing with the urinary tract, which is not always sterile in women with prolapse.

Hysterectomy

If the cervix is seen emanating through the vaginal opening, a hysterectomy may be beneficial. If the cervix has come all the way through the vagina, efforts to preserve the uterus through a suspension are not usually successful. The uterus is so small in most women with uterine prolapse that it is basically out of the body by the time the cervix is seen. The back of the vagina is pulled down with the cervix, foreshortening the vagina as well. Removing the uterus will allow for better lengthening of the vaginal canal and support of the other structures than if the uterus were preserved and suspended. I am not a big fan of hysterectomies, but in the case of a total prolapse, it may be the best way to approach the repair.

Any prolapse of the uterus short of it totally falling into the canal can allow for uterine preservation. The cervix can be supported vaginally to prevent further descent. Repair of the bladder and rectal descent will also change the angle of the vagina which helps to guard against further uterine prolapse.

If a hysterectomy is planned, it is done first. When a vaginal hysterectomy is performed, a small opening in the abdominal cavity through the very deepest part of the canal has to be made to remove the organ. That opening needs to be closed in order to prevent the bowel from ultimately pushing through the top of the vagina, resulting in an enterocele. This is a common problem that is often seen years after a hysterectomy. The length of the vagina should not be compromised by a vaginal hysterectomy. Adequate depth for intercourse can be obtained in every woman who undergoes a vaginal repair. After the uterus is removed, attention can then turn to the bladder repair.

Cystocele (Bladder) Repair

The cystocele repair is done the same way no matter what other repairs need to be done at the same time. The vaginal skin overlying the dropped bladder is opened from the urethra to the cervix. The vaginal tissues are dissected off of the underlying support muscles, which are weakened and stretched

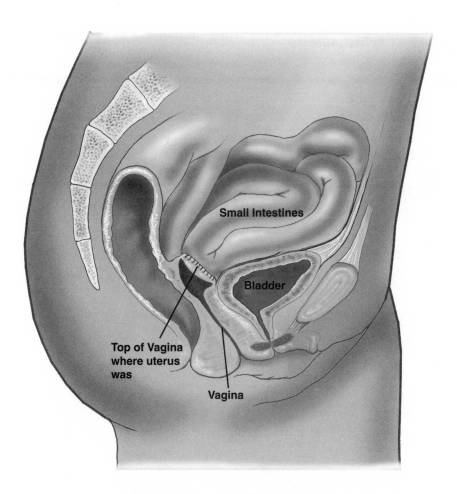

Small Intestines

Bladder

Top of Vagina
where uterus
was

Vagina

FIGURE 9. *After Hysterectomy.*

A. Exposure

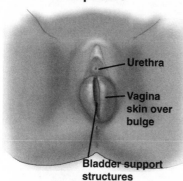

- Urethra
- Vagina skin over bulge
- Bladder support structures

B. Ligaments Exposed

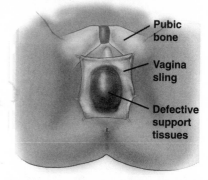

- Pubic bone
- Vagina sling
- Defective support tissues

C. Mesh positioned

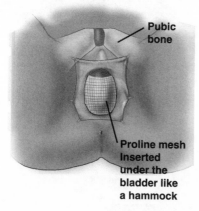

- Pubic bone
- Proline mesh Inserted under the bladder like a hammock

D. After Repair

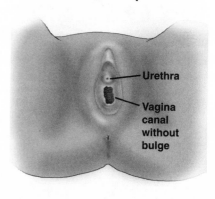

- Urethra
- Vagina canal without bulge

FIGURE 10. *Cystocele Repair.*

out of shape. The bladder is then pushed up and a mesh hammock is placed under the bladder and attached to the pelvic side wall. The back of the mesh can be attached to the cervix and its support structures, or, if the cervix has been removed, it can be attached to stronger ligaments in the vagina. The skin is then closed over the hammock.

Different materials are available for making the hammock. Some surgeons use the tissues native to the patient, other surgeons use donated cadaveric materials; others use processed animal tissues, while I and many other surgeons use synthetic mesh. Synthetic mesh is used in most hernia surgeries. A vast experience exists for the use of synthetic materials in the human body. The application of these tissues to vaginal surgery is fairly new. The most commonly used material is nylon, (called proline) which is durable, strong, resistant to infection, and not reactive with the body. My opinion is that this repair should last a lifetime. A material that disintegrates will leave you at risk for recurrence of your prolapse. Synthetic materials will certainly last. They are safe and effective. The concern lies with the risk of infection and of rejection (see Chapter 4 for a discussion of materials).

MATERIALS USED TO SUPPORT THE BLADDER IN A CYSTOCELE REPAIR

Your own tissues
Tissues from human cadavers
Tissues processed from animals
Synthetic material—usually nylon

The main concern with using synthetic mesh is infection. If the material becomes infected, it will be rejected by the body. The woman who has this problem will present to her physician with a persistent vaginal discharge, which is usually slightly bloody and malodorous. When examined, the mesh will be seen or felt emanating from an opening in the vaginal skin. The treatment is a trial of antibiotics first, often accompanied with estrogen cream in the postmenopausal woman. If this conservative treatment fails, removal of the piece of infected, rejected mesh is warranted, usually under sedation in an ambulatory surgery setting. Although inconvenient, this complication is impossible to predict and easily remedied. Most women with rejected mesh will not need further repair of the prolapse after the smell infected area is removed.

Incidents of synthetic mesh being found in the bladder have been reported. This is very rare and only occurs if proper surgical technique is not adhered to. Part of any prolapse surgery will involve cystoscopy, which is where the inside lining of the bladder is visualized with a scope after the mesh is inserted. Cystoscopy will identify bladder injuries and misplaced mesh, which can be removed and replaced immediately at the time of surgery without any untoward effects.

Should Incontinence Surgery Be Performed at the Time of Prolapse Repair?
Performing an incontinence surgery at the time of a prolapse repair remains a debatable topic. Many surgeons feel that raising the bladder in a woman with weakened tissue will predispose her to the development of stress incontinence, which is caused by weakened tissue supporting the urethra. In other words, the same underlying weakness that caused the bladder to fall will lead to stress incontinence, which is caused by weakened support under the urethra. Placing a sling under the urethra to support it, just as the hammock supports the bladder, will not only guard against stress incontinence, but it may save you from another operation. The sling adds about five minutes to the operation and very little increase in risk. Those surgeons who do not perform an incontinence procedure at the same time feel that any risk that is added to the surgery is too much for a problem that is not present.

My feeling is that an incontinence surgery should be done if the bladder is lifted. The risk of developing stress incontinence either immediately after surgery or in the near future is great enough to warrant an extra five minutes to put in a support sling under the urethra. I want this to be the only surgery that my patients ever need to treat prolapse and stress incontinence. The plan to put in a sling or not should be discussed before the surgery is done.

Rectocele and Enterocele Repair
Rectocele surgery is done in nearly the identical manner as cystocele surgery. Different surgeons champion different techniques, but the idea is the same. An incision is made in the vaginal skin overlying the bulging rectal wall. The bulging tissue that is exposed is pushed down and the muscle is pulled over the defect. Some surgeons will place a piece of reinforcing mesh over the weakened muscle that is filling in the defect before the skin is closed.

After childbirth, the episiotomy is closed at the vaginal opening, while the tears in the muscle deep in the vagina are left open. These tears do not heal together, leaving a space through which the rectal wall herniates. The diameter of the vaginal canal is widened by the tears as well. You will

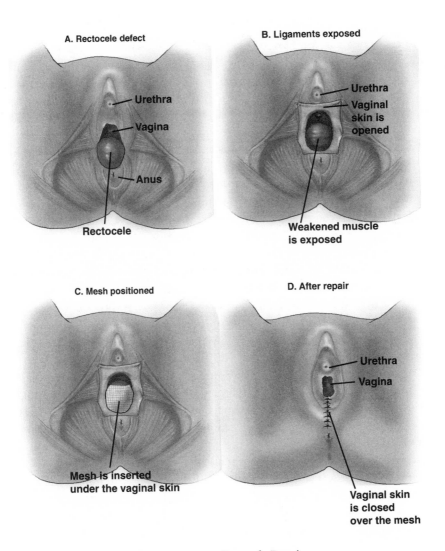

A. Rectocele defect

Urethra

Vagina

Anus

Rectocele

B. Ligaments exposed

Urethra

Vaginal
skin is
opened

Weakened muscle
is exposed

C. Mesh positioned

Mesh is inserted
under the vaginal skin

D. After repair

Urethra

Vagina

Vaginal skin
is closed
over the mesh

FIGURE 11. *Rectocele Repair.*

report that your vagina feels capacious and open. Pulling the back wall of the vagina together will help to close the gaping cavity that many women feel in the back of the vaginal canal.

Enterocele repairs are performed only in women who have had previous hysterectomies. The intestines cannot fall into the vaginal cavity unless the uterus is removed. Again, the vaginal skin is opened to expose the underlying tissues. If small intestine is seen, an entercele is present and needs to be repaired. The abdominal cavity is opened and the intestines are pushed back inside. The sack that holds the intestines in place is closed to prevent a recurrence of the enterocele. If an enterocele is missed because it is sitting behind a large cystocele, it will present as a persistent bulge after surgery.

The Postoperative Course

After surgery, you will awaken from anesthesia with a vaginal packing in place and a catheter in the bladder just as A. did. These will stay in for a day or two, depending on the length of the surgery, the amount of blood loss, and the preference of the surgeon. Pain medication will be dispensed as needed. The first day or days after the surgery, most women feel like they have just been run over by a truck. It is a difficult operation to endure because not only is there a fair amount of trauma to the body, but the work is done internally. No incisions are visible because they are inside the vagina. You will look down and won't see anything, but you feel miserable. It is a strange sensation.

Once the catheter and packing come out, recovery can ensue in earnest. Bladder function may take a few days to a few weeks to return to normal. Slow flow, incomplete emptying, and frequency are common for the first week or two after a prolapse repair. Some women have urgency with urge incontinence immediately after the catheter is removed. Occasionally, a woman will not be able to urinate at all after the catheter is removed. It will need to be reinserted for a few days before another attempt is made to remove it. All of these experiences are normal in the first few days after surgery

The stay in the hospital lasts anywhere from one to four days. Some surgeons will discharge their patients on the same day if only a bladder repair is done. You will go home with a catheter that is removed in the office the next day, or you can remove it yourself at home. If it is desirable to remain in the hospital overnight because of sick family members or children are at home, be sure to request that of the physician. I think that an overnight stay will expedite recovery. A good immediate postoperative period that allows for rest will make a big difference. Any woman with medical problems must stay in the hospital overnight to monitor her vital signs after anesthesia. These details are discussed before the surgery is scheduled.

Showering can begin 48 hours after surgery. I do not impose any restrictions on my prolapse patients. This is fairly unorthodox. Most physicians request that you refrain from lifting heavy objects or taxing yourself for 4 to 6 weeks after surgery. Because the repair that I perform relies on the nylon mesh, nothing that you do should destroy the repair. The whole point of the surgery is to increase your activity level, not limit it. Therefore, if it doesn't hurt, it can be done. Any activity that causes pain should be abstained from until it doesn't hurt.

Vaginal spotting of blood will occur for a few days or even a week after surgery. Pads will need to be worn to protect undergarments from the blood. Discharge may persist for longer because the stitches that are placed vaginally will create discharge that helps them to dissolve. It is a copious, yellowish white discharge that should not have a foul odor. It persists for about one month, which is how long it takes for the stitches to dissolve. Occasionally a drop of blood may be seen after the spotting has ceased. As a stitch loosens and falls out, it may take a drop of blood with it.

Nothing should be inserted into the vagina for one month after the surgery. The stitches need to dissolve before intercourse can resume. Not only will the stitches be uncomfortable for the partner, but there is a risk that they will rip the skin of the vagina and expose the mesh. Exposed mesh becomes infected and will need to be removed. Tampons should also be avoided until at least one month after the surgery, as well.

I ask my patients to come back to the office two weeks, six weeks, and three months after the operation. It takes about three months to fully recover and know what the permanent results of the repair will be. Some women bounce back more quickly than others, but long-term results appear at about three months. The average amount of time that I recommend that women take off from work is two weeks. Sometimes, a woman will be able to go back earlier, but the pressure to get better and get back to work can slow down healing. If the time is available to get better, your progress is usually faster. At each postoperative visit, I measure the post-void residual urine as well as check the urine for infection. Each visit requires an examination of the operative site to check the wounds for healing. All of the stitches are absorbable, so nothing will need to be removed.

The Finances of Surgery

Although it is elective surgery, prolapse repair is covered by insurance. It is considered an operation of medical necessity. Preoperative authorization will need to be obtained before the surgery in order for the insurance company to pay for it. Most medical offices are familiar with this process and can take care of this for you. The insurance company usually approves the surgery and a certain number of days in the hospital. Any additional days are granted if a problem comes up that requires extra attention. The allotted number of days is nearly always enough to ensure proper convalescence. Not all physicians accept all insurance. You must inquire with the doctor's office or your insurance company regarding coverage, co-payments, and deductibles. Each person's policy is different.

Complications

Complications of prolapse surgery fall into four different categories: problems related to the bladder, the prolapse repair, the anesthesia, and the pain medications. Of course, the risk and type of problems that may be expected depend on which organs are involved in the repair. Bowel injuries, for example, are only an issue if the abdominal cavity is opened for a hysterectomy or enterocele repair. In bladder repairs done vaginally, the bowel is nowhere in sight, so the risk of injury is pretty much zero.

Cystocele repairs are the most common prolapse surgeries that are performed, since the bladder is the most common organ to prolapse and it is the most symptomatic prolapse. In women with bladder prolapse, the prolapse itself can be unpleasant, but so can the derangements to bladder function that the prolapse creates. For these reasons, postoperative bladder problems are the most common. To actually call these complications implies that they are present because of a surgical problem. In fact, these outcomes may be unavoidable. No matter how much preoperative testing is done or how well the surgery is performed, some of these complaints are unpredictable. All of them can be treated effectively to ultimately ensure a good outcome.

COMPLICATIONS OF PROLAPSE SURGERY

Related to the Bladder
Stress urinary incontinence
Urge urinary incontinence
Urinary retention

COMPLICATIONS OF PROLAPSE SURGERY—continued

Urinary tract infection
Mesh erosion
Recurrence of prolapse
Bladder-vaginal fistula
Related to the Prolapse Repair
  Bleeding
  Ureteral injury
  Recurrent prolapse
  Other prolapse
  Bowel injury
  Rectovaginal fistula
Related to Anesthesia
  See chapter 11
Related to pain Medication
  See chapter 11

Problems Related to the Bladder

Stress Incontinence

Stress incontinence can present after prolapse surgery. Once the bladder is pushed back up into the pelvis, the kink that was present between the urethra and the bladder is no longer causing blockage of urine. With removal of the obstruction, weakness of the support under the urethra may be unmasked, resulting in leakage with coughing, laughing, or sneezing. Many vaginal surgeons will place a support material under the urethra at the time of the bladder repair to prevent the onset of stress incontinence after a prolapse repair. Other surgeons will not, claiming that unnecessary procedures should not be done. If a sling is not inserted under the urethra routinely, patients should ask if the surgeon has tested for the possibility of stress incontinence resulting after the repair. Many practitioners will place a pessary in the vagina during urodynamic testing to push the bladder up and elicit stress incontinence. The pessary mimics the prolapse repair, so underlying stress incontinence will be revealed.

Treatment of stress incontinence is either pelvic muscle exercise, infection of a bulking agent, or the insertion of a pubovaginal sling (see Chapter 4). There is a high likelihood that another surgery will be needed to cure the stress incontinence. Women with weak pelvic tissues who suffer from pelvic-floor prolapse are at high risk of either having stress incontinence at the time of their original surgeries, or of developing stress incontinence in the future due to their predisposition. However, this opinion is not universal. Physicians who elect not to do slings at the time of surgery cannot be faulted for their choices. Every added procedure has its potential downside.

Urge Incontinence and Prolapse

Urge urinary incontinence is another story. Besides stress incontinence, urge incontinence is the other most common cause of urinary incontinence in women, which may or may not have been present before the prolapse surgery was performed. Many women with bladder prolapse will report frequency of urination, urgency of urination, and leakage with the urge to urinate. These problems are not surgically correctable in most instances. There are women in whom correction of the prolapse will result in resolution of the urge incontinence, but it cannot be an expected outcome. Most of the time, medication will need to be added postoperatively to treat this problem (see Chapter 5).

There is a small group of women, approximately 8% of those undergoing prolapse surgery, who will develop urge incontinence after surgery, having no symptoms before surgery. Although rare, it does occur and can be very bothersome to those women who ultimately suffer from these symptoms. Urgency and urge incontinence can be treated effectively with medications. No further surgery will be necessary.

Urinary Retention

Temporary postoperative urinary retention is common. Permanent urinary retention is rare. Immediately after surgery, especially if the prolapse was bad, most women will have difficulty emptying their bladders. They may have urgency of urination, frequency, and incomplete emptying. Over the course of a few weeks, the urination will return to normal. Occasionally, a woman will not be able to urinate at all. She will have the urge to empty her bladder but no urine will come out. This problem is handled differently by different physicians. One option is to reinsert a catheter into the urethra and leave it there for a few days. The catheter is connected to a bag that is attached to one of your legs. The urine will drain into the leg bag continuously. A week or so later, the tube is removed in the doctor's office or by you at home, and a trial to urinate will ensue. After a few more days of healing, the swelling should be reduced and urination should not be a problem.

Another option is to teach you how to insert a catheter into your urethra to drain the urine yourself. A small plastic tube can be directed into the urethra, a hole above the vagina through which the urine is released.

When the flow stops, the tube is removed. Before inserting the tube again at the next urge to urinate, an attempt to empty spontaneously can be made. Whatever comes out is flushed away, while the amount that comes out through the tube is recorded. When the residual urine, the amount that comes out of the tube, falls to 100 cc ($3\frac{1}{2}$ ounces of urine), the catheterizations can be discontinued. This method of treating urinary retention is called self-catheterization.

Rarely, the post-void residual urine that is measured with the catheter remains above 100 cc. If three months after the surgery, you are still catheterizing, then you are in urinary retention and will need to have revision of the surgery. Some women do not want to wait this long to stop catheterizing. Although it is a nuisance, postoperative urinary retention can be corrected. Another surgery to remove the mesh and the scar tissue can be performed. A new mesh may be inserted at the same time, or at third surgery, if it is necessary. The scar tissue that remains often holds the prolapsed tissue in place. This condition usually occurs if an incontinence surgery is performed, although it may result from a prolapse repair alone.

Infections after Prolapse Surgery

A cluster of urinary tract infections can result after prolapse surgery. Women are concerned that a foreign material was left in the bladder, causing the infections. However, most of us perform cystoscopy at the time of the surgery to ensure that no foreign material is present. With a perfectly normal bladder, these infections cannot be explained. Perhaps the surgery, anesthesia, and perioperative antibiotics suppress the immune system which leads to infections in women who are prone to them.

The symptoms are obvious. They include frequency of urination, burning with urination, and pelvic discomfort. Sometimes, blood can be seen in the urine. Treatment is oral antibiotics. Some of you will experience flank pain, which does not mean that a kidney infection has resulted. Kidney infections include fevers over 101.5°F and an elevation of the infection count in the blood. Urinary tract infections are treated with three to five days of antibiotics by mouth. Rarely, a woman will have so many infections that a daily suppression dose of antibiotics will be recommended (see Chapter 8).

Mesh Erosion

Extrusion of the material that is placed under the bladder to support the pelvic structures can result. This usually only happens if synthetic material is used. If you get this, you will present with persistent vaginal discharge, usually yellow with a tinge of pink. It may have a foul odor, and it usually is copious enough to require a minipad. When examined, you will be found to have a piece of mesh exposed through the vaginal skin. It may be just a tiny hole.

The first attempt at solving the rejection of the mesh is to apply vaginal estrogen cream and antibiotics. The piece of exposed mesh is usually infected and will need to be sterilized with the antibiotics. The estrogen cream increases the blood flow to the vaginal tissues to help heal the area. After a few weeks, if the hole has still not closed, it will need to be repaired in the operating room in an ambulatory setting. The piece of mesh is removed and the opening is sewn closed. If a large piece of mesh needs to be removed, then a new piece may eventually need to be reinserted. I recommend inserting the new piece at a later time when the area has had a chance to heal. Mesh erosions do not occur if biodegradable material is used or if a patient's own tissues are used in the suspension.

The advantage to using the patient's own tissues or tissues from animal is that the material will not erode. However, the durability of these products is probably not as long as it is with synthetic. In choosing a reinforcing material, the advantages and disadvantages of each option need to be weighed. The risk of erosion is low. The permanence of the synthetic mesh and the durability of the response outweigh the risk of erosion. I encourage the use of synthetic materials for prolapse repairs.

Fistulas

The development of a fistula between the bladder and vagina after a cystocele repair is a devastating and extremely rare event. A fistula is a hole that joins two organs that normally do not communicate. In this case, the hole is between the bladder and the vagina. Fistulas occur when an injury results to one organ, and abnormal healing ensues. In nearly all healthy women, the hole will close normally, even if the injury to the bladder is not recognized at the time of the surgery. A fistula forms if an infection occurs in that area, if stitches or mesh prevents the bladder hole from closing, or if there is a history of pelvic radiation.

You will know if you have a fistula pretty quickly. Urine leaks constantly through the vagina. Depending on the size of the hole and its location, the bladder may or may not fill with urine. A tiny hole will result in leakage, but also normal bladder activity. A large hole will prevent the bladder from filling because all of the urine is exiting through the hole. You will not have the urge to urinate, but are always wet.

Fistulas can be repaired successfully in nearly every case. Although a short course of conservative management can be attempted, the treatment is usually surgical. A catheter is inserted into the bladder and left to drainage for a few days. Not only will this keep you dry for hygiene purposes, but it may help with the closure. If this fails, which it usually does, surgery should be scheduled as soon as possible. During the operation, if a foreign material is preventing the bladder from healing, the material must be removed. If infection is the problem, the infected tissue should be excised and the hole closed. Very rarely, the presence of a tumor is the source of the fistula. The tumor will need to be removed in the same fashion as the other causative agents.

Fistula repair is a surgical undertaking. Sometimes the operation can be done through a vaginal approach. If it is deep in the vagina, some surgeons feel more comfortable approaching it abdominally. The most important thing is for the hole to be closed. Whichever approach the surgeon feels more comfortable with is the approach of choice. Fortunately, this complication is a rare one.

Problems Related to the Prolapse Repair

Complications related to repairing the prolapse are distinguished from problems that arise within the bladder after surgery. Dissection of the tissues surrounding the prolapsed organ can result in excessive bleeding and possible injury to the nearby structures.

Bleeding

Excessive bleeding is often difficult to control. The best management is working rapidly, closing the incisions, and applying pressure to stop the hemorrhage. Occasionally, a blood transfusion will be needed. Because the spaces in which the bleeding occurs are small, the bleeding will be self-contained and will stop on its own. A large hematoma, or blood clot, may form behind the bladder before the bleeding stops. Large blood clots can push against the bladder or kidney, affecting the flow of urine through that side of the urinary system. A stent, or flexible plastic tube, may need to be inserted between the kidney and bladder to insure adequate drainage while the hematoma dissolved on its own. These large blood clots can be very unpleasant, causing pressure and pain until they are reabsorbed by the body. Complete reabsorption of the blood clot may take up to six months.

It is rare that a woman needs to be taken back to the operating room to stop heavy bleeding. When this happens, an incision is usually made abdominally to get the best exposure. If the surgeon feels that this intervention is indicated, no other choice is available. Sometimes it is better to go back and control the hemorrhage before it is too late, than it is to try to wait it out. A potential risk in any operation, excessive bleeding is an extremely rare complication.

Injury Caused by Surgery
Injury to the ureters, the tubes that drain the kidneys into the bladder, can result from placing stitches in the wrong position or from bunching up tissue that causes a kink in these structures. The kink will prevent adequate drainage of the affected side, causing blockage of the kidney. Sudden onset of kidney blockage will present with pain in the back under the ribs. If both sides are tied off or kinked, neither kidney will drain, resulting in no urine output after the operation.

During surgery, most surgeons will give an injection of blue dye into your intravenous line. The dye will turn the urine blue, so that it can be seen in the bladder. If both systems are working well, the blue dye will be visualized squirting into the bladder from each kidney through a cystoscope. If no dye is seen coming through one or the other ureter, the repair will be immediately taken down and redone. Rarely, blue dye will be seen in spite of a ureteral injury. The dye will be eliminated, but over a few hours, the swelling around the area will close off the ureter and block it. It is important for the surgeon to know if a woman is missing a kidney or has only one functioning kidney. There are few things more frustrating than looking for blue dye only to find out that no kidney is present on the side in

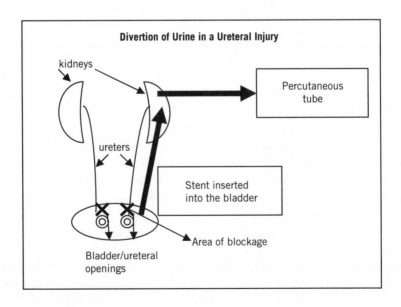

question. I do kidney ultrasounds on all my surgical patients for just that reason.

If an injury is suspected after surgery, an ultrasound can be done to evaluate the kidney in question. If urine is building up in the kidney, blockage is suggested. It may take a day or two for the kidney to back up enough for a diagnosis on an ultrasound study. Once the diagnosis is made, intervention should take place immediately. Two options are available at this point. One choice is to go in through the bladder and try to insert a tube between the bladder and the kidney on the affected side. This small tube is called a *stent*. It will bypass the blockage and allow the kidney to drain until the sutures dissolve and the kink relaxes or the injury heals. The stent may be slightly irritating to the bladder lining, but medications can be given to suppress this discomfort. It usually stays for six weeks and is removed in the office through an office cystoscopy.

The second option is to insert a tube into the kidney through a puncture in the back. This is called a *percutaneous nephrostomy tube*. The tube will bypass the bladder and the ureter, protecting the kidney by draining urine into a bag attached to the tube going through the back. Once the kidney is draining well and recovers its function, a stent can be inserted from above through the kidney and into the bladder, as opposed to through the bladder up to the kidney.

Once the tube is placed in either position, the kidney is unblocked and urine will drain. The pain will subside, and the kidney is protected. At that point, a decision can be made regarding how to manage the blockage. If taking down the repair is necessary, it can be done at that time, or later. If synthetic mesh is used, it may be better to repair the injury immediately by going back in vaginally and taking down the mesh, and releasing the ureter in question. New material can be inserted and the repair completed. This way, the ureter will be sure to heal and the surgery will be completed.

Other surgeons may prefer to wait a few weeks for things to heal and for you to recover before you are subjected to another operation. In many cases, the blockage resolves itself once the swelling goes down and the sutures heal. These decisions are made on a case by case basis.

Recurrent Prolapse
Recurrent prolapse rates are variable. Early recurrences, those that occur within weeks of the original surgery, differ from late recurrences, ones that occur within years of the original surgery. Early recurrences occur because of technical error, infection, or failure to recognize all of the defects.

Sometimes a small cystocele or rectocele will not be repaired at the time of other repairs, such as a hysterectomy or enterocele repair. If you have no symptoms and the defect is small, the surgeon may choose not to repair that defect. However, within a few months, this small cystocele or rectocele gets larger and needs to be repaired. In many cases it is better to only repair what needs to be addressed at the time. Although not ideal, another prolapse can always be fixed when it needs to be.

Late recurrences are fairly common, especially if reinforcing materials are not used. In the past, repairs involved pulling the muscles together and closing the vaginal skin. The same weak tissues that led to the problem in the beginning were being used to hold up the organs. The risk of recurrence in this setting would undoubtedly be high. With reinforcement of the woman's native tissue with other materials, the repair should be stronger and last longer. The recurrent rates of pelvic-floor prolapse in which synthetic mesh has been used are just being published now. We generally consider five years to be the first point at which data are useful. Recurrences at five years seem much lower in women in whom synthetic mesh has been implanted. Theoretically, the recurrence rate should be close to zero if nylon mesh is used because the mesh is holding up the repair, and it does not weaken or disintegrate over time. No surgery is 100% reliable or free of complications, but the risk of recurrence is much lower than it has been in the past.

Bowel Injuries
Bowel injuries during prolapse repair are exceedingly uncommon but very dangerous. The bowel is exposed in enterocele surgery and in a hysterectomy. The abdominal cavity is actually entered through the vagina in these surgeries. If recognized at the time of injury, a small tear or knick in the small intestine can be repaired without any problems. If the injury is not recognized immediately, intestinal fluid may leak into the abdomen, causing an infection or blockage in the bowel. Sometimes conservative management will suffice. Refraining from eating and decompressing the intestines with a tube through the nose will allow the hole to close. Reoperation to repair the injury and remove the damaged piece of intestine may be necessary.

Rectal Injuries
Injuries to the rectum can occur during rectocele surgery. A small hole in the rectum is closed immediately without any problems. An unrecognized rectal injury can result in a permanent hole between the rectum and the

vagina. Called a rectovaginal fistula it is recognized when a woman complains of stool in her vagina. This unpleasant complication is repaired surgically through the vagina. If mesh is used at the original repair, the mesh must be removed to insure adequate healing. Precautions against rectal injury include packing the rectum with gauze prior to initiating the repair and careful dissection. Many surgeons require bowel cleaning with an enema before surgery.

Anesthesia Complications and Problems Related to Pain Medications
Anesthetic complications and problems related to pain medications are addressed in detail in Chapter 11. Competent surgeons, anesthesiologists, and support staff will help avert any untoward events, but every surgery includes risks. An old adage says that a surgeon is only as good as his complications. In other words, not only does a surgeon need to be good at performing the surgery, but he has to be able to handle the complications associated with that surgery. Access to the surgeon is essential. He must take all complaints and concerns seriously in order to recognize when a problem has arisen. Communication between patient and doctor is essential to ensure a good outcome.

Reviewing all of the potential complications of prolaspe surgery is enough to deter even the most determined patient. It is important to recognize that these operations are real surgeries, not "procedures." Adherence to all the instructions that you are given is imperative to a safe and satisfying result. All operations have risks, which none of us wants to face. Knowing what they are will help you to communicate promptly with your surgeon if anything seems out of the ordinary.

SUMMARY

Pelvic organ prolapse is a complicated problem for both women and their doctors. For women, the shame, embarrassment, and belief that nothing can be done prevent them from seeking treatment. Physicians often don't recognize a prolapse when they examine a patient, or they don't know where to send patients when they do. Gynecologists and urologists with special training in the management of prolapse are sprouting up all over the country (see Chapter 3). As we all get older, our bodies change, often resulting in problems that interfere with a healthy lifestyle. Treatment of these debilitating conditions will help women return to the social and physical activities that are essential for us, regardless of our age. No one is too old or too young to have pelvic-floor prolapse and its associated urinary issues.

Nor is anyone too old or too young to seek treatment. Both surgical and nonsurgical choices are available and nearly all evaluation and management is covered by conventional insurance. See a physician, get examined, gather information, and then make an informed decision regarding your own condition. You will be surprised at how much this small step will change your life!

PART FOUR

THE PAINFUL BLADDER

CHAPTER 8

Urinary Tract Infections

SYNONYMS

Cystitis
Bladder infection
UTI

SYMPTOMS (NOT ALL WILL BE PRESENT)

Frequency
Urgency
Burning with urination
Blood in the urine
Back pain
Groin pain
Cloudy, smelly urine

Those of you who have been plagued with recurrent urinary tract infections will be able to relate to the following story:

A. just got promoted at work. Five years with the company and her boss finally recognized her ability. Of course this meant more responsibility and more stress, but she was up for the challenge. On the day her new position was to begin, A. woke up with mild lower back pain, abdominal pain, and burning when she went to the bathroom. The day went well. She received lots of congratulations and began organizing her strategies. By the time she got home that night, the burning got worse and the constant need to urinate was driving her crazy. She was too tired to deal with this; she thought that maybe her body would just give her a break and fight this off by itself.

By 11:00 that night she had been to the bathroom about 25 times and could not get to sleep. She called the doctor's on-call number and the nurse practitioner answered. Amy was told to go to the emergency room and drop off a sample of urine before picking up a prescription for antibiotics. After three hours in the ER, she arrived home exhausted. Her new job was starting out just great!

About one month later, she went out on a blind date that one of her friends set up. For a blind date, it went extremely well. After getting to know each other over the next few weeks, they decided it was time to move the relationship to the next level. Having not had sex in over a year, A. was no longer on the birth control pill. She dusted off her diaphragm, checked it for holes, and bought some new spermicidal jelly. The morning after their first encounter, the all-too-familiar back pain, stomach pain, and burning with urination returned. Of course it was Sunday, and she would have to go back to the emergency room. This time she knew better that to sit there and wait to be seen by a doctor. She dropped off the urine and picked up a prescription. This time it only took an hour and a half. She slept most of the afternoon.

Her quarterly report was due on her boss's desk by Monday morning. During the entire last week, she had been crunching numbers and making graphs on the computer. This was her first presentation in her new position. She was nervous. That morning, she woke up with very mild back pain, but no burning and no frequency. She chalked it up to nerves. The presentation went well, but by the time it was over, her back pain was worse, she had lower abdominal pains, she was nauseated, and she was dying to get to the toilet. When she sat down to go, she could barely squeeze anything out. She was in agony. She thought that she had seen some blood on the toilet paper. That was the last straw. She needed to see the doctor.

She left work early because the doctor could see her that afternoon. He collected a sample of urine and confirmed that she had another infection. After taking a thorough history, he performed a physical examination. He asked her whether or not she wet the bed or had urinary tract infections as a child. He was also interested in whether or not her mother had a problem with infections. They discussed methods of birth control and her sexual activity. He prescribed another course of the same antibi-

otic and a sent her home to bed with reassurances that "everything would be fine."

After three infections in the same number of months, she decided to come to see me to get some information and find out what she could do about this problem. After hearing her story and examining her, I analyzed the urine sample she left. It was completely normal, with no blood, white blood cells, or bacteria present. We sat down to talk.

I explained to her that we don't know why certain women get urinary tract infections and others do not. Without a history of childhood infections or high fevers (over 101.5°F), an exhaustive evaluation is not necessary. She can be spared x-rays and cystoscopy because her urine is completely normal between infections. After each episode, her bladder heals, leaving no residual scarring or damage. These infections will not lead to a small contracted bladder or incontinence later in life. They have absolutely no effect on her kidneys. They are extremely painful and upsetting, but they are not harmful or dangerous.

Clusters of infections are common. A series of three or four infections in a row may then be followed by a period of calm that could last one or two years. Even though it feels like the infection won't go away, each one actually resolves and a new one begins. Periods of normalcy between infections, even if they last for two or three days, indicate that the last infection resolved before the new one began.

Since we don't know why they happen, we cannot prevent them. What we can do, however, is come up with a better strategy for managing them when they do occur. We discussed three methods of treatment: 1) self-medication, where she takes three days of antibiotics when her symptoms arise; 2) the postcoital pill, where she takes one pill within 24 hours of having sex; or 3) suppression, where she takes a tiny dose of an antibiotic every day for three to six months to prevent infections. She chose the self-medication program.

I sent her home with a prescription for antibiotics which she will fill immediately. If the symptoms begin, she can start the medication right away for a short, three-day course. Excessive water and cranberry juice will not help her once her symptoms begin. A healthy lifestyle is her best defense: a good diet, exercise, and a decent night sleep.

Much relieved, A. filled the prescription on her way home. She has had one infection in the last six months, which responded to the self-medication program beautifully. Her job is going really well, and she recently got engaged to the guy she met on the blind date.

One out of three women will experience a urinary tract infection during her lifetime. Twenty-five percent of women between the ages of 20 and 40 have already had a urinary tract infection. In the United States, one million hospital admissions per year are due to infections in the urinary tract alone. At a cost of $1 billion per year, *urinary tract infections account for seven million outpatient office visits annually and remain the most common cause of infection in hospitalized patients.*

Urinary tract infections (UTI) occur in all age groups, from newborn infants to the elderly in nursing homes. In children, the rate of infections is equal between the sexes, occurring in approximately 2% of children under the age of 10. Once in adulthood, women develop infections at a rate eight times that of men. By old age, the incidence, again, becomes equal. In both pre- and postmenopausal sexually active women, UTIs are one of the most common causes of visits to physicians' offices. Infections in these women are very different than those in children and the elderly. The causes of this painful, disruptive, and, often, debilitating problem remain elusive in sexually-active, otherwise healthy women.

Most women who get infections develop one isolated infection that is easily treated with a single course of antibiotics. About 20% of you will have a recurrence after the full course of antibiotics is completed. A subset of you will suffer frequent, disabling, recurrent UTIs. As in A.'s case, the infections occur in clusters, where one, two, three, four, or even five infections will occur per year over a year or two, followed by long periods of remission, before the cycle recurs.

In 1863 Louis Pasteur proved that bacteria grow in urine. This discovery led to the realization that bladder symptoms are related to the presence of bacteria in the urine. Normally, the urine is sterile—no bacteria live in the bladder or the urethra, the tube that drains urine from the bladder out of the body. However, bacteria *do* live in the vagina and the rectum and serve to protect these organs from becoming infected with pathogenic, or bad, organisms. In the vagina, these protective bacteria are called lactobacilli, and in the rectum, they are called diphtheroids. These organisms grow poorly in the bladder, and do not cause UTIs. Therefore, if a culture result shows either diphtheroids or lactobacilli, it is not a UTI. Bacteria in the rectum that migrate to the vagina do not belong in the vagina. These stray organisms can then travel the short distance from the vagina into the urethra, which gives them easy access into the bladder.

The reason urinary tract infections occur much more frequently in women than in men lies with the differences in the anatomy of the urinary tract between the two sexes. We have short urethras, which allow bacteria

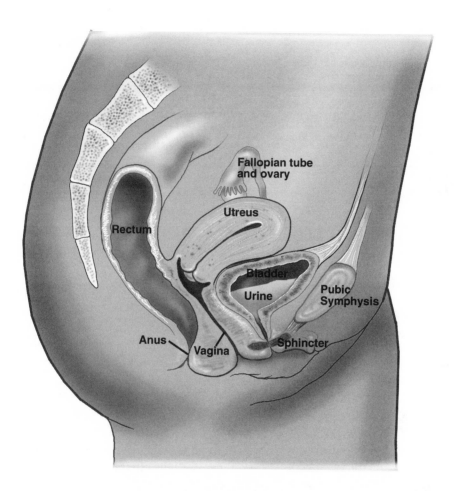

FIGURE 1. *Normal Female Anatomy.*

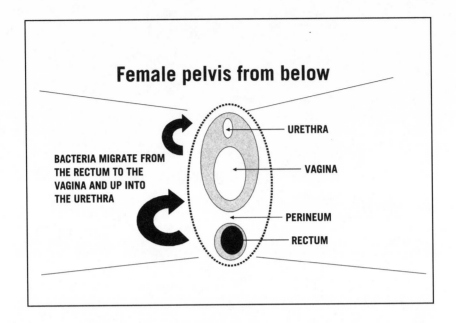

FIGURE 2.

to enter the bladder once the urinary tract is accessed. The moist haven of the vagina allows bacteria to grow and flourish before they make the short ascent into the urethra and then the bladder. Men have no reservoir for bacteria to multiply between the rectum and the urethra. In addition, the male urethra is longer than the female. It extends the entire length of the penis and courses behind the pubic bone before it finally meets the bladder. Even if tenacious bacteria are allowed to find their way from the rectum to the tip of the penis, the long journey into the bladder is usually interrupted by a strong gush of urine during urination, which washes away the organisms. For this reason, men with urinary tract infections often have an abnormal anatomy, like a large prostate, or a medical condition, like diabetes. Women who develop recurrent infections, on the other hand, usually have normal urinary tracts and have no medical problems that increase their risk of problems. This chapter defines the terminology related to urinary tract infections and addresses the causes of urinary tract infections in healthy women, the need for evaluation, including when extensive testing is warranted, the treatment of existing infections, including the risks and benefits of antibiotic therapy, and the prevention of further infections.

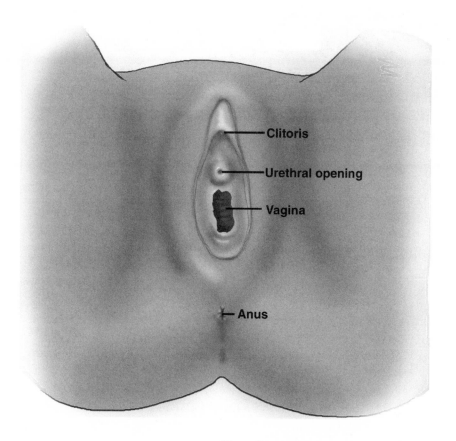

FIGURE 2A. *View of Perineum.*

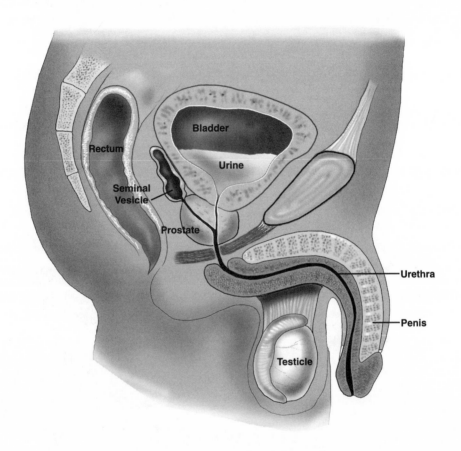

FIGURE 3. *Normal Male Anatomy.*

DEFINITIONS

CYSTITIS = Inflammation +/− Bacteria
UTI = Inflammation + Bacteria
BACTERIURIA = Bacteria − Inflammation

Cystitis is defined as an inflammatory response of the bladder wall to an irritant. The irritant may be a chemical, such as food; it may be radiation treatment for pelvic organ cancer; or it may be bacteria. A **urinary tract infection** is cystitis caused by bacteria. If bacteria are found in the bladder, but you *do not have* symptoms of cystitis, then you have **bacteriuria**. Cystitis and urinary tract infections are not normal. Bacteriuria is normal. One percent of adolescent girls and 5% of young women have bacteria in their urine with no symptoms of an infection. As girls grow up, the incidence of bacteriuria increases 2% per decade. Over 50% of elderly institutionalized women live with bacteria in their urine. Whether bacteria in the urine will eventually cause a symptomatic infection remains unpredictable. Over half of us who have bacteriuria at any given time will clear it from the urinary tracts without ever taking antibiotics. But, if a woman is followed for one year with bacteria in her urine, there is a 30% chance that she will develop a symptomatic infection at some point during that year. In spite of her developing an infection, her kidneys will never be negatively impacted by the presence of bacteria in her bladder. So, this begs the question: "If the doctor finds bacteria in my bladder on a routine urine test, should I be treated with antibiotics?" The answer is no, not until you develop symptoms, unless, of course, a complicating factor is introduced into the equation, such as pregnancy, diabetes mellitus, or an abnormal urinary tract.

Pyuria is the presence of white blood cells in the urine. White blood cells fight infection and combat irritation all over the body. They are intimately involved in the immune response. Their presence indicates bladder irritability, but not necessarily infection. Pyuria is especially significant in women who have recently been treated with antibiotics for a UTI, and still have symptoms. The bacteria may be gone, but the bladder may still be inflamed and irritated, which would account for the persistent symptoms. The continued inflammation will be evident by the pyuria, but the actual infection will have been successfully treated.

UTIs are divided into uncomplicated and complicated infections. **Uncomplicated** UTI refers to infections in a structurally and functionally normal urinary tract. In other words, the urine drains from the kidneys to the bladder and out through the urethra without some of it going in the wrong direction (from the bladder to the kidneys, which is called reflux); the bladder empties completely when urinating; and only one kidney and one ureter exist on each side of the body.

Complicated infections refer to infections that occur in women with abnormal urinary tracts, which you were either born with, or they develop as a result of a medical problem. The two medical problems that most commonly cause urinary tract infections include diabetes mellitus and neurological diseases, such as multiple sclerosis, Parkinson's disease, stroke, and paralysis. Pregnancy-related UTIs are also characterized as complicated. The reason that the distinction is made between complicated and uncomplicated infections is that the treatments and the consequences of failing to treat differ between the two. Complicated infections, as one would suspect, need more aggressive therapy.

UNCOMPLICATED URINARY TRACT INFECTIONS

- **Simple**
  - **First infection goes away**
- **Recurrent**
  - — **Reinfection**
    - **First infection goes away but returns**
  - — **Unresolved/persistent**
    - **First infection nerver goes away**
- **Pyelonephritis**
  - **Infection in the kidney**

Most sexually active, healthy women develop the uncomplicated type of urinary tract infection. These infections are due to a narrow spectrum of bacteria and are treated with short-term, inexpensive medications taken by mouth. Even in women with recurrent, bothersome problems, like those described in A., the organisms are mild, meaning that they do not injure the urinary tract permanently and do not need heavy-duty antibiotics to cure.

Uncomplicated Urinary Tract Infections
The different types of uncomplicated urinary tract infections are 1) simple infections, 2) recurrent infections, and 3)kidney infections, also called pyelonephritis. The simplest and most common type is a single infection,

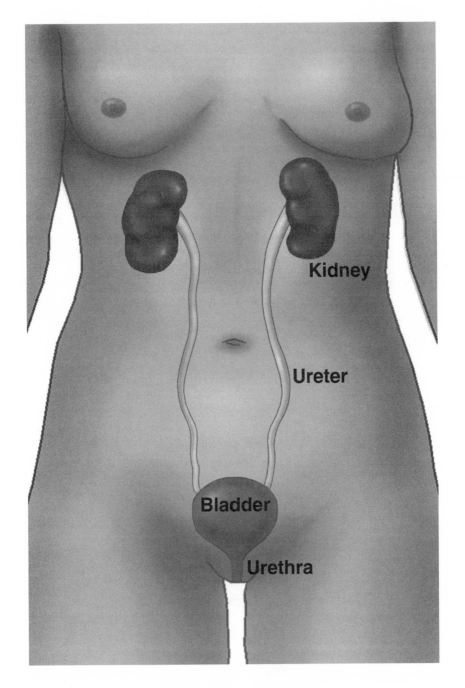

FIGURE 4. *Female Urinary Tract.*

which is treated once, and does not come back in less than six months. If the infection goes away, but returns again in *less than six months*, you have been **reinfected.** A urologist would call this a recurrent infection due to *reinfection* as opposed to an unresolved infection. Ninety-five percent of recurrent urinary tract infections are due to reinfections, and they occur at varying intervals of time.

Although terribly unpleasant, the frequency of recurrent, uncomplicated infections will not increase the risk of injury to the kidneys, nor does it mean that a problem within the urinary tract exists. Usually, no evaluation needs to be initiated if you suffer from recurrent urinary tract infections.

Recurrences due to bacteria that never were cleared from the urinary tract are called **unresolved** infections. Unresolved infections are caused by inadequate therapy, either because of resistant bacteria that the antibiotic cannot kill, or because you are not taking the medication correctly. Occasionally, an unresolved infection will be due to **bacterial persistence,** which is caused by a collection of bacteria that cannot be killed by antibiotics alone. The causes of bacteria persistence include kidney stones and foreign bodies, such as a catheter, in the urinary tract. Infections caused by bacterial persistence must then be reclassified as complicated UTIs if a kidney stone or foreign material is identified.

The final type of uncomplicated urinary tract infection is **pyelonephritis,** or a kidney infection. Rarely, a bladder infection will work its way up the ureter, into the kidney, causing back pain and fever, as well as the typical urinary symptoms of cystitis. Again, you may be a perfectly healthy woman whose infection spreads rapidly. No investigation of the urinary tract is necessary, but therapy must be instituted for a longer period of time than is necessary for the other types of uncomplicated UTIs.

Complicated Urinary Tract Infections
Complicated infections occur in women who have undergone:

- Recent surgery
- Recent instrumentation of the urinary tract
- Immunosuppression
- Treatment for diabetes mellitus
- Recent hospitalization
- Recent use of antibiotics

If any of the following conditions exist, kidney damage can result:

- Reflux of urine
- Infections caused by the organism Proteus (will promote stone formation)
- Infection in the presence of a blocked kidney
- Infection in a paralyzed patient
- Infection in the presence of pregnancy

Women with these conditions must seek medical advice immediately upon developing symptoms, and cannot be treated without a diagnosis through a urine culture and sensitivity test (see Diagnosis and Evaluation section).

CAUSES OF URINARY TRACT INFECTIONS

The reason that some women spend their adult lives plagued with infections and other women never experience a single episode remains unknown. However, many things are known about the propensity of certain bacteria for the cozy environment of certain urinary tracts. Multiple theories abound, some of which make no sense. The myths and realities that we will review in this section regarding the causes of UTIs include:

- **Personal hygiene**: Bathing, bubble baths, and bathroom habits
- The ability of **the bladder to defend** itself against infection
- The ability of **bacteria to adhere** to the tissues of some women
- The effects of **hormones, menstruation, and menopause**
- **Sex, spermacides, and contraception**
- Abnormal **anatomy**
- **Medical illnesses**

Over 80% of urinary tract infections occurring in sexually active women are caused by the organism *E. coli*. The other 20% are caused by *Staphylococcus saprophyticus* (staph), *Proteus mirabilis*, *Klebsiella pneumoniae*, and *Enterococcus faecalis*. The bacteria migrate from the anal canal, through the vagina, and up into the urethra. In women with recurrent infections, a single vaginal culture may be absent of the offending bacteria, indicating that these organisms are not harbored by the vagina continuously. They are cleared by the natural defenses of the body or by antibiotics periodically, only to return and attempt their descent up the urinary tract again. The process of colonization (the presence of bacteria on a tissue bed without evidence of their presence, such as burning, itching, or pain) and infection (the presence of bacteria *with* evidence of their presence) is dynamic. In other words, a swab at the physician's office may be negative one day and positive the next.

Personal Hygiene: Bathing, Bubble Baths, and Bathroom Habits
The issue of cleanliness and hygiene remains controversial and highly sensitive. Women who get infections are not dirty. The susceptibility to developing this painful problem has nothing to do with how often or how thoroughly one women cleans her vagina versus another women. Douching every day, versus once per week versus once per month will not alter the recurrence rate of infections. In general, douching is not a good idea, because it upsets the balance of bacteria and yeast in the vagina. The vagina has its own ability to cleanse itself of bacteria and dirt. Part of this natural cleansing process involves the presence of good bacteria, called lactobacilli. Lactobacilli police the vagina for bacteria that do not belong in that region, thus protecting against invasion of evil *E. coli*, staphylococcus, and yeast. If the vagina is aggressively cleaned too often, these good bacteria will be washed away, leaving the environment defenseless against yeast and fecal organisms that travel from the rectum between washings. On the whole, **douching is not good**, and should be avoided, especially in women prone to infection. Showering and cleaning the vagina with warm water once a day will maintain excellent hygiene without exposure to increased infection.

Bubble baths have also been implicated in causing infections. In general, bathing is not bad for the natural vaginal flora. Bath oils, soaps, perfumes, and bubbles may promote skin irritation that may mimic an infection, but they will not increase the risk of a problem. A good rule of thumb is to avoid any chemical that causes irritation, including laundry detergents, lotions, and underwear fabrics. Nylon undergarments will not increase the risk of infection, but they may increase the temperature and moisture of the vagina, which will promote growth of bad bacteria that are already present. If the environment is less friendly to the bacteria, they may not be inclined to reproduce so rapidly. For this reason, cotton-crotch underwear, which does not lock in moisture, is recommended. Along the same line, tight pants can aggravate problems, but will not *cause* problems. Because exercise leads to sweating and moisture in the crotch, patients may be inclined to limit this activity. However, exercise is excellent for overall health and immune function and should in no way be limited because of concerns about acquiring a urinary tract infection. If there are concerns, wear loose clothes that can breath while exercising, thus reducing the temperature and moisture in the genital area.

Finally, the issue of wiping from front to back in the toilet needs to be addressed. Intuitively, it makes sense to clean the genitalia from front to back after urinating in order to avoid spreading bacteria from the rectum toward the vagina. However, no study has ever proven that bacteria will spread through improper wiping techniques. Many women and girls dab the vaginal area from the front and never develop infections. In my opinion, wiping technique has little impact on the susceptibility to infection.

Natural Bladder Defenses
The bladder contains natural defense mechanisms that protect it from constant invasion by bacteria. The principle defense mechanism is the washing effect of the urine. The urine cascades out of the bladder and down the urethra, taking anything in its path. Unless the bacteria can attach themselves to the wall of the urethra or the bladder, they will be washed away. If the bacteria are able to survive the urinary stream, they are prevented from sticking to the bladder wall by a second level of defense: a layer of slime, called the glycosaminoglycan layer. This slippery layer contains proteins that will trap the bacteria and evacuate it, in a similar way that the nose is lined by mucus. Women with recurrent infections may have a problem with this protein layer. If the layer is not intact or if the proteins are not sticky enough, the bacteria will be allowed to sit in the bladder and reproduce.

Ability of the Bacteria to Stick to Your Cells
In order for bacteria to migrate from the rectum to the vagina, reproduce, and then move into the urethra and ultimately wind up in the bladder, they must be able to hold on to the surface of the tissues over which they travel.

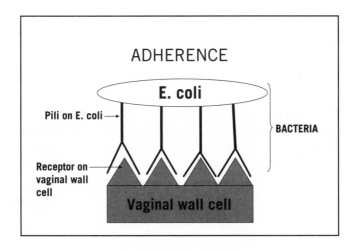

The bacteria must be hearty enough to survive wiping after urinating, rubbing from clothing, and washing from urinary streams. This ability of bacteria to stick to tissues is called *adherence*. *E. coli* have tentacles, called pili, which they use to hold onto the vaginal and bladder walls. The vaginal tissues of some women have receptors onto which the pili can adhere with considerable strength. The presence of the pili on the *E. coli* organism may be the reason that of all of the intestinal bacteria, it is the most often the cause of urinary tract infections. This adherence phenomenon identified in *E. coli* allows it to travel from the rectum to the bladder without destruction.

Women with recurrent UTIs often suffer from recurrent sinus infections and problems with cavities, which are infections of the teeth. If the vaginal and cheek cells from women with recurrent UTIs are grown in culture media laden with *E. coli*, the cells will be covered with bacteria. Vaginal and cheek cells from women who do not get UTIs will have no adhering bacteria. Even between infections, the women with recurrent infections will have bacteria sitting in the vaginal opening, holding fast to the tissue until the opportunity is ripe to ascend the urinary tract. In women with occasional infections, there are no bacteria being harbored by the vaginal tissues.

This predilection for bacterial adherence may be genetic. Receptors on the vaginal cells may be genetically programmed, which accounts for women whose mother's suffered with the same problem. Women over the age of 65 have greater bacterial adherence than menstruating women between the ages of 18 and 40. The adherence phenomenon does not appear to be related to estrogen and it is in no way determined by hygiene.

Hormones, Menstruation, and Menopause
Estrogen plays a role in the development of recurrent infections. However, what that role is, remains unclear. Postmenopausal and premenopausal women develop different types of infections. Postmenopausal women may have two or three bacteria causing the infections, whereas younger women have a single causative organism. Staph infections are rare in older women. Premenopausal women with recurrent infections usually have the same species of organism causing the problem each time, whereas postmenopausal women have different organisms with each episode.

Explanations for these differences are limited but a few observations have been made regarding the differences in the vaginal environment in pre- and postmenopausal women. Postmenopausal women have less acidic vaginal secretions, probably due to the lack of estrogen. Bacteria grow in

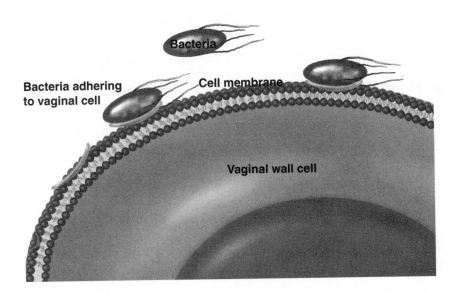

FIGURE 5. *Adherence.*

high pH fluid, so the more acidic (low pH) the environment, the less they will grow. Premenopausal women have a vaginal pH of about 4, compared with a pH of anywhere from 5.4 to 7.0 in postmenopausal women. This difference will increase adherence of bacteria by at least three times. The lack of estrogen may also create other problems that allow for bacterial growth. Estrogen encourages the colonization of the vagina with lactobacilli, the good bacteria that ward off infection. Less estrogen means less lactobacilli, which means fewer police-organisms warding off infection.

Sex, Spermicides, and Contraception

Urinary tract infections are *not* sexually transmitted diseases. If a woman has a UTI and has sex with a man, he will not get her infection, nor will she get a urinary tract infection from him if he has one. Urinary tract infections are caused by one's own intestinal bacteria, not by someone else's. So, do not send your partner to the urologist if your problem is recurrent urinary tract infections. However, yeast infections and vaginitis, caused by trichomonas or gardinerella, are sexually transmitted. Symptoms of vaginitis include vaginal discharge, vaginal itching, and vaginal odor. You may experience burning upon urination from vaginal skin irritation, but the symptoms of frequency, urgency, and pelvic pain are usually absent. If any question exists, you should consult a health-care professional for diagnosis and treatment.

Spermicidal jelly containing nonoxynol-9 will decrease the lactobacilli colonization and increase the bacterial adherence in the vagina, thus promoting urinary tract infections. The use of the diaphragm for contraception has also been implicated in the development of UTIs. An ill-fitting diaphragm can block the bladder and prevent proper emptying during urination. The residual puddle of urine will allow bacteria to fester and grow. If you have a problem with urinary tract infections related to intercourse, it is wise for you to use a different form of birth control. Condoms and birth control pills have not been shown to increase the occurrence of UTIs in women.

Anatomical Abnormalities

There is a small group of women with recurrent infections who have structurally abnormal urinary tracts. These conditions can be either congenital (a person is born with it) or acquired (it develops after birth). Often, women who were born with slight defects in their urinary tracts will have lived their entire lives without knowing that they had a problem. The only reason the abnormality becomes an issue is the recurrent infections. In the

Diagnosis and Evaluation section later in this chapter, the issue regarding who should be concerned about anatomical defects and how they are detected will be addressed.

The most common anatomical defects that cause infections are:

- Urethral diverticula
- Kidney stones
- Pelvic-floor prolapse
- Foreign body
- Vesicoureteral reflux

A urethral diverticulum (diverticula is plural) is a defect that is acquired; you are not born with it. A urethral diverticulum is a pocket that sits below the urethra and has a neck that drains into the urethra. Urine can enter the pocket but cannot leave because of the narrow neck. The urine sits there and becomes infected. The bacteria sit in the pocket, like the pouch of a pelican, and reproduce without recourse. Antibiotics cannot access the pouch, so the bacteria are not cleared with medication. These must be surgically removed.

Kidney stones occur more often in men than in women; however, they do occur in women, especially if there is a family history of stone disease. Not always painful, kidney stones can sit in the urinary tract and grow without being noticed. Most kidney stones harbor bacteria and serve as a constant reservoir of infection.

Pelvic-floor prolapse has been addressed in detail in Chapter 7. When the bladder sags into the vaginal canal (cystocele), it may not empty completely during urination. The incomplete emptying results in stagnant urine that will not clear bacterial invasion. The bladder becomes like a bathtub with a faulty drain. The murky water serves as a breeding ground for bacteria.

Foreign bodies in the bladder are not normal. They are inadvertently left there during surgery or a procedure. Sometimes, suture material or graft material can wind up in the bladder after different bladder or gynecological operations. They must be removed.

Vesicoureteral reflux is a fancy name for a condition in which some of the urine travels in the wrong direction in the urinary tract. Instead of it passing from the bladder into the urethra, it "refluxes" from the bladder into the ureters, and occasionally makes its way up into the kidney. This condition can be either inherited or acquired, and it may be silent. It is not usually dangerous, unless you develop an infection that travels into the kidney. Most

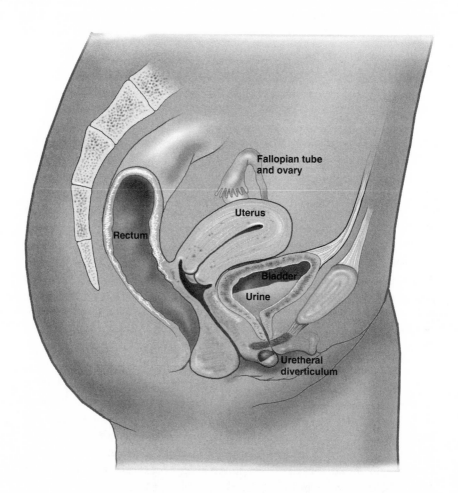

FIGURE 6. *Urethral Diverticulum.*

of the time, this condition is detected in childhood, when the infant or toddler develops a urinary tract infection. Routine evaluation will identify the reflux and it can be dealt with at that time. If a woman presents with persistent bacteria in her urine and recurrent infections, it is possible that she has reflux that has never been identified. Reflux does not *develop* in adults unless neurological disease (paralysis or multiple sclerosis, for example) is present.

Medical Conditions

A few medical conditions that affect the entire body can contribute to the development of urinary tract infections. The most common illness is diabetes mellitus. Diabetes mellitus, often referred to as sugar diabetes, wreaks havoc on the entire body, without sparing the urinary tract. If the blood sugar is well controlled through compliance with medications and diet, less damage will occur. Diabetics spill sugar into their urine, which serves as a culture media in which bacteria can flourish. In addition, long-standing diabetes can cause nerve injury to the bladder, just like it causes nerve injury to the feet and toes. The nerve injury results in a bladder that does not completely empty, so the sweet urine left behind serves as a warm, welcoming home to bacteria.

Immunosuppression also predisposes people to infection. Immunosuppression refers to using medication to decrease the body's ability to fight infection. Transplant recipients are aggressively immunosuppressed because if the immune system is allowed to fight foreign invaders, the transplanted organ will be the target. Women with a transplant frequently suffer from UTIs. Cancer sufferers on chemotherapy also are immunosuppressed and easily contract urinary tract infections. Less obvious immunosuppressed people are asthmatics who take steroids for flare-ups of their asthma. Steroids, like prednisone, will decrease the surveillance of the bladder for bad organisms. For example, if you are taking a 5- or 10-day course of steroids for an asthma attack, you may develop an infection that will need treatment with antibiotics, but was most likely caused by being on steroids. Inhaled steroids can also cause immunosuppression.

DIAGNOSIS AND EVALUATION

Women who have experienced a UTI know when there is a problem. Those of you who have gotten them know the symptoms well: pelvic pain and pressure, a constant urge to go to the bathroom, occasionally blood in the urine, and burning with urination. The symptoms are horrendous.

However, symptoms alone do not make the diagnosis of a UTI. There are other syndromes that present with the same symptoms as an infection, but there are no bacteria in the bladder. For this reason, a proper diagnosis should be obtained, especially if this is your first infection. If you develop a recurrent problem, a formal diagnosis does not need to be made before initiating treatment for each episode.

The first step in making an accurate diagnosis of a urinary tract infection is the collection of a urine sample, called a **clean-catch specimen**. Clean-catch urine is collected after you clean the vaginal area with a swab and let a few drops of urine empty into the toilet before collecting the remainder in the specimen container. The reason for the clean-catch technique is to eliminate collecting bacteria that sit in the vagina or the perineum, but are not in the bladder. If the area is not cleaned first, these bacteria will be washed into the specimen container by the urine stream and a false positive diagnosis will be made. As was mentioned earlier, many women have bacteria in their vaginas without having bacteria in their bladders. Generally, there is no need to catheterize the bladder to obtain a specimen. In a woman with an infection, this maneuver is painful, irritating, and unnecessary if she can do a clean-catch collection.

The simplest, least expensive, and quickest test to suggest an infection in the bladder is a **urinalysis**. It is done in the doctor's office, and although it does not *make* the diagnosis, it will suggest the presence of an infection before more definitive diagnostic tools are used. Treatment can begin immediately based on the results of the urinalysis and altered, based on the results of the culture and sensitivity that will be obtained two to four days later. Two methods of urinalysis are available. One is the **dipstick method** and the other is the **microscopic analysis**. For the dipstick method, after collecting a clean-catch specimen, a strip with color-coated reagents is dipped into the container by the technician in the office. The different reagents will turn colors if certain abnormalities are present in the urine. For microscopic analysis, after a clean-catch urine is collected, it is poured into a test tube, spun down in a centrifuge, and the liquid is poured off. The pellet that collects on the bottom of the tube is suspended in a drop of urine and poured onto a microscope slide. The doctor can then view the specimen under magnification. The **presence of bacteria** under the microscope strongly suggests that an infection is present. Unfortunately, the dipstick urinalysis does not directly identify bacteria. Both methods will detect the presence of **white blood cells**, which are present in bladders that are infected or irritated. White blood cells fight infection all over the body. The presence of white blood cells in the urine does not automatically make the diagnosis of an infection; however, if no white cells are in the urine, it is unlikely that an infection exists. In other words, absence of white blood cells is a more reliable finding for *ruling out* an infection than the presence of white blood cells is for *ruling in* an infection.

The dipstick analysis is more commonly performed. It is automated, faster to do, and technically less demanding. The dipstick analysis measures the presence of a number of enzymes that cannot be detected by the microscopic exam. **Leukocyte esterase** (LE) is an enzyme that is released by white blood cells that are fighting an infection. The presence of LE in the urine on the dipstick analysis is 75% accurate in diagnosing a UTI. **Nitrates** are produced by bacteria as they grow and multiply. Again, the presence of nitrates on the urinalysis will detect an infection about 75% of the time. If the urinalysis suggests the presence if a UTI, either by bacteria or white blood cells visualized under the microscope, or the presence of LE and nitrates on the dipstick, a urine culture should be performed with the urine that was collected for the urinalysis.

Traditionally, a urinary tract infection is *diagnosed* when a culture of the patient's **clean-catch urine grows 100,000 colony forming units (CFU) of bacteria per ml**. "Colony forming units" is a measure of the number of bacteria in the bladder. Because bacteria are tiny, they are tedious and time consuming to count on an individual basis. A method of quantifying their numbers was developed. After collection, the urine is refrigerated until it can be transported to the laboratory. In the lab, it is spun down in a centrifuge and one milliliter of urine is poured onto a culture plate. A culture plate is a soft bed of gel infused with nutrients that the bacteria need to grow and reproduce. The culture plate is placed in a warm, dark, moist environment to incubate for 24 hours. The bacteria grow and replicate in clusters or colonies. After 24 hours, a technician or machine can count the number of colonies on the plate. If there are over 100,000 colonies present on the plate, the diagnosis of a UTI is made. Over one quarter to one half of you with symptoms of a UTI will have colony counts of less than 100,000 CFUs. Therefore, the current definition of "*over* 100,000 CFU/ml" will under-diagnose as many as 50 percent of UTIs in women with acute bacterial cystitis. The bottom line is: **if symptoms are present, be sure to ask the lab to report on** *any* **growth because a symptomatic UTI can be caused by as few as 5000 CFU/ml.**

Urine cultures should be done in anyone with sporadic infections; that is, either a first time infection or an infection that has not occurred within the last six months. Other women who should have pretreatment cultures include women over the age of 65, pregnant women, diabetics, and women with symptoms that persist after seven days of treatment with antibiotics. If you have recurrent infections (more than two infections in six months or three infections in one year), you do not need to have a urine culture done before you begin treatment. If you develop symptoms, you can treat yourself without having a urine culture done first.

If you have recurrent infections, cultures can be done routinely in one of two ways. The most accurate way is to deliver the clean-catch specimen to a lab or to a doctor's office and have it done there. A simpler, less reliable technique is called the **dipslide culture** or Uricult®. You can buy the culture tube that contains a gel-coated slide in a pharmacy. You dip the slide into your urine and seal it. You then deliver it to the lab or the doctor's office for incubation. For infections in which over 100,000 colonies grow, the dipslide method is fine, but if fewer colonies grow, these home methods are less sensitive. In addition, the dipslide technique does not allow for antibiotic sensitivity testing.

In addition to identifying the presence and the number of colonies of bacteria, urine cultures can determine the type of bacteria that is growing and the susceptibility of the bacteria to different antibiotics. The antibiotic susceptibility is called **sensitivity testing**. Discs soaked in different antibiotic solutions are dropped onto the culture plate and the plate is incubated. After 24 hours, the plate is removed from the incubator, and if the bacteria are sensitive to the antibiotic, there will be no colonies growing around that disc. If the bacteria are not sensitive, they will ignore the disc and grow next to it or even over it. This technique allows the physician to identify the best antibiotic with which to treat you.

Once the culture and sensitivity results are obtained, you can begin treatment, and that is the end of the story. No further evaluation should be done; no x-rays or follow-up cultures need to be ordered in most women. There are a few groups of women who *do* need further investigation. The question is: who, and is that me?

Patients who need to be evaluated by a specialist, such as a urologist or a women's health expert, include:

- Women who develop recurrent infections with the **same organism** over a short period of time
- Women who develop more than **five infections** in one year
- Women who have **medical conditions** that can cause infections (see "Causes" section)
- Women who are **pregnant**
- Women with **neurological impairments**

Those of you who **do not need** to be evaluated with further tests include:

- Women who get infections with intercourse
- Women with up to three infections per year
- Women with infections caused by multiple organisms
- Women over the age of 65 with up to three infections per year
- Women with infections whose mothers' also had infections

Evaluation of the urinary tract can be extensive. Many different tests will define the anatomy of the kidneys, bladder, and ureters. Not all of these tests need to be done. In spite of an exhaustive workup, most of you will wind up with no identifiable cause for your infections. The only reason to do radiographic tests is to be sure that no anatomical abnormalities are the cause of these infections. A poorly developed urinary tract may need to be surgically corrected or a stone may need to be removed. Less than 10% of healthy women with recurrent infections will have a surgically correctable cause for their problem. If you have a history of infections as a child or if you get high fevers with your infections, then your urinary tract needs to be studied thoroughly. Women with infections caused by intercourse almost *never* have any identifiable reason for their problem. Even women with up to five infections per year will have no findings on x-ray. Reassuringly enough, most of these women will have normal urinary tracts with no evidence of scarring or injury as a result of recurrent infection and inflammation.

The two least-invasive tests are ultrasound (same as a sonogram) and magnetic resonance imaging (MRI). Both will delineate the anatomy of the urinary tract. Ultrasound will not test kidney function, whereas MRI will, if a contrast material is injected into the bloodstream during the test. Neither test uses radiation. Many centers, however, do not have MRI machines available for studying the urinary tract. An intravenous pyelogram (IVP) tests both function and anatomy, but it involves giving an injection of an iodine-based dye into the arm. It is also time consuming and involves radiation exposure. Computer-assisted tomography (CAT) scanning is excellent for showing anatomy and function; however, it, too, requires an injection of dye and radiation exposure. The pictures that are taken before the injection is done are excellent for finding kidney stones. Once the referral is made to the urologist, he will order the test that he feels is most appropriate to your situation. Each test provides excellent information.

Occasionally, cystoscopy is necessary. This procedure is done in the doctor's office by either a urologist or a gynecologist with specialty training in disorders of the urinary tract. It involves having you put your legs up in stirrups and injecting a local anesthetic agent, in the form of a gel, into the urethra. The scope is about $1\frac{1}{2}$ feet long, but only about 3 inches gets inserted into the urethra and the bladder (see Chapter 12 or more details). The doctor can see the inside of the bladder and the bladder wall, as well as the urethra. Foreign bodies, stones, and tumors can be detected, as well as urethral diverticula and infected urethral glands. All of these conditions are very unlikely causes of urinary tract infections, but they do occur, and should be investigated in indicated patients.

TREATMENT

General Approaches

Antibiotics are the mainstay of treatment for urinary tract infections. Before the myriad issues regarding antibiotics are addressed, good urinary habits, the length of antibiotic treatment, preventive measures to avoid recurrent infections, and the promise of vaccines will be discussed.

Some general principles of good urinary habits that may help ward off infections before they become symptomatic include:

1. Drinking four glasses of water a day to irrigate bacteria out of the bladder
2. Urinating regularly during the day and emptying completely with each visit to the bathroom to purge the bladder of bacteria.
3. Urinating after sex, before falling asleep, may help in women who have a problems with post-intercourse infections.

Although these minor behavioral interventions may be helpful, they should not be taken to an extreme. Too much water consumption will result in frequency of urination that may drive you crazy. Jumping out of bed to empty your bladder after intercourse may spoil a very intimate moment. You will need to take a short course of antibiotics no matter what you do, so don't let these suggestions spoil your quality of life.

Treatment of Recurrent Uncomplicated Urinary Tract Infections

There are three ways of approaching the treatment of recurrent infections in healthy women of any age:

- Self-medication
- Prophylaxis
- Postcoital pill

Self-Medication

In those of you with a first-time infection or the first infection within the last six months, a urinalysis, and culture and sensitivity study are done, and you are started on a course of antibiotics. Ideally, your doctor can provide you with a prescription of antibiotics that you should fill and keep available for later use if your symptoms return. **Three days of full-dose treatment** is all that is necessary in a healthy woman with no medical problems, no fever with the infection, and no history of childhood infections. Seven days of treatment is routinely prescribed, but the added four days of treatment does not clear the urinary tract more thoroughly of bacteria. The extra four days *will* increase the cost of treatment and the risk of developing side effects from the antibiotics. Usually, the symptoms begin to abate one day into treatment, which is also when 90% of the bacteria have been destroyed. No post-treatment cultures need to be obtained.

In those of you with recurrent infections, each infection that causes symptoms, including burning with urination, frequent urges to urinate, and pelvic pain, should be treated with a three-day course of full-dose antibiotics, just like in women with a first-time infection. However, unlike women with their first infections, patients with recurrent infections must obtain post-treatment cultures, at least after the first few infections, to be sure that the bacteria are cleared with the antibiotic. Ten percent of women with recurrent problems have *unresolved or persistent infections*, where the bacteria never get cleared from the bladder. Persistently positive urine cultures occur because the wrong antibiotic is being used or you are taking the medication incorrectly (unresolved infection), or you have an anatomical defect (bacterial persistence), which needs to be treated surgically. Ninety percent of recurrent problems in which the urine culture remains positive are due to unresolved infection.

Even though it would seem that women with recurrent infections would have more difficult infections to treat, in reality, each infection is easy to treat. The problem is keeping the bacteria from returning to the bladder. In women with recurrent infections, immediate post-treatment swabs of the vagina and perineum are free of offending bacteria, indicating that the antibiotics clear the bladder and the vagina of organisms. However, within a few days after completion of the antibiotics, the bacteria have returned. If you are one of these women, preventive measures can be taken *between* infections to keep the vagina and the bladder as free of bacteria as possible.

Prophylaxis

Prophylactic treatment begins by first treating the current, active infection with three days of full-dose antibiotics. Once the urine culture is clear of bacteria, you start a long-term program of taking a quarter of the therapeutic dose every night at bedtime for the next three to six months, depending on what you and your physician decide. After the three or six months, the antibiotic is stopped. The idea is to allow your body to heal from the relentless series of infections. Even when it is discontinued, prophylaxis will reduce the risk of recurrent infections by 90% in most women.

Each low-dose antibiotic tablet should be taken at night because that will allow the drug to dwell in a full bladder for the longest period of time. During the day, we tend to urinate more frequently, which will eliminate the antibiotic. The key to choosing the best prophylactic medication is finding an antibiotic that will not impact on the normal intestinal and vaginal bacteria that serve to protect the body from invading organisms. Many of these antibiotics are available and will be described in the next section. Prophylactic treatment will not become less effective over time, nor will it select out for resistant bacteria to grow. Even in women who have been on prophylaxis for five years, resistant infections do not become a problem. Extensive research has been done by microbiologists, as well as drug companies, on this issue. The only disadvantages of prophylaxis are inconvenience and the cost of medication.

Postcoital Pill

Postcoital therapy involves taking a single pill immediately after intercourse (coitus, in Latin). This strategy is used in women who can identify sexual relations as the cause of their problem. The frequency of intercourse has no bearing on the therapy. If you are having relations once a week, five times per week, or once a year, if you feel that intercourse leads to infections, you can take a pill after sex.

Non-Antibiotic Interventions

Other agents besides antibiotics are available for prevention. The efficacy of these interventions does not approach that of antibiotics, but many women do not like the idea of taking antibiotics as frequently as may be necessary with treatments that were just discussed. The two most commonly used agents are methenamine mandelate (Mendelamine®) and hippurate. They alter the urinary environment in such a way that the bacteria do not want to grow in the bladder. Each of these medications comes in pill form and needs to be taken two to three times a day. They will not cure a full-blown infection, and their ability to ward off infection is questionable. At worst, they are harmless.

Estrogen may have a preventive impact on UTIs. Postmenopausal women who suffer from recurrent infections can decrease the pH of the vagina by applying $\frac{1}{2}$ applicator of vaginal estrogen cream, such as Premarin, Dienestrol, or Estrase, one to three times per week. Women with a history of heart disease or breast cancer must consult a physician before using estrogen creams. They are not supposed to get absorbed into the circulation, but some physicians feel that they can negatively affect an existing problem. Once the pH of the vaginal secretions is reduced to 4.0, the number of bad bacteria in the vagina will be significantly reduced.

Cranberry juice is commonly used to prevent infections. Studies have been done that both support and negate the effect of cranberry juice on UTIs. Theoretically, cranberries have an enzyme that prevents the attachment of the pili on the E. coli bacteria to the bladder wall. Many women drink cranberry juice because they think it acidifies the urine, which it may also do, but that is not its main mechanism of action in preventing infections. Blueberries do the same thing as cranberries.

Treatment of UTIs

Type of infection	Treatment	Antibiotic
First infection resolves simple	3 days of antibiotics	1. TMP-SMX 2. Nitrofurantoin 3. Fluoroquinolone
First infection resolves but returns RECURRENT: reinfection	3 days of antibiotics followed by: 1. prophylaxis 2. post-intercourse pill 3. self-start	1. TMP-SMX 2. Nitrofurantoin
First infection does not go away RECURRENT: unresolved	Reculture and change antibiotic	Fluoroquinolone
Kidney infection pyelonephritis	10–14 days of oral antibiotics	1. TMP-SMX 2. Fluoroquinolone

The problem with cranberry juice is that it is all sugar, even the unsweetened variety. All juice is fructose, which is a form of sugar. Acting as a diuretic, sugar pulls fluid out of your system and dehydrates you. If you want to flush the system, water would be a better choice. No studies have looked at the effectiveness of cranberry pills. The manufacturing of supplements is not regulated, so you don't know what you are purchasing. Although not dangerous, I question their usefulness.

Kidney Infections

Infections that ascend the urinary tract and settle into the kidney are much more painful and require more aggressive treatment. Instead of three days of antibiotics, women with kidney infections need 10 days to two weeks of therapy. Fevers accompany kidney infections, so absence of a fever for 24 hours signals that the infection is being effectively treated. Pretreatment and post-treatment cultures should be obtained. Although these infections are debilitating, they do not cause long-term injury to the kidneys or the bladder in women with normal urinary tracts who seek prompt treatment.

Vaccines Against Recurrent Infections

Studies are currently being done to look at the use of vaccines in the prevention of urinary tract infections. Vaccinations work by priming the immune system to fight a foreign invader, which is introduced in a tiny quantity through the vaccine. A number of different strategies are being investigated. One method is to inject pili from the *E. coli* bacteria into the woman whose immune system will make antibodies to them. The pili act as adhering agents, thus allowing the bacteria to climb into the bladder. Without the pili, the bacteria won't be able to travel into the urinary tract. Another method is to inject a larger number of lactobacilli, the good bacteria normally found in the vagina.

The problems with the concept of a vaccine for UTI prevention are 1) too many bacterial strains and different bacterial species cause infection to include in any single vaccine and 2) many of the bacteria strains that cause infection are normally found in the body, they just happen to be in the wrong place at the wrong time. The entire body does not need to get rid of them, just the bladder. No vaccination is on the horizon.

Antibiotics

Since the discovery of penicillin over 50 years ago, antibiotics have revolutionized modern medicine. Urinary tract infections used to be lethal diseases, causing kidney damage, septic shock, and often death. As with many innovations, antibiotics have their drawbacks as well as their benefits. The industry surrounding antibiotics has grown into a competitive, highly profitable business, resulting in a mind-boggling selection of medications from which to choose. Fifty percent of the cost of evaluating and treating urinary tract infections goes into paying for antibiotics alone. This section is dedicated to sorting out the multitudes of medications that have been touted as the best treatment for uncomplicated urinary tract infections.

First, the basic concepts behind choosing the best antibiotic will be discussed, followed by a review of the major classes of medication now available on the market. Finally, the serious complications that can result from antibiotic use, including the development of resistance, will be addressed.

Basic Concepts Behind Choosing an Antibiotic for Treatment

Characteristics of the best antibiotic to treat an uncomplicated urinary tract infection in a healthy woman include:

1. **Specificity:** The most specific antibiotic for the offending bacteria should be used.
2. **Low GI absorption:** The antibiotic should not be excessively absorbed by the gastrointestinal (GI) tract, thus winding up in high levels in the bloodstream. If high levels enter the bloodstream, the antibiotic will circulate into other tissues in the body and kill the good bacteria that protect other organs, like the mouth, the vagina, and the GI tract. Killing good bacteria will result in more side effects.
3. **High excretion into the urine:** Since the target bacteria are in the urine, the ideal antibiotic will concentrate in the urine without being changed into a different form by the liver or the kidneys.
4. **Selective killing pattern:** Antibiotics that kill all the bacteria in their tracks will also harm the good bacteria that colonize the vagina and the GI tract. We don't want this.
5. **Cost:** A good drug is not exorbitantly expensive so that those who need it can afford to buy it.

Antibiotics, like many prescription medications, have two names: a generic name and a trade name. The generic name refers to the scientific name. It cannot be owned or copyrighted. The trade name is the name that a company gives to the drug under which it is sold. The company owns the name and, possibly, the recipe for mixing the ingredients for the drug. For example, chocolate cake is a type of cake: the generic name. There is German chocolate cake and Flourless chocolate cake: these cakes can be the trade names or proprietary names. One generic drug may have many trade names because many different pharmaceutical companies make the same drug and each sells it under its own trade name.

Many classes of antibiotics have been discovered and developed. Most of the earlier antibiotics were discovered as natural products, but nearly all of them are now synthetically produced. It is cheaper and safer, with a lower incidence of allergic reactions, to manufacture antibiotics using genetic engineering. Antibiotic classes are divided by the way in which the antibiotic kills the bacteria. Some antibiotics destroy the bacterial cell wall, others insinuate themselves into the bacterial DNA so that the bacteria cannot reproduce. The method of killing is not important in choosing a drug, but it is important in determining which drugs will become resistant to bacterial killing. Traditionally, the first-line antibiotics for use in urinary tract infections were the sulfa-based drugs; second, was nitrofurantoin; and, third was the fluoroquinolones. The sulfa drugs have become resistant to over 30% of the most common organisms that cause uncomplicated UTIs, so many physicians do not use them as first-line treatment anymore. Penicillins are used less and less because of the large number of resistant strains of bacteria. Finally, the cephalosporins can be used, but they are mostly saved for serious infections requiring hospitalization.

Classes of Antibiotics
Sulfa-Based Drugs

Sulfa-Based Drugs

Trade Name	Generic Name	Frequency	Formulation
Gantanol®	Sulfamethoxazole	3 or 4 times per day	Tablets
Trimpex®	Trimethoprim	2 times per day	Tablets
Bactrim™	Trimethoprim and sulfamethoxazole	2 times per day	Tablets and suspension
Gantrisin®	Sulfamethoxazole	4 times per day	Suspension
Proloprim®	Trimethoprim	2 times per day	Tablets
Septra®	Trimethoprim and sulfamethoxazole	2 times per day	Tablets and suspension

Sulfa drugs were among the first successful treatments for urinary tract infections. Many women who are in their 70s and 80s today remember taking Gantrocin, which was an early, very effective way to get rid of bladder infections. Trimethoprim-sulfamethoxizole (TMP-SMX) is the sulfa pill that is available today. Sulfamethoxazole is a sulfa-based antibiotic which is mixed with trimethoprim, an agent that slows down the multiplication of the bacteria. It is highly effective against *E. coli*, which is the most common cause of urinary tract infections. TMP-SMX is excreted mostly in the urine, with very little absorption through the GI tract. It is also inexpensive.

On the down side, TMP-SMX will not kill *Enterococcus* or *Pseudomonas* species, two organisms that are seen more commonly in catheterized and elderly patients than healthy, sexually active women. It is also highly allergenic. Many patients develop allergies to the sulfa component of the antibiotic, especially after repeated use. Allergic reactions include nausea, vomiting, and skin rashes.

TMP-SMX is effective as both treatment for acute infections and prevention against future infections. Because allergies to the sulfamethoxazole component can develop, many practitioners will prescribe only the trimethoprim component of the combination for prevention. Although trimethoprim is not as effective as the combination for treatment, it may work in prevention.

Nitrofurantoins

Nitrofurantoin is the second choice, after TMP-SMX, for the treatment and prevention of UTIs in healthy young women only because of cost. It is slightly more expensive than the generic sulfa-based medications. Excreted unchanged in the urine, nitrofurantoin effectively sterilizes the urine within the first few doses. It is poorly absorbed by the GI tract, resulting in low levels in the bloodstream, thus low levels in the vaginal and rectal tissues. If these tissues are saturated with antibiotic, their good bacteria will be killed, causing yeast infections and diarrhea. The nitrofurantoins specifically kill *E. coli* and *Enterococcus* species, the most common causes of UTIs. Most impressively, bacteria have not become resistant to the drug over the 30 years that it has been in use. As a preventive medicine, nitrofurantoin is as highly effective. It is used for both post-coital therapy and prophylaxis.

Nitrofurantoin

Trade Name	Generic Name	Frequency	Formulation
Furoxone®	Nitrofurantoin	4 times per day	Tablets or suspension
Macrobid®	Nitrofurantoin	2 times per day	Tablets
Macrodantin®	Nitrofurantoin	4 times per day	Capsules or suspension

Side effects do occur, especially in the generic formulation. The most common problem is nausea, vomiting, and an upset stomach. The more expensive trade formulations cause fewer problems.

Fluoroquinolones

The fluoroquinolones revolutionized the antibiotic industry when they were introduced. They were touted as a wonder treatment for serious, complicated infections with the oral formulation working as effectively as the intravenous treatment. They are concentrated in the urine, so infections are treated rapidly and effectively. They selectively kill the bad bacteria and spare the good. At that time, little resistance had developed to the fluoroquinolones. The market for this class of antibiotics exploded. Practitioners began prescribing these wonder drugs routinely, not saving them for treating the complicated infections for which they were so useful. Recently, many important strains of bacteria that cause urinary tract infections have become resistant to the fluoroquinolones. The high resistance is thought to be due to overuse. This development is problematic because many of these resistant strains can now only be treated with intravenous antibiotics, requiring hospitalizations for infections that used to be treated at home.

Fluoroquinolones

Trade Name	Generic Name	Frequency	Formulation
Maxaquin®	Lomefloxin	1 time per day	Tablets
Floxin®	Ofloxacin	2 times per day	Tablets
Cipro®	Ciprofloxacin	2 times per day	Tablets or intravenous
Levoquin™	Levofloxacin	1 time per day	Tablets
Neogram®	Nalidixic acid	4 times per day	Suspension or capsules
Noroxin®	Norfloxacin	2 times per day	Tablets
Penetrex®	Enoxacin	2 times per day	Tablets

The fluoroquinolones are an excellent class of antibiotic, but as effective as they are in treating complicated infections, they are like using a sledgehammer to kill an ant for uncomplicated infections. The fluoroquinolones have many side effects that occur in a large number of patients who take the medication. The side effects are not rare. **If an infection is resistant to sulfa or nitrofurantoin, then you should take a fluorquinolone.** The benefits outweigh the risks. If a milder medication will offer the same cure with fewer side effects, you should be spared the potential side-effects and expense of a fluoroquinolone.

Fluoroquinolones can cause nausea, vomiting, abdominal discomfort, headaches, restlessness, depression, hallucinations, and seizures. They also interact with other drugs, specifically Tagamet® (cimetidine), so the practitioner must know what medications you are taking. Many flouroquinolones cannot be taken with antacid liquids like Maalox® and Mylanta® because the antibiotic will not be absorbed. Two hours must transpire between the time the antibiotic is taken and the antacid is consumed.

Fluoroquinolones should not be used in children if another antibiotic will work equally as effectively because they will interfere with cartilage formation. Finally, the fluoroquinolones are very expensive.

I must stress that in the correct setting, the fluoroquinolones are an excellent choice of antibiotic. However, for the treatment of acute cystitis or the prevention of recurrent infections in healthy women, either a sulfa-based drug or nitrofurantoin should be used if possible. The fluoroquinolones can be reserved for more difficult treatment problems.

Penecillins

Penecillins

Trade Name	Generic Name	Frequency	Formulation
Amoxil®	Amoxicillin	3 times per day	Tablets or suspension
Augmentin®	Amoxicillin and clavulanate	2 or 3 times per day	Tablets or suspension
Geocillin®	Carbenicillin	4 times per day	Tablets
Lorabid®	Laracef	2 times per day	Tablets or suspension
Omnipen®	Ampicillin	4 times per day	Capsules

Penecillin is the prototype antibiotic. For many years it was an effective agent for the treatment of simple urinary tract infection. However, for multiple reasons, it is no longer useful. Over 30% of bacteria that cause simple infections are resistant to penicillin and its derivatives. Approximately 70 to 80% of the drug will enter the GI tract, which will potentially alter the fecal bacteria, causing diarrhea. The natural vaginal flora is also disrupted, resulting in over 25% of patients contracting a yeast infection while taking penicillin. In addition, from 3 to 10% of the population is allergic to penicillin. The allergies range from mild skin reactions to serious life-threatening throat constriction, called anaphylaxis. Since newer medications are available that do not have these problems, the penicillins are generally not used as first-line treatment for UTIs. If you are taking penicillin for a skin or a sinus infection and also have a urinary tract infection, penicillin is usually an acceptable treatment. However, for treatment specifically of urinary tract problems, penicillin is not adequate therapy.

Mild penicillin allergies involve development of itching, skin rashes, and fevers. Usually, the allergy will not appear upon first taking the drug. The second course of antibiotics will trigger the allergic reaction. Less than one-tenth of one percent of patients who take penicillin will experience anaphylactic shock, where your throat tightens up and you can't breathe. Less than 10% of these people will die as a result of a penicillin allergy. Anaphylaxis begins with a sudden onset of itching, redness, and swelling of the skin all over the body. It progresses to difficulty breathing, a drop in the blood pressure, and eventually shock, and death. Although the risk of anaphylaxis is small, and death, even smaller, it seems unnecessary to take even this tiny risk when numerous other medications are available that do a better job without these problems. The reason penicillin is mentioned in this section is that it is still widely used for other infections, especially in the mouth and on the skin, and you need to know its limitations in the urinary tract.

The problem with resistance to penicillin has been addressed by combining different agents with penicillin. Aumentin® is a combination penicillin that is very effective for urinary tract infections, but should be reserved for complicated problems, and not be used in routine, simple infections. The side effects of penicillin are still present in the combination agents. The most effective agent against urinary tract infections that is available on the market is Imipenem-cilistatin®, a combination intravenous penicillin that will kill almost any bacteria. This agent is only used in severely ill, hospitalized people in whom no other intravenous or oral medication works.

Efforts are being made in many hospitals to limit the use of Imipenem because once bacteria become resistant to this medication, they are unstoppable.

Cephalosporins

Cephalosporins			
Trade Name	Generic Name	Frequency	Formulation
Ceclor®	Cefaclor	3 or 4 times per day	Tablets, capsules, suspension
Ceftin®	Cefuroxime	2 times per day	Tablets, intravenous, suspension
Keflex® Keftab®	Cephalexin	3 or 4 times per day	Tablet or suspension
Duracef®	Cefadroxil	1 or 2 times per day	Tablet or suspension
Vantin®	Cefpodroxil	2 times per day	Tablet or suspension
Fortaz® Tazidime®	Ceftazidime	2 or 3 times per day	Intramuscular or intravenous
Cefizox®	Cefizoxime	1 or 2 times per day	Intramuscular or intravenous
Rocephin®	Ceftriaxone	1 or 2 times per day	Intramuscular or intravenous
Claforan®	Cefotaxime	3 times per day	Intramuscular or intravenous
Cefobid®	Cefoperazone		Intravenous
Maxipine®	Cefipime		Intravenous
Cefotan®	Cefotetan		Intravenous
	Cefixime	1 or 2 times per day	Tablet or suspension
	Cefalothin	4 times per day	Intravenous
	Cefazolin	3 times per day	Intramuscular or intravenous

Cephalosporins are an expensive, broad-spectrum antibiotic distantly related to the penicillin family. "Broad-spectrum" means that it targets many different types of bacteria. In women with infections caused by multiple bacteria, having a broad spectrum is desirable. However, most women with simple and uncomplicated recurrent urinary tract infections have only a single offending organism. Postmenopausal women who are not on estrogen replacement therapy are more likely to have many offending bacteria in the urine.

Four different "generations" of cephalosporins have been developed. The generations refer to the spectrum of activity and when the formulation was developed. The higher the generation, the newer the drug, the broader the spectrum, and the stronger the medication. It will also be more expensive. The most virulent infections are treated with a third or fourth generation cephalosporin.

Derived from penicillin, cephalosporins have similar but less serious toxicities than the penicillins. Most commonly, they cause skin irritation, rashes, and itching, as well as vaginal yeast infections. About 10% of people who are allergic to penicillin will also be allergic to the cephalosporins. Very rarely, cephalosporins will cause problems with bleeding. This usually only happens with the intravenous formulations and after the second week of use.

The cephalosporins are still commonly used, especially the first-generation oral agents. Although they do kill many types of offending bacteria, they target the most common, including staphylococcus and *E. coli*. They are very good agents for both the treatment and the prevention of urinary tract infections in healthy, sexually active women. They would be higher on the list if they weren't so expensive.

Tetracyclines

The tetracycline class of antibiotics is not commonly used for urinary tract infections because of the high incidence of resistance of bacteria to the effects. They will be mentioned here because sometimes tetracycline is prescribed in women who have severe allergies to other antibiotics. These antibiotics cannot be used in children or pregnant women.

Tetracyclines

Trade Name	Generic Name	Frequency	Formulation
Minocin®	Tetracycline	1 time per day	Capsule
Vibramycin®	Doxycyeline	2 times per day	Tablets, capsules, and suspension
Zithromax®	Azythromycin	1 time per day	Tablets, capsules, and suspension

Common Side Effects of Antibiotics

Side Effects of Antibiotics

Antibiotic	Minor Side Effects	Major Side Effects
TMP-SMX	Mild skin rash (hives)	Severe skin rash
Nitrofurantoin	Nausea and vomiting	Numbness in fingers and toes
		Lung infection
Fluoroquinolones	Nausea and vomiting	Seizures
	Diarrhea	Joint degeneration
	Abdominal pain	Hallucinations
	Skin rash	
Cephalosporins	Mild skin rash (hives)	Liver disease
Penicillins	Mild skin rash (hives)	Severe skin rash
	Vaginal yeast infection	Throat constriction
		Severe diarrhea
Tetracyclines	Nausea and vomiting	Liver disease
	Skin rash (hives)	Kidney disease
	Vaginal yeast infection	

Resistance

Resistance of bacteria to an antibiotic can be **within an individual person or within a population of people**. For example, you may have an infection in which the urine culture and sensitivity test reports sensitivity of the bacteria to a certain antibiotic. After taking the medication for a few days, you do not get better and a second culture reports that the bacteria are no longer sensitive to that drug. You are now, *temporarily*, resistant to that antibiotic. The next infection may very well be sensitive to that antibiotic. In population-based resistance, a bacteria that has developed resistance to an antibiotic has now infected a population, usually within a hospital or a nursing home. In population-based resistance, entire classes or antibiotics become useless.

Resistance develops in three ways:

1. **Natural resistance:** An organism was never sensitive to the antibiotic.
2. **Mutation of bacteria:** A bacteria changes so that the antibiotic becomes ineffective.

3. **Plasmid-mediated resistance:** The bacteria acquires a weapon (the plasmid) against the antibiotic.

An example of natural resistance is nitrofurantoin and its inability to destroy the bacteria *Proteus* (an organism found, often, in people with kidney stones). The antibiotic never had the ability to destroy the organism, so the use of nitrofurantoin in women with *Proteus* UTIs is fruitless. These bacteria would be able to grow and multiply without recourse if there were no other antibiotics available to combat the organism. Eventually, the bacteria would spread throughout the population with abandon. However, other antibiotics are available to kill *Proteus*, so it is not a problem.

Selection of mutated species is a much bigger problem. In this case, the antibiotic kills all of the bacteria that it can, and leaves behind the few organisms that are able to resist the demise. These few organisms then reproduce, populating the bladder with bacteria that are resistant to the antibiotic. The resistant strain began as a small colony of organisms and grew into a giant population that is not able to be killed by the antibiotic. Some strains of *E. coli* are becoming resistant to the fluoroquinolones, the class of antibiotics reserved for the most serious outpatient infections. Selection of mutated species can occur in individual patients, where it can be treated by changing the antibiotic; or in communities, where it may not be treated. There are strains of bacteria that are emerging that are resistant to nearly every antibiotic available.

Before the discovery of the fluoroquinolones, plasmid-mediated immunity used to be a terrible problem, especially within the penicillin family. In plasmid-mediated immunity, the bacteria acquire a piece of DNA that gives it instructions (the plasmid) on how to block the antibiotic attack. Recently, scientists have discovered a way to block the transfer of the plasmid information between bacteria. The combination penecillins, like Imipenem, and Augmentin were developed to retain the benefits of penicillin with the addition of the ability to block plasmid activity.

Although resistance is a serious community concern, if you have an infection requiring strong antibiotics, development of resistance should not determine the antibiotic that you are given. The main goal of treatment is cure. The most effective antibiotic for each situation should be used. However, overtreatment will not help you either. If too strong an antibiotic is prescribed, neither you nor the community will benefit. Finally, prophylaxis (see above) will not lead to the development of resistant strains. The low dose of the medication (only $\frac{1}{4}$ of the treatment dose is used) and the choice of the medication prevents the selection of resistant organism.

The nitrofurantoins and sulfa-based drugs are an excellent choice for prophylaxis because they cannot induce plasmid-mediated resistance or the selection of mutated strains.

Diarrhea

Antibiotic-induced diarrhea can be a mild self-limited problem, or it can be a life-threatening catastrophe. Most antibiotics cause some GI upset through the effect of killing the good bacteria in the intestine that help absorb water and food across the wall of the gut. Once the antibiotic is stopped, the good bacteria repopulate the intestine within a day or two, absorption of water improves, and the diarrhea stops. Occasionally, a more serious form of diarrhea can occur, resulting in serious fluid losses, dehydration, and in severe, untreated circumstances, death. This is called **Clostridium difficile (C. diff.) colitis.**

    C. diff. colitis can be caused by any antibiotic, topical, oral, or intravenous. Most patients who contract the problem are on intravenous antibiotics in the hospital, but that does not have to be the case. *C. difficile* is an organism that normally inhabits the GI tract in 5% of healthy people and 20% of hospitalized patients. It is easily transmitted from patient to patient in the hospital, which leads to outbreaks of C. diff. diarrhea on hospital wards. The antibiotics kill the normal bacteria that usually keep the *C. difficile* in check. The result is that the *C. difficile* grows uncontrollably, releasing its toxin, which causes the copious diarrhea. The diarrhea is watery, green in color, and foul smelling, usually accompanied by abdominal cramps. The diagnosis is made through a stool culture. Usually, merely stopping the antibiotic and getting hydrated with intravenous fluids will cure the problem. More serious cases need the institution of vancomycin, an intravenous antibiotic that, if given orally, will kill the *C. difficile* organisms. Although C. diff. colitis is rare, it *does* occur and must be recognized if you are on antibiotics and have debilitating diarrhea.

Yeast Infections

Women who take antibiotics on a regular basis are well aware of the risk of getting yeast infections. Yeast infections occur because, again, the antibiotic upsets the balance of flora within an area of the body. In the vagina, bacteria and yeast coexist happily, maintaining vaginal secretions and the proper acidity. When antibiotics kill some of the bacteria, the balance is upset and the yeast multiply out of control. The result is a thick, white discharge which produces a terrible itch and a beefy red discoloration of the vaginal opening. Treatment is either vaginal creams, which can be purchased over-the-counter, or Diflucan (fluconazole is the generic name) in tablet form. Only one tablet is taken, which works over a five-day period.

Prevention of yeast infections is the same as the prevention of the other side effects of antibiotics: short courses of low-dose pills. An uncomplicated urinary tract infection does not need more than three-days of treatment in most cases. Longer courses of antibiotics will not do a better job of getting rid of the infection, and may lead to yeast infections. Generally, a three-day course of any antibiotic will not cause a yeast infection. If it does, it will be a mild problem which usually does not need treatment. Leaving everything alone for a few days will allow the vagina to re-colonized with good bacteria and the yeast will come under control.

Eating yogurt will not help in preventing a yeast infection because the acidophilus in the yogurt will not make it that far. It will get taken up by the intestines before it reaches the vagina. The same is true for acidophilus that comes from the health food store. Putting plain yogurt in the vagina is the only way to provide the area with good bacteria while the antibiotic is doing its job. It may be less messy to just limit the use of antibiotics and take Diflucan if necessary.

Kidney Infections

Kidney infections (pyelonephritis) cause chills, fever (temperature over 101.5°F) and flank pain (back pain). Many women will have burning with urination, frequency, and pelvic pain as well, but not all do. Sometimes, the only symptoms will be a fever and back pain. Although as many as 20% of women with pyelonephritis will have less than 100,000 CFU of bacteria per ml, positive urine cultures usually clinch the diagnosis. The most common offending organism is E. coli, the causative agent in simple urinary tract infections. These infections occur if bacteria travel up the ureters from the bladder into the kidneys. In acute cystitis, the tissues around the ureteric orifices swell, allowing the bacteria to gain access into the upper tracts.

In healthy, nonpregnant women, TMP-SMX for 14 days will usually eradicate the infection. Nowadays because of resistance issues, most physicians will use a fluoroquinolone to treat kidney infections. Generally, you can be treated at home with oral medication. Hospitalization is indicated if you cannot eat or drink, have severe pain requiring intravenous pain medication, cannot be effectively treated by oral medication, or have vesicoureteral reflux, a kidney stone, or diabetes mellitus.

If your fever does not come back to normal within three days of being on antibiotics, further testing must be done to look for problems that are not being treated by the antibiotics. The most conclusive radiographic test

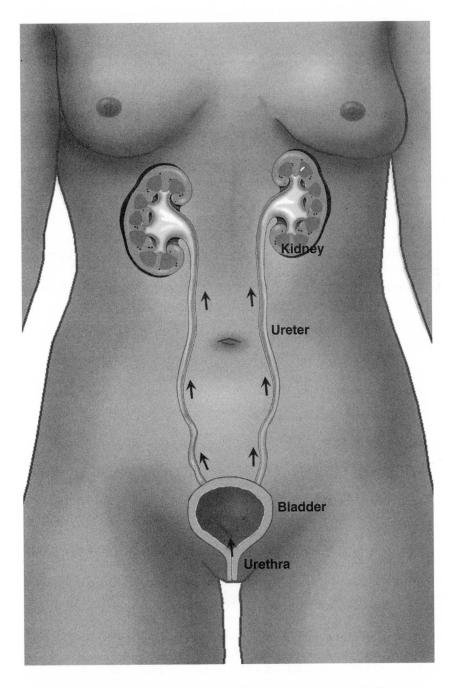

FIGURE 7. *How infections reach the kidneys from the bladder.*

is a CT scan, which can look for a collection of pus around the kidney, called an abscess. If an abscess is present, you will be sent to the hospital for further intervention.

Approximately 10 to 30% of patients with kidney infections will relapse following a two-week course of treatment. If you develop a recurrent problem, six weeks of oral antibiotics should be prescribed to be sure that all of the offending organisms are eliminated. Follow-up cultures must be done to confirm resolution.

Urinary Tract Infections in the Pregnant Woman

Pregnant women need to be screened for bacteria in their urine at the first prenatal visit. If bacteria are identified, treatment must ensue *whether symptoms are present or not*. Untreated infections during pregnancy increase the risk of complications for both the mother and the fetus. Penicillins, cephalosporins, and nitrofurantoin are the safest drugs to be used during pregnancy. **Fluoroquinolones, tetracyclines, and sulfa drugs are to be avoided.** Not necessarily more common during pregnancy, bacteria in the urine is more dangerous at that time, and therefore, should be treated.

If a kidney infection develops, intravenous antibiotics will need to be administered. The oral medications that are safe to take during pregnancy are not strong enough to combat a kidney infection. Once the fever goes down, oral antibiotics can be prescribed for 14 additional days of treatment. You may then be placed on preventive treatment for the remainder of the pregnancy, depending on what your obstetrician thinks is safest. Low-birth-weight infants and the induction of preterm labor result from kidney infections.

Urinary Tract Infections in the Elderly Woman

Infections in the elderly woman are more complex to *diagnose*, but not to treat. Bacteria in the urine (bacteriuria) occurs more frequently in the elderly, whose infections usually result from multiple species of organisms. Decreased immune status, poor bladder function resulting in incomplete emptying and stagnant urine, urinary and fecal incontinence, and pelvic-floor prolapse all contribute to the increased infection rate in this population.

Frequently, elderly women have vague symptoms. Unlike young women who may complain of burning with urination and frequent urination, older women may have no symptoms related to their bladders. They may display confusion and disorientation, poor appetite, apathy and malaise, urinary incontinence, and nausea and vomiting. When these signs are overlooked, the diagnosis is delayed. Thus, many elderly women become very sick before a urinary tract infection is recognized. Once the condition is suspected, the same diagnostic evaluation and treatment regimen is implemented. Unlike in pregnant women, the elderly with bacteria in their urine but no symptoms of an infection should not be treated.

Catheter-Associated Infections

All people with catheters in their bladders will become colonized with bacteria in the urine within one week because:

1. Bacteria can be introduced when the catheter is placed in the bladder.
2. Organisms can gain entry into the bladder through the urethra, stick to the catheter, and multiply.
3. Bacteria can crawl along the catheter itself. The coating of bacteria over the catheter is called biofilm.

Cleanliness and hygiene play little role in preventing colonization of bacteria. Usually, no symptoms occur and you should not be treated.

If you spike a fever or develop pain and irritation secondary to the catheter, antibiotics should be given and the catheter changed. If infections causing symptoms occur repeatedly, the catheter should be removed and another method of bladder drainage can be considered, such an intermittent catheterization or surgery to allow the urine to drain into a bag attached to the skin. Intermittent catheterization is when a catheter is inserted into the bladder through the urethra when the bladder is full. The catheter is removed after the bladder is drained, and is reinserted three or four hours later when the bladder refills. Although neither solution is ideal, these are sometimes the only options available to those of you who require constant catheterization.

Nonbacterial Cystitis

Sometimes, women who have had urinary tract infections in the past develop burning, frequency, and pelvic pain without having bacteria in their bladders. Non-bacterial cystitis is a syndrome that consists of the signs and symptoms of an infection, but no bacteria are identified in the urine. On physical examination, the urethra is exquisitely tender to touch. The urinalysis will often be completely negative, or it may show a few white blood cells in the urine, indicating the presence of inflammation. Although it may last for months, this painful and frustrating condition will usually resolve spontaneously. Aggravating the condition, however, practitioners often erroneously prescribe antibiotics for lack of a better treatment. Behavioral modification, including diet control, can often help reduce the symptoms. Sometimes urethral dilatations are done to try to relieve the pressure and pelvic pain. This maneuver is usually painful and fruitless. For more information on this problem, see Chapter 9.

SUMMARY

Urinary tract infections are by no means a problem exclusive to healthy, sexually active women. Children and men certainly suffer the wrath of bacterial invasion into the normally sterile urine. However, women have a propensity to develop infections in the urine more so than men because of their unique anatomy. Those of you who are plagued with infections know how frustrating and painful they can be, especially when treatment is delayed because antibiotics are not accessible. Although the cause of recurrent infections is not understood, management is possible. Self-medication, postcoital therapy and prophylaxis can be effective as both prevention and treatment of this problem. It is important to know when to seek professional help because a more serious problem exists. Urinary tract infections should not control or ruin a productive life. Over time, our understanding of the causes of UTIs will evolve. Once we know why they occur, prevention and cure will be imminent.

CHAPTER 9

Interstitial Cystitis and Pelvic Pain Syndromes

N. recently started dating J., whom she met through some friends. He's attractive, smart, fun, and has a good job. Of course, money isn't that important, but stability and ambition are certainly attractive in a man. It has been nearly eight months since N. has dated anyone seriously. Dating and intimacy are difficult under any circumstance, but for N., sex takes on a new level of anxiety with which most women don't have to deal.

In her 20s, N. had a problem with urinary tract infections. Every month or two, she had burning, frequency of urination, and urgency. When she got to the bathroom, nothing came out. She was on the phone with the doctor's office so frequently that she had him on speed dial. She took antibiotics for nearly 10 days every month over about a three-month period.

Finally, her gynecologist sent her to a urologist, who did a whole battery of tests on her, many of which were not pleasant. He put tubes in her urethra to collect urine and a scope with a light on it to look at the bladder wall. Everything looked good except that N.'s urethra was too narrow. He suggested that she have her urethra dilated in an effort to reduce the number of bladder infections.

Except for a little lidocaine that he squirted into her urethra immediately before the procedure, no anesthesia was used. He used metal rods in a sequential manner to widen the opening through which N. urinates. Although he was as gentle as he could be under the circumstances, the procedure hurt so much that N. felt like she was being split into two. When she got up from the table to get dressed, she had tears from the pain and the burning. A little blood dripped into the toilet when she urinated before leaving the doctor's office. He gave her some antibiotic tablets to take over the next few days and a prescription for painkillers to help her get through the night.

At the doctor's suggestion, she went in for dilations about three more times over the next 18 months just to keep everything open. Surprisingly, her infections stopped completely during the next three years. As unpleasant as the dilations were, they seemed to helped with her problem. She continued to go to the bathroom frequently, awaking up about twice a night to empty her bladder. Because of the history of infections, she drank about three large bottles of water every day to keep her bladder clean. These minor inconveniences were nothing compared with what she was used to with the infections. At least the burning and pain were gone.

During her later 20s, Nicole developed some pain and bloating in her abdomen and pelvis. She felt gassy and had trouble making bowel movements. Some days she would go four times and other days she wouldn't be able to go at all. Now that the bladder problem was solved, another problem had to crop up. Stress probably accounted for most of her symptoms. With her new job, she was working harder and traveling more. Her diet was inconsistent, and really not as healthful as it should be. Her periods had become irregular at the same time, so maybe there was a correlation.

Nicole reported all of her symptoms to her gynecologist, who prescribed birth control pills to regulate her period. She recommended a gastroenterologist (a GI doctor) for the bloating and bowel problems. A routine urine sample revealed a few bacteria in her bladder, so, of course, she went on a 10-day course of antibiotics. Now her bowels really went haywire, and she developed a raging yeast infection. She got a prescription for the treatment of her yeast infection as well.

The GI doctor examined her and her stool sample. Based on her symptoms, he diagnosed N. with irritable bowel syndrome, a common disorder that ranges from mild abdominal discomfort and bloating to serious constipation and diarrhea requiring potent medication. N.'s condition was pretty mild. Some dietary and lifestyle changes would help alleviate the majority of her complaints. She needed to cut out dairy products and wheat products. Lactose intolerance and difficulty digesting wheat and yeast were at the root of her problem. The doctor explained that she is basically allergic to these two food groups. Fruits, vegetables, non-wheat grains, and fish should be the mainstay of her diet. Daily exercise and lots of water would round out her program. On days in which the constipation is bad, a laxative can be used, but only under dire circumstances. Well, she will at least be healthy, and maybe even lose a few pounds in the process!

With her new program underway, N. finished the antibiotics that the gynecologist gave her, treated her yeast infection, and felt well for about a month. On the lactose- and wheat-free diet, Nicole felt better in the bowel department, but her bladder was acting up again. She had burning, frequency, pain, and urgency all of the time. The urine tests at the gynecologist's office were negative. *The doctor recommended another course of antibiotics even with a negative culture, which N. took religiously. She finished a two-week prescription this time around, but her symptoms never changed. If anything, the pelvic pain got worse and the frequency got a little better. At least she only got up twice a night instead of the six times she was getting up when her symptoms were bad.*

The doctor performed a transvaginal ultrasound in her office which showed an ovarian cyst on the right side, which was sort of where the pain was. Since the pains got worse just before N.'s period, the doctor thought maybe her problem was the cyst or possibly endometriosis. The best way to evaluate the situation was through a laparoscopy. The doctor explained that laparoscopy is a surgical procedure in which scopes are inserted into the pelvis through tiny holes in the abdomen. Requiring general anesthesia, it takes about an hour and N. can go home the same day or stay overnight, depending on how she feels.

The laparoscopy went well. The cyst was removed, and it turned out to be benign. Some abnormal areas that looked like endometriosis were removed, but otherwise, according to the doctor, N.'s pelvis looked very healthy. Because the pelvic pain remained in spite of the interventions, N. tried a few other brands of birth control pills to try to control this cyclic problem. Neither she nor her doctor was totally convinced that this was endometriosis, but, what else could be wrong?

Over the next few months, the pain continued to escalate. She maintained strict dietary and exercise regimens to keep the irritable bowel syndrome under control. She drank copious amounts of water, and kept her genital area meticulously clean, to hold the infections at bay. No matter what she did, the pain remained. She urinated every hour to keep her bladder empty, and even woke up at night a few times to be sure that no urine was sitting there waiting to get infected. Her bowels and bladder began to rule her life. The pain ruled her life. This was getting ridiculous!

N. decided to take matters into her own hands. Through the internet, she learned everything she could about endometriosis, irritable bowel syndrome, and urinary tract infections. Those were the three conditions for which she had a diagnosis. Often contradictory, the literature on all three topics was scant. What was available was frustrating and confusing. Finally, she came upon an interesting website that discussed "pelvic pain syndromes," including endometriosis and irritable bowel syndrome. The authors felt that the two conditions were related and really were part of a similar entity that included urinary, vaginal, and bowel problems. Called interstitial cystitis, *the urinary component manifested itself with urgency and frequency, but no burning. The frequency can occur up to every five minutes, and relieves some of the pelvic pain. Unbelievable! N. just diagnosed herself. Now, she just had to find a doctor who would get her some relief.*

N. discussed her research with both the gastroenterologist and the gynecologist. Neither one knew much about interstitial cystitis or pelvic pain syndromes. She was referred to me, since the condition relates to urination. Immediately, she felt comfortable because she saw women in the waiting room, which was not the case with the last urologist she went to. After listening to her history, I examined her thoroughly, including performing a gentle pelvic exam. Her urine test revealed a few bacteria and some blood. The ultrasound of her bladder showed that she was emptying well.

Based on her history, I suspected interstitial cystitis. There is no way to make a definitive diagnosis of this condition. The closest we can come is to perform a cystoscopy with hydrodistention under anesthesia. While she was asleep, N.'s bladder was filled with water to see how much it could hold and how the wall responded to the distention. The walls cracked and bled after being distended, confirming the diagnosis of interstitial cystitis. Sometimes the hydrodistention helps relieve the symptoms temporarily, as well.

The first thing we did was put her on an interstitial cystitis diet that eliminated citrus fruits, tomatoes, bananas, spicy foods, alcohol, and caffeine. I prescribed some medications to help with the urgency at night and the frequency during the day. We also started her on a new medication, called Elmiron® that was recently approved for the treatment of interstitial cystitis. Unfortunately, it would take about three months for this medication to help.

Just having a diagnosis and an understanding doctor to consult when flares occurred helped calm N. She felt much better already. The diet helped considerably, and the medications got her through four hours of sound sleep at night helping her cope better during the day. After a *few months, she felt that the Elmiron was beginning to repair her damaged bladder.*

J. had stuck with her through these tough few months. They even started to have sex on a semi-regular basis. Although she wouldn't call it pleasurable yet, she thought that she would eventually get to a point where she would enjoy it again. She missed so much work through this whole ordeal that she was laid off. She was looking for something a little less stressful to help her cope better with her condition. Now on a different path, the future seemed brighter, and maybe even pain-free.

Interstitial cystitis and pelvic pain syndromes have long been ignored by physicians. Patient demand for research and treatment has forced urologists, gynecologists, and gastroenterologists to focus on the diagnosis and treatment of these increasingly more-pervasive conditions. More common in women, all of these syndromes range from annoying to debilitating, disabling the victims and destroying their relationships. In a large number of cases, the diagnosis is not made for years. Women are sent for psychiatric evaluation because they are perceived as hysterical and unstable. Perhaps some of these women become hysterical and unstable from pain, lack of sleep, anger, frustration, and despondence at the lack of help from the medical community. Unrecognized, unvalidated, untreated illness can drive anyone to desperate ends.

PELVIC PAIN SYNDROMES

Interstitial cystitis (IC)
Irritable bowel syndrome (IBS)
Endometriosis

INTERSTITIAL CYSTITIS

Definition and Symptoms

Interstitial cystitis is a *syndrome*, a constellation of symptoms that make up the diagnosis. The main problem is pelvic pain, which is relieved with urination. The urge to empty the bladder in order to gain some relief from the pain becomes so overwhelming that a woman will be driven to urinate every 5 or 10 minutes both day and night. In 1987, a group of patients, physicians, and investigators was organized by the National Institutes of Diabetes and Digestive and Kidney Diseases (NIDDK), a research branch of the NIH, to establish the criteria needed to make a diagnosis of Interstitial Cystitis. The NIDDK criteria were not meant for diagnostic purposes, but because the disease description is so vague, they have become the standard inclusion criteria used to make a diagnosis. Meant for research purposes, they have become the definition of the disease for clinical purposes as well.

Most of the data used to establish the criteria came from 200 patients. Any variable in which 90% of the patients were positive or negative was included in the definition. Because of these strict inclusion criteria, more symptoms that exclude the diagnosis were identified than those that include it. In other words, it is easier to eliminate the diagnosis than it is to actually make a positive identification. Strict adherence to this definition of interstitial cystitis will exclude many women from obtaining a diagnosis, subjecting them to years of searching for a label for their problem. Most of us get tremendous relief from the recognition and acknowledgment of our problem. One of the most frustrating answers that people hear from a doctor is: I don't know what is wrong with you. Not that we necessarily want to have a chronic, debilitating illness, but we want to know that our problem is not in our heads.

SYMPTOMS THAT DEFINE DIAGNOSIS OF INTERSTITIAL CYSTITIS

Inclusion criteria
Ulcers in the bladder
Pain in pelvis and vagina
Findings on cystoscopy

Exclusion criteria
Less than 18 years old
Bladder tumors
History of radiation
History of tuberculosis
Active urinary tract infection
Active vaginal infection
History of chemotherapy
Urethral cyst or diverticulum
Gynecological cancer
Active herpes zoster
Bladder or urteral stones
Frequency less than 5x/day
Waking up less than 2x/night
Duration less than 12 months
Unstable bladder on urodynamics
Bladder can hold more than 12 oz.

Presentation of this disease comes in a spectrum. Some of you will have full-blown symptoms, while others will have a mild form. When you consult with a physician and tell your story, a certain gestalt about the description will ring a bell with the doctor. That is not the most confidence-inducing way to diagnose a major illness, but for now, that is the best we can offer most people. The truth is: just like Nicole, many of you will diagnose yourselves.

For a poorly defined syndrome, the symptoms of interstitial cystitis are surprisingly consistent from person to person. The symptoms come on so abruptly that many women can pinpoint the week that the symptoms began. Although many of you go even *more* often, you must report the urge to urinate at least eight times in a 12-hour period and at least three times per night for the diagnosis to be made. You are actually awakened from sleep with an overwhelming urge to urinate. No burning accompanies the frequent urination. Burning on urination is associated with other disorders, such as recurrent urinary tract infections, urethral syndrome, and urethral diverticula.

As bad as the frequent urination is, the overwhelming symptom is pain. Pain can be present above the pubic bone, in the vagina, between the vagina and the rectum (the perineum), in the lower back, and in the inside of the thigh. In the beginning, many women describe the pain as being relieved by urinating. It gets worse with bladder filling, compelling you to empty your bladder for relief. Although intertwined to some degree, the voiding problems and the pain are separate entities. If one is corrected, the other one will persist until it, too, can be treated. Many women report worsening of the symptoms the week before and during menstruation. Sexual relations exacerbate both the pain and the frequency, usually immediately after the encounter. The symptoms can persist for days before they begin to let up.

For women with full-blown interstitial cystitis, the quality of their lives is worse than the same age-group on hemodialysis, the regimen of thrice-weekly three-hour sessions hooked to a blood-cleansing machine needed by people with end-stage kidney disease. As those of you in this category know, you cannot sleep, work, have sex, or carry on normal lives. Most of you have had some history of urological problems in the past. Urinary tract infections and childhood bladder problems, such as bed wetting, are more common among interstitial cystitis sufferers. The average time of symptom onset to diagnosis is two to four years. During this time, over 50% of you will experience periods of remission for an average of eight months.

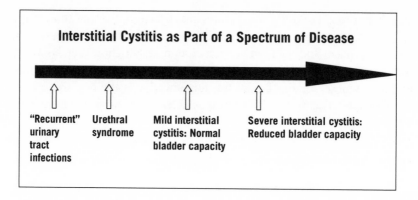

Practitioners who see a large number of women with intersitial cystitis feel that it is part of a spectrum of disease that begins with a diagnosis of recurrent urinary tract infections that are treated with antibtiotics. It starts with mild symptoms. Many people improve after a few years of mild symptoms, but a small number will get progressively worse.

Urethral Syndrome
Urethral syndrome is another catch-all term for a series of symptoms that include pain and discomfort in the pelvis behind the pubic bone, frequency of urination, incomplete emptying, and occasional burning after urination. Some women will describe difficulty initiating the flow, an intermittent stream during urination, and dribbling after they urinate. Urine cultures will be negative for infection and the physical examination is usually normal, with very little tenderness when the urethra and vagina are examined.

A typical story is what N. experienced: you begin with burning, frequency, and urgency of urination, which will be interpreted as a urinary tract infection, even if the urine culture is negative. Antibiotics will be prescribed and the symptoms will improve during the course of treatment. Most antibiotics have an antiinflammatory agent mixed into the tablet to help soothe the bladder during its recovery. The antiinflammatory component of the medication will alleviate the symptoms for a few days. Once the antibiotic is discontinued, the symptoms of burning, frequency, and urgency return.

The physician thinks that perhaps the infection was not completely treated, so another course of antibiotics is prescribed. Usually, the second course is given for a longer period of time to "be sure that the infection is totally gone." This cycle may go on for two, three, or fours courses of medication over a few months. The symptoms were present before the antibiotics were given, so the antibiotics did not cause the symptoms. The symptoms have persisted in spite of the multiple courses of antibiotics. (Lesson: if you are not prone to urinary tract infections, do not start antibiotics without seeing a doctor and providing a urine sample for culture.) Eventually, the idea of an infection is no longer entertained, so a diagnosis of *urethral syndrome* is given to the condition.

The urethral syndrome is caused by spasms of the muscles that line the pelvic floor. No bones support the bottom of the pelvis, only muscles do. These muscles are perforated by three structures, the anus, the vagina, and the urethra. If one of these muscles goes into spasm, similar to the way the back can go into spasm, symptoms will occur depending on which structure is being irritated by the muscle in spasm. If the muscles that surround the urethra spasm, then we call this the "urethral syndrome." Spasms around the vagina will cause painful intercourse. Spasms around the rectum and anus will cause defecation problems.

A short-lived problem, urethral syndrome lasts about six months on average. Many physicians will continue to prescribe antibiotics to try to alleviate the persistent symptoms. Of course, the antibiotics will do very little. Treatment of the urethral syndrome is mostly supportive: symptom relief until the spasm goes away on its own. Warm baths, antiinflammatory agents, such as ibuprofen, as well as bladder anesthetics, such as pyridium, will help. The mainstay of treatment is physical therapy of the pelvic floor. Innovative techniques have been developed by physical therapists to alleviate the spasm. Massage, stretching exercises, vaginal weights, electrical stimulation, and biofeedback are all used to help relieve the symptoms.

If the syndrome does not go away on its own or with physical therapy, it may progress to mild interstitial cystitis. The majority of you will have resolution of the symptoms permanently by six months. Rarely, the condition will progress. If it does, you may be suffering from interstitial cystitis at this point. Perhaps the entire pelvic floor is in spasm, which is why you have pain with intercourse and vaginal exams. Because this spectrum of presentations exists, some of you will be labeled as interstitial cystitis sufferers earlier than others. It may take you years to be given a diagnosis. Partly, this delay is due to ignorance on the part of physicians, but some of it is due to the fact that the symptoms change over time.

Epidemiology
First described in 1907, interstitial cystitis occurs more commonly in women than in men at a rate of nine women for every man. Approximately 90,000 cases have been identified since the NIH criteria for this symptom

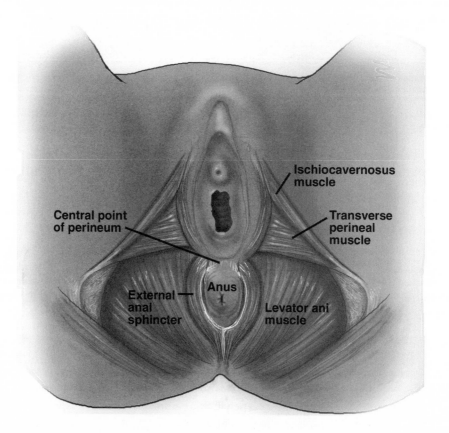

FIGURE 1. *Pelvic Floor Muscles.*

complex were first developed. Of course, many more people may have it than are recognized because the diagnosis is so difficult to make. The annual incidence of new diagnoses remains at 1.2 patients per 100,000 people. The average age of presentation is from 42 to 46 years old and it is predominately diagnosed in Caucasian women.

Major deterioration of bladder function is the exception more than the rule. Only 10% of sufferers will eventually develop the severe form of the disease. Most women peak with the worst symptoms quickly, and then rapidly stabilize or go into remission. All of the information regarding the frequency of the disease has been obtained over the last 13 years by the NIDDK research group. It is possible that many more women suffer from this disorder than we actually recognize.

Causes

The reason that some women develop interstitial cystitis and others do not remains a mystery. Because so little is understood about this debilitating disorder, a number of theories regarding its cause have remained under debate for years. Many of the theories seem reasonable; some seem unlikely. However, none have been dismissed yet because not enough data have been gathered to substantiate any one. Many of us who treat women with interstitial cystitis agree that more than one problem leads to the persistence of the symptoms. One event does not cause this disease. It is multifactorial in origin, meaning that many different events come into play.

SUSPECTED CAUSES OF INTERSTITIAL CYSTITIS

Infection
  Bacteria
  Virus
Defect in the bladder lining
Allergic or autoimmune problems
Neurological defect
Psychosomatic causes
Other
  Food intolerance
  Endocrine problems

Infection

Infection as a cause of interstitial cystitis remains one of the most popular theories among both patients and practitioners. The fact that many women begin with symptoms suggestive of a urinary tract infection and take multiple courses of antibiotics leads many of us to suspect a relationship between the two conditions. An atypical bacterium that is not eliminated by traditional medications may be the cause, leading investigators to search for this elusive bug.

The idea is not novel. Our experience with peptic ulcer disease has taught us to be tolerant of any idea until it has been disproved. For many years, peptic ulcer disease was thought to come from the overproduction of acid in the stomach, often stimulated by stress. A small group of investigators found that peptic ulcer disease is actually caused by a bacterium called *Helicobacter pylori*, which is easily treated by conventional antibiotics. The treatment of peptic ulcer disease was revolutionized by this discovery. Perhaps interstitial cystitis is also caused by a yet-undiagnosed virus or bacteria.

Adherence Theory

One of the more popular theories suggests that the cause of interstitial cystitis is the **breakdown of the lining of the bladder wall**. The bladder wall is composed of cells that expand at the top like an umbrella. These umbrella cells overlap one another to seal the spaces that normally exist between cells. A slimy sealant called, the GAG layer, cements the umbrella cells together to reinforce the impermeability of the cells. The tightly closed spaces prevent toxins from the urine from penetrating the top layer of cells and seeping into the deep wall of the bladder. Underneath the layer of umbrella cells, the nerves and blood vessels that supply the bladder provide nourishment and sensation to the organ. If the toxins are able to irritate these structures, symptoms will occur.

With leaking between the cells, potassium from the urine can enter the wall of the bladder and cause muscle spasms. Potassium induces muscle spasms all over the body, especially in the heart muscle. Laboratory testing has shown that bladder muscle is also sensitive to potassium. The muscle cells of women with interstitial cystitis are especially sensitive to the effects of potassium, which may irritate the muscle and nerves below the surface.

Autoimmune Disease

These days, the **allergy/autoimmune** theory remains another popular theory. During evaluation under anesthesia, a biopsy is often done of the bladder wall. The biopsy specimen in women with interstitial cystitis usually

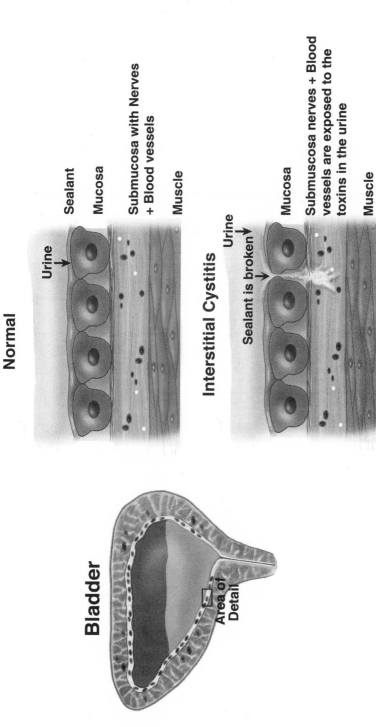

FIGURE 2. *Breakdown of Bladder Lining as Cause of Interstitial Cystitis.*

contains *mast cells*. Mast cells congregate in areas in which an allergic reaction is occurring. These cells contain packages of histamine, which burst open and attack the offending agent. In interstitial cystitis, the mast cells with the histamine packets may be attacking the bladder wall itself. The cells "think" that the bladder wall is the foreign agent and attack it. When the body sees itself as foreign and attacks its own tissues, we call this an "autoimmune" response. "Auto" means self. It is an immune reaction against itself.

This theory is intriguing for a number of reasons. First of all, mast cells are seen frequently in the bladders of women who fit the NIDDK criteria for a diagnosis of interstitial cystitis. Not all of you will have mast cells on the biopsy, but most of you will. Secondly, many of the other disorders from which interstitial cystitis women suffer are also thought to be autoimmune in origin. These disorders include fibromyalgia, irritable bowel syndrome, chronic fatigue syndrome, and migraines. Medications that inhibit the mast cell/histamine response appear to help alleviate some of the symptoms. Opponents of the allergy/autoimmune theory speculate that the mast cell release of histamines may be a *response* to infection, trauma, stress, toxins, medication, or neurological problems. Like the infection theory, the allergy/autoimmune theory may be missing the actual *cause* of the problem, and only looking at the effect.

Nerve Damage
Neurological impairment is another theory regarding the etiology of interstitial cystitis. An unknown toxin can causes the nerves of the bladder wall to fire uncontrollably. When they fire, they release substances called neuropeptides that affect other nerves, which, in turn, will alter the blood vessels around the area. The blood vessels go into spasm and prevent oxygen from getting to the bladder muscle, causing pain. Similar to the way lack of oxygen to the heart causes chest pain. Neuropeptides are protein particles that send messages between nerves. They will tell the other nerves that an irritant is around and is causing problems. The irritant needs to be eliminated through the recruitment of blood cells that fight inflammation.

The irritant may be anything from a bacteria or a virus, to an allergen, or a food substance. Each person with interstitial cystitis may have her own irritant. The response to the irritant is what is abnormal. The reaction of the nerve leads to the overproduction of neuropeptides, which induces a cascade of reactions that becomes more toxic to the bladder than the original irritant. This theory is similar to the autoimmune theory in that the

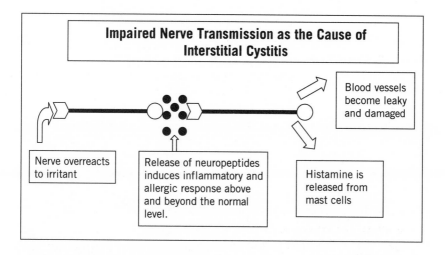

Impaired Nerve Transmission as the Cause of Interstitial Cystitis

Nerve overreacts to irritant

Release of neuropeptides induces inflammatory and allergic response above and beyond the normal level.

Blood vessels become leaky and damaged

Histamine is released from mast cells

response to the irritant is the actual problem, not the irritant itself. In the autoimmune model, the inflammatory cells go crazy. In the neurological model, it is the neurological response that is at fault.

Mental Illness

Psychosomatic causes of interstitial cystitis should be disregarded entirely. This is a true disease with clear symptoms and objective findings although I think the symptoms can drive people crazy if they go untreated. Those of you who present with the disorder are not crazy. Lack of sleep and the constant urge to urinate mixed with sharp, agonizing pain in the pelvis can certainly create terrible psychic distress. That is not the same as saying that the cause of the problem is psychological. The cause is organic, physical, and real, but you can become very distressed by the symptoms and the lack of compassion that the disease often fosters.

Allergies

Food intolerance and endocrine disorders seem like rather simplistic causes of this problem. Many of you, like N., find that avoiding certain foods helps minimize the symptoms. For this reason, the food-induced theory of interstitial cystitis was popular for a short time. Endocrine imbalances, such as a thyroid or hormone problems were considered because the symptoms seem to be affected by the menstrual cycle in some women. Perhaps hormonal changes throughout the month exacerbate or alleviate the symptoms, but a cause-and-effect relationship seems unlikely.

Normal Blood Vessel

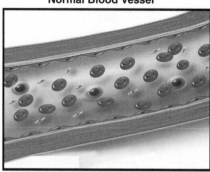

**Bladder
Nerves, Arteries and Veins**

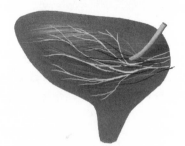

Damaged Blood Vessel

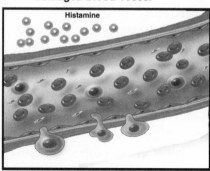

FIGURE 3. *Neurological Impairment as Cause of Interstitial Cystitis.*

Integrated Theory

As I have mentioned before, one theory probably does not account for all of the symptoms that are caused by interstitial cystitis. This disease results from a combination of injury and abnormal response to that injury. In order for you to develop interstitial cystitis, you need to have a predisposition that causes your bladder to overreact to that injury. Most of us would heal from the insult and move on with a normal bladder. Those of you with interstitial cystitis suffer from a cascade effect involving many faulty mechanisms. The integrated theory of interstitial cystitis that makes the most sense to me is illustrated in the accompanying diagram.

The diagram incorporates many different theories regarding the cause of interstitial cystitis. An unknown injury, such as a series of infections or courses of antibiotics, induces an autoimmune response. An abnormal response by the mast cells results in a release of granules of histamine that damage the protective covering over the umbrella cells of the bladder wall. With the damage to the protective layer, potassium can leak between the cells into the deep wall of the bladder, causing spasms of the muscle. The spasms and irritation to the whole wall set off the nerves beneath the surface of the bladder. These nerves fire away and release neuropeptides that then induce a pain response in the entire pelvic floor. The cycle continues despite the fact that the insult may no longer be present. The cycle has begun and will continue without any further exposure to the original problem.

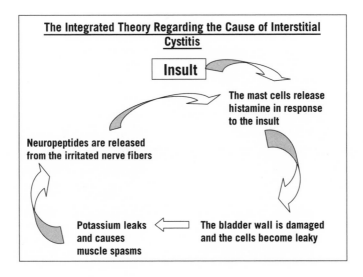

The Integrated Theory Regarding the Cause of Interstitial Cystitis

Insult

The mast cells release histamine in response to the insult

The bladder wall is damaged and the cells become leaky

Potassium leaks and causes muscle spasms

Neuropeptides are released from the irritated nerve fibers

Depending on your predisposition toward this disease, you will have part or all of this response. The worse the symptoms, the more reactive each aspect of the cascade is in your bladder. In some of you, the cycle is self-limited and the symptoms will resolve on their own. In others, the cycle continues until it is broken by an outside force. In any case, this multifactorial theory of the cause of interstitial cystitis helps to explain why so many different treatments help control the symptoms.

Evaluation of the Suspected Interstitial Cystitis Patient
Before a diagnosis of interstitial cystitis can be considered, other causes of frequency and urgency need to be eliminated. During the initial consultation, the physician should obtain a thorough history. As I have mentioned over and over again, the history will make a diagnosis over 50% of the time. With the right questions and accurate answers, the physician will know if the diagnosis can even be considered. The physical exam and urine tests are done mostly to eliminate other causes of similar symptoms.

CAUSES OF FREQUENCY AND URGENCY

Urinary tract infection
Large fluid intake
Pregnancy
Kidney or bladder stone
Urethral cyst
Genital infections: herpes
Diabetes mellitus
Chemical irritants: spermacides, douches

The physical exam will consist of an abdominal exam and a pelvic exam. The physician is feeling for abdominal masses that may suggest another diagnosis. The pelvic exam is done to identify masses in the urethral and vaginal wall, which can mimic the symptoms of interstitial cystitis. Burning, frequency, and urgency will result from an infected cyst under the urethra. This lesion can be seen easily during the exam. Many of you with interstitial cystitis will experience intense pain and spasms from the pelvic exam. The physician needs to be gentle, patient, and sensitive in order to minimize the trauma that an exam can cause to those of you with vaginal symptoms as well. However, it is imperative that the exam be done. No instruments, such as speculums or catheters, need to be used; just a single finger is inserted in the vaginal canal. The examiner needs to feel for masses in the ovaries and the uterus, as well as the muscles of the pelvic floor. The entire process should take less than one minute to complete. Some of you absolutely cannot undergo a pelvic exam. In these cases, the examination can be done under anesthesia when the rest of the evaluation is completed.

A urine specimen is collected to test for bacteria, protein, and blood, as well as white blood cells and glucose. Bacteria imply that an infection is present. The specimen will be sent for a urine culture to identify the type of bacteria and its sensitivity to antibiotics. **If an infection is found in the urine, interstitial cystitis cannot be diagnosed.** Protein suggests kidney problems. If protein is found, a 24-hour urine collection will be ordered to assess the amount of protein and other electrolytes excreted into the urine by the kidneys. Blood in the urine is often seen in women with interstitial cystitis, due to the irritation to the bladder lining from the disease. If blood is seen in the urine, a kidney x-ray, either an ultrasound or a CAT scan, may need to be done to look for stones and masses. Glucose, or sugar, in the blood implies that diabetes is present. Blood tests will confirm a diagnosis.

A bladder ultrasound (same as a sonogram) can be done in most urologists' offices. The amount of urine that is left in the bladder after you urinate is called the post-void residual urine (PVR). This noninvasive test is done be placing a small metal probe with lubrication on the tip on the abdominal wall over the pubic bone. An image is generated on a computer screen. The volume of urine can be calculated from the image. The test is not painful, even if you have severe interstitial cystitis. An elevated post-void residual (over 200 cc) suggests that a diagnosis other than interstitial cystitis should be considered.

Catheterizing the bladder for sterile urine samples causes unnecessary discomfort. A clean-catch specimen is usually accurate enough to eliminate many of the diagnoses listed above. Any instrumentation should be avoided in those of you suspected of having interstitial cystitis. It is extremely painful, creating horrible spasms and pain for days with very little yield in terms of information.

A three-day voiding diary can be helpful in objectively assessing your symptoms as well as providing a foundation to which treatment can be compared. During any three-day period, you record the time you void, the volume you void, and your level of pain during urination on a 10-point scale (1 = no pain and 10 = horrible pain). The days do not have to be consecutive, and one should be on a weekend and one during the week. Sometimes certain situations will cause more problems than others. The average woman with interstitial cystitis urinates 8 to 16 times per day and empties only 2 to 3 ounces (normal bladder volume is 10 to 12 ounces) with each urination.

Most of the other causes of frequency, urgency, and pelvic pain can be eliminated by this point. If interstitial cystitis is still suspected, the next step is called *cystoscopy with hydrodistention under anesthesia*. Over half of you with interstitial cystitis will not need to undergo this procedure because your symptoms will have improved by this stage of the evaluation. Of the half of you that do submit to it, 50% will actually have relief as a direct result of the test. Although it is done to make a more-definitive diagnosis, it can also be therapeutic. There are women in whom the procedure relieves the pain. It can be repeated whenever the symptoms return.

You will need anesthesia because instrumentation in women with interstitial cystitis is so painful that false results will be obtained unless you are given some medication. The procedure has three parts. The first part is the visualization of the urethra and the bladder wall. The second part involves filling the bladder with fluid and distending the walls to see how the tissue reacts. The third part includes a biopsy of the bladder wall to check for mast cells. After you are brought into the operating room, anesthesia is induced. A cystoscope is placed into the bladder through the urethra and the walls are inspected. Some women with interstitial cystitis have normal-looking walls upon first inserting the scope. The initial inspection will not help diagnose interstitial cystitis, but it will exclude other diagnoses, like bladder stones and tumors. In less than 10% of the women, a red patch will be seen on the bladder wall. This lesion, called a *Hunner's ulcer*, is the only finding in the entire evaluation that is only seen in interstitial cystitis. All of the other findings *suggest* a diagnosis. The Hunner's ulcer confirms it, undoubtedly. Not a true ulcer, Hunner's ulcers are rarely seen and cannot be relied on to make a diagnosis.

The bladder is then filled passively with water that is drained slowly from a level of 80 cm above the bladder. When the bladder can no longer hold any more fluid, the water will automatically stop draining. The volume that enters the bladder is then measured by emptying the water into a basin through the scope. This volume is extremely important in determining the severity of the disease. The average bladder capacity in a woman with interstitial cystitis under anesthesia is between 550 and 650 cc or 16 to 20 ounces. Smaller volumes of 350 cc (11 ounces) usually correlate with a more severe form of the disease. Women without interstitial cystitis will be able to hold 800 cc or 25 ounces of water. After the water is drained, if you have interstitial cystitis, regardless of the volume of water that the bladder can hold, you will have cracking and bleeding of the bladder wall.

Post-distention cystocopy is done to evaluate the bladder wall. *Glomerulations* are seen in interstitial cystitis. These are dots of blood speckled throughout the bladder wall. These glomerations indicate that the tiny blood vessels on the bladder wall have bled and are now clotted from the trauma of the procedure. Not specific to interstitial cystitis, like Hunner's ulcers, glomerulations are seen in other disorders, so we cannot use this finding alone to make a diagnosis. Radiation injury to the bladder wall, diffuse cancer, and chemical injury to the bladder can all damage the wall and create the same predisposition to the development of glomerulations as interstitial cystitis.

Biopsies are often done once the bladder has been emptied. Not all clinicians will opt to do a biopsy because they do not think the findings will contribute to the information. Other physicians feel that all the information that they can get during the procedure will help with the diagnosis, treatment, and prognostication of each woman's disease. A small piece of tissue can be removed from different areas of the bladder wall through the cystoscope. No incisions are made in the skin to access the bladder. The pathologist looks under the microscope at the tissue to see if any mast cells are present. Mast cells are not always seen in the bladder with interstitial cystitis, but they often are. Mast cells can be found if inflammation is present. They react to foreign and irritating substances all over the body. Researchers are looking for specific markers that could be tested for in the the urine than may be helpful in diagnosing interstitial cystitis, and eliminating other diseases, like bladder cancer.

Except for the presence of a Hunner's ulcer, no single finding on cystoscopy, hydrodistention, or biopsy will make a diagnosis of interstitial cystitis. A number of different bits of information gleaned from the procedures above will help to confirm an already suspected diagnosis from the history and physical exam.

FINDINGS ON CYSTOSCOPY, HYDRODISTENTION, AND BLADDER BIOPSY UNDER ANESTHESIA THAT SUGGEST A DIAGNOSIS OF INTERSTITIAL CYSTITIS

Normal bladder wall
Hunner's ulcer—atypical
Reduced bladder volume (<650 cc)
Post-distention bleeding
Glomerulations
Mast cells on biopsy

Treatment of Interstitial Cystitis

Once the diagnosis is made, treatment can begin. Most of the treatments for interstitial cystitis are not curative; they merely relieve the symptoms until the disease goes away by itself. You will need to accept the fact that this problem may be with you for a long time. However, management of the frequency, urgency, and pain can be very effective. If a flare-up occurs, you will know what works for you to keep the symptoms controlled, even if you cannot eliminate them completely.

Treatments can be broken down into behavioral modification, the instillation of medication directly into the bladder through a catheter, oral medications, nerve modulators, and surgery. As with all interventions, the least-invasive therapy should be tried first, with progressively more-aggressive methods introduced as required. Frequently, a baseline combination of medications will keep the symptoms at bay, with stronger ones available when they are needed. Every woman with interstitial cystitis is different in terms of her response to treatment. By the time the disease is diagnosed, you are very familiar with your symptoms and your body. I listen closely to the reports from the women and work with them to come up with a reasonable way to control this horrible problem.

AVAILABLE TREATMENTS FOR INTERSTITIAL CYSTITIS

Behavioral
  Diet modification
  Physical therapy

Bladder Instillation
  DMSO (Rimso®)
  Marcaine
  Heparin
  Steroids
  Sodium bicarbonate
  BCG

Nerve Modulators
  TENS unit
  Nerve stimulator

Surgery
  Hydrodistention
  Botox injections
  Bladder removal

ORAL MEDICATIONS

Antihistamines	**Narcotic Painkillers**
Atarax/Vistaril	Darvocet
	Vicodin/Vicoprofen
Antispasmotics	Oxycontin
Baclofen	Norco
Valium	
Flexeril	
Antidepressants	**Antiinflammatories**
Elavil	Ibuprofen
Pamelar	Celebrex
Paxil	Uricept
Prozac	Bextra
Zoloft	
Effexor	
Other	
Elmiron	
Neurontin	

Whenever I see a list of treatments this long and this diverse, I immediately think that we don't have a handle on the disease in question. Clearly, this is the case with interstitial cystitis. Because the cause of the disease is unknown, all we can offer is symptomatic relief. Actual cure cannot be expected when the root of the illness is unknown. However, the treatment options for the symptoms hold hope for the sufferers. Nearly everyone will get some, if not complete, resolution of her pain, frequency, and urgency through using one or more of the methods listed. Some of you will get permanent improvement, while others will get temporary help. In all cases, some benefit will be gained by trying different interventions until the correct combination is found.

Behavioral Modifications

In general, I recommend that you begin with the least-invasive treatments first. Just because an intervention involves alterations in lifestyle, does not mean that it will be less effective than a pill. Pills can be good, but other options can be just as good. For a chronic disease like interstitial cystitis, dietary modifications, voiding diaries, and physical therapy can have longer lasting effects than medications. In addition, these lifestyle changes can be implemented in addition to taking medications when the symptoms get considerably worse.

Dietary Changes

Dietary modifications remain one of the mainstays of treatment for interstitial cystitis. The theory behind altering the food that you consume lies with the deterioration of the bladder wall hypothesis for the cause of interstitial cystitis. Acidic foods, spicy foods, alcohol, and caffeine are thought to irritate the lining of the bladder. Avoiding citrus fruit, coffee, wine, and peppery items may help to soothe the bladder during especially unpleasant periods. The list of foods is exhaustive. The best way to determine which foods irritate your bladder is to eliminate foods within the acidic, spicy, alcoholic, and caffeinated food groups altogether. Then, reintroduce each group one at a time. The effect of the food will be noted within a day. If the burning returns after the introduction of a particular food, then that food is an irritant.

A food additive, called Prelief®, will neutralize the urine and may allow you to eat those forbidden foods on special occasions. Prelief is not a medication, so no prescription is needed to purchase it. It comes in pill and powder forms, and can be purchased at supermarkets, pharmacies, and health food stores.

Voiding Diary

Voiding diaries can help you follow your progress after initiating treatment. Diaries are especially helpful in bladder retraining efforts. You keep track of the number of times you urinate within a day and the volume that you eliminate with each void. This information is written down on a piece of paper over a three-day period. At the end of the three days, an assessment can be made regarding the pattern of urination. For example, you may urinate frequently during the day, but only once or twice at night. Or you may go frequently but only empty very small amounts each time. In general, if you urinate often only during the day, and not at night, no serious pathology exists, like bladder cancer. Of course, it may be annoying, warranting treatment, but no serious hormonal or metabolic problems will be the cause of the frequency. If you urinate large volumes with every time you to the bathroom, that is suggestive of a metabolic disorder, such as diabetes mellitus. In this case, a 24-hour urine collection should be done to measure electrolyte content and creatinine, which is a blood test that checks for kidney function.

Once the voiding diary is analyzed, therapy can be instituted as long as no medical problem is suspected. After therapy, the voiding log can be repeated. You should see changes in the number of urinations and the volumes that are eliminated. The diary can be an effective reenforcement of the treatment.

Bladder Training

Bladder training involves learning to hold urine for longer and longer periods of time before responding to the urge to urinate. When the need to empty comes on, you will count to 10 or 20 before you head to the bathroom. Eventually, you may be able to hold it for 5 minutes, then 10 minutes, then 20 minutes, and so on. Slow progress will eventually turn into a major change in the frequency. Once you get the reassurance that it is safe to hold it and you learn not to respond so quickly to the urges, you may be able to retrain your bladder to hold it for longer.

Women with interstitial cystitis will often not do well with bladder training because of the pain component of the disease. The pelvis actually hurts when you hold urine for longer than the urge permits. Even though no leakage will result if you hold it, the pain will become overwhelming. Bladder training can be used in conjunction with other techniques to reduce the frequency.

Physical Therapy

Physical therapy is one of the most important treatment options for those of you with interstitial cystitis. A well-trained physical therapist, familiar with both the disease and the techniques used to treat it, can be a lifesaver. Compassionate and patient, physical therapists can offer support as well as relief for suffering women. I recommend that you consult with a woman therapist, since many of the techniques involve intravaginal work.

Each therapist will tailor her treatment to your individual needs. Many different techniques are used, including massage, stretching exercises, hot and cold, packs vaginal weights, electrical stimulation and biofeedback. Massage therapy involves gently putting pressure on the pelvic-floor muscles that are in spasm, as a result of the pain and clenching that patients do to deal with the urgency and frequency. Sometimes the massage therapy is painful, but relief can be detected within a few hours of the first session. Some of you will need many sessions to even begin to do the deep massage that is needed to release the spasms even partially. Some women are so tight that only a single digit can be inserted vaginally at the first visit. Although it sounds horrifying, pelvic massage can be an excellent relief for some of the spasms.

Stretching exercises can be done at home. Spreading the legs out on the floor and leaning into the center will pull the inner thigh muscles at the pubic bone. Many women will find that doing this simple stretch will give them an urge to urinate. If that is the case, the correct exercise is being done. Vaginal weights are mostly used to strengthen the pelvic floor muscles in women with incontinence, but some physical therapists feel that strength will prevent tensing of some muscles to compensate for weaker ones. Electrical stimulation is a passive way to contract a muscle. A machine will cause the muscle to twitch. It can be used to help you to identify certain muscles, as well as to exercise weak muscles that need a little help before you can do it voluntarily.

Biofeedback is a method of exercising specific muscle groups through visual feedback. A sticky pad with a wire attached to it connects the muscle to a device that will respond to the correct movement. This method allows you to see, visually, whether or not you are exercising the right muscle.

Pelvic-floor physical therapy offers a number of benefits to interstitial cystitis women. First of all, you have contact with a health care provider on a regular basis to answer questions and offer support. Secondly, it will help alleviate the secondary muscle spasms that are seen in interstitial cystitis. Lastly, it is a non-medicinal therapeutic modality that can be re-instituted during flare-ups in those of you who have this chronic condition. You need to accept that this problem may be with you for many years.

Bladder Instillations

Bladder instillations have been one of the mainstays of treatment for interstitial cystitis for decades. Through a small catheter that is introduced into the urethra, different medications can be delivered directly into the bladder. You can be taught to catheterize yourself, giving you the freedom to treat yourself whenever you think it is needed. Horrified by the idea of self-catheterizing at first, most women find relief with the method and some comfort in knowing that they can deliver the medication on their own.

Many different agents have been used in the past, some of which have been abandoned and some that we still use today. Silver nitrate was popular years ago, but it causes painful scarring and bleeding of the bladder wall in some women and needs to be instilled under anesthesia due to pain. We no longer use it. Clorpactin (oxychlorosene), a highly reactive chemical compound, has also been replaced by some of the newer medications It works by liberating hydrochloric acid, which oxidizes the tissues and exerts a detergent effect on the bladder wall.

The mainstay of intravesical instillations is a medication called **DMSO** (dimethyl sulfoxide) or **Rimso®**. It was first approved for use in interstitial cystitis in 1977; however, no controlled clinical trials have yet been conducted to evaluate its effect. It works by penetrating the wall of the bladder and enhancing the absorption of other medications that can be instilled at the same time. It is thought to exert antiinflammatory effects, numb the bladder for pain relief, induce muscle relaxation, and inhibit mast-cell release. Whether or not it actually has any of these effects has not been proven. In this treatment, 50 cc of 50% DMSO is instilled into the bladder through a catheter and the liquid is left in there for 10 to 20 minutes. Six to eight weekly instillations are usually recommended to determine if the treatment relieves the symptoms. If it works, it may provide relief for up to six months. DMSO has been shown to induce cataracts in lab animals. No cataracts have been reported in human subjects. It leaves a garlicky taste on the breath immediately after instillation. That unpleasant sensation passes within a few minutes. Occasionally, DMSO can cause tremendous pain, requiring an injection of pain medication.

Many practitioners instill a cocktail of medications with the DMSO, to broaden the effect of the DMSO on the bladder lining. **Marcaine** and **lidocaine** are local anesthetic agents that can numb the bladder when instilled. **Steroids**, such as cortisone, will reduce the inflammation created by both the disease and the medications used for treatment. **Heparin** is a blood thinner that may help restore the bladder lining when injected directly into the bladder. It is not absorbed through the bladder wall, so no side effects will occur. **Sodium bicarbonate** is the same as baking soda. It will turn acidic urine into a basic pH, which may decrease the amount of stinging and burning. Some women even take a teaspoon of baking soda dissolved in a glass of water every day to try to decrease the acidity of the urine. The efficacy of all of these interventions is not proven. At this point, most of us will try different treatments until you respond to something. No controlled clinical trials have been done on any of these treatments to justify their use.

BCG has recently been investigated as a treatment for interstitial cystitis. BCG stands for bacille Calmette-Guérin and is a dead tuberculosis organism that is used to vaccinate against tuberculosis, mostly in Europe and Asia. This agent has been successfully used to treat bladder cancer for years. The exact mechanism of effect is not clear, but it seems to induce an inflammatory and then healing reaction in the bladder. Controlled, double-blind studies have been conducted using BCG for interstitial cystitis, but the numbers are small and the follow-up period has been short.

Oral Medications

Most medications that have been used for interstitial cystitis have developed out of desperation to help women get relief until the symptoms spontaneously resolve. Few studies have been conducted to evaluate the efficacy of these choices, and none have been done using a control group. There is some rationale, however, for the selection of medications that have been applied to this disease. Trial and error, mixed with faith and patience, will help find a successful program for each you.

Antihistamines are thought to stabilize mast cells, which explode when we are exposed to an allergen. The contents of the mast cells create an autoimmune reaction that can be the beginning of the cascade that leads to the symptoms of interstitial cystitis. Stabilizing the mast cell and preventing the release of it's contents may inhibit the cascade. The most commonly used antihistamine for interstitial cystitis is hydroxyzine (Vistaril® or Atarax®). It can be taken every six hours, only as needed, and is particularly effective in conjunction with other medications. It will rarely provide relief on its own. The main side effect is sedatiom; many of you will get drowsy on hydoxyzine.

Antispasmodics prevent the bladder from going into spasm. For a long time, many physicians who treated this disease felt that bladder spasms played an important role in the symptoms. However, few women respond to any type of antispasmodic medications. **Baclofen** is used to treat spasms in people with spinal cord injureis. It seldom helps relieve the urgency and frequency seen in intersitial cystitis. Diazepam (**Valium®**) and **Flexeril** are both skeletal muscle relaxants that can be very effective in patients with back spasms and pelvic-floor spasms. Since many of you suffer from pelvic-floor spasms in addition to the bladder condition, these medications can offer secondary relief. Diazepam is sedating and has an addicting quality to it. It is important to take it prudently since this is a chronic condition that may require long-term management.

Antidepressants have become a mainstay of oral treatment in interstitial cysititis. There actually is some rationale for their use. Many different classes of antidepressants are now available to patients. The two classes that work the best are the tricyclic antidepressants, such as **amitriptyline** (**Elavil** and **Imiprimine**) and **nortriptyline** (**Pamelor**), and selective seratonin reuptake inhibitors (SSRIs), such as **Effexor**, **Paxil**, **Prozac**, and **Zoloft**.

Amitriptyline and nortriptyline exert their effects both in the brain and at the level of the bladder. In the brain, they alleviate depression that is brought on by lack of sleep and pain. In the bladder, they directly affect neurotransmitters to induce bladder relaxation. They may have the secondary effect of stabilizing mast cells and inhibiting the autoimmune response that results from mast-cell degranulation. In addition, they create an antispasmodic effect. The dose begins low, at 10 to 25 mg and can then be increased up to 75 or 100 mg depending on the response. The most common side effect of these medications is sedation. Many of you will only be able to tolerate them at night.

The SSRIs have only recently been used to treat interstitial cystitis. Very little literature has been published supporting the use of these agents specifically for this problem. All four of the medications listed effect the brain chemistry through increasing the levels of seratonin, a neurotransmitter that mediates mood. However, they also have secondary effects that act as antispasmodics and as tricyclic antidepressants, both of which affect the bladder directly. They are not sedating, which has been the major limitation of nearly all of the other medications.

Narcotic painkillers, unfortunately, need to be used at some point in most women with severe interstitial cystitis. All narcotics are derivatives of opium, the natural product after which morphine was modeled. Morphine is one of the most potent and effective painkillers available, however it has a number of drawbacks that have spawned the development of the newer generation of pain products. Many of the newer drugs have smaller amounts of narcotic in them and offer a great deal of relief. Used judiciously, they can be lifesavers in times of terrible pain and distress. A small dose will often break the pain cycle and allow you to sleep, which will make you feel better, reduce your pain, and give you the strength to cope with the condition. It is a good idea to keep a supply of pain medication at home to deal with the worst symptoms.

New medications are always on the horizon. Most are a combination of narcotic (such as codeine, oxycodone, or hydrocodone) mixed with either aspirin, Tylenol, or an antiinflammatory agent, such a ibuprofen. If you are allergic to the additive (Tylenol, ibuprofen, or aspirin) be sure to tell your doctor because many of these are combination mediations. Some of you may be allergic to certain types of narcotics as well. For example, you may be allergic to codeine, but not to hydrocodone. Be sure to mention all drug reactions to your physician.

Each state has its own regulations on controlled substances, which all narcotic drugs are considered. In the state of New York, a physician cannot write hydrocodone on a regular prescription. It has to be written on a special triplicate form that is hand-delivered to the pharmacist. No call-in prescriptions. However, in Connecticut, certain doses of hydrocodone can be

written on a regular prescription pad and mailed into the pharmacy. Whatever the case, a supply of emergency pain medication is very important to
have available in case a terrible cycle of pain hits and no other relief can be
found. Taking a strong painkiller may be the best way to put you to sleep
to begin recovery quickly.

Antiinflammatory agents have emerged as the second coming for all
pain conditions, especially arthritis. Patients who used to suffer with severe
joint pain can now walk, and even dance. Because these are the first strong
pain medications that are not narcotic-based, they are being applied to all
sorts of chronic pain conditions. The most common short-acting antiinflammatory agent is ibuprofen, which is the chemical name for the active
ingredient in Advil, Motrin, Aleve, and Naproxyn. All of these medications
have to be taken several times per day because they are metabolized by the
liver and the kidney and leave the body within 4 to 6 hours. The newer formulations, such as **Mobic®**, **Celebrex®**, **Uricept®**, **Bextra®**, and **Anaprox®**
all work for at least 12 hours at a time. They have greater potency with fewer
side effects and need to be taken less often than the older agents. The differences among the agents are subtle. If one brand does not agree with you,
then another may. The most common side effect with all of these agents is
an upset stomach. They can make gastritis and reflux disease worse, so you
need to report all side effects to the prescriber. Recently, some of the long-
acting antiinflammatory agents have come under attack for affecting the
heart. Long-term use of these agents is not recommended.

I find that women will often do well with a combination of medications, such as a narcotic and an antiinflammatory agent. They will accen-
tuate each other's effects so smaller doses of each medication can be used.
Generally, these drugs are only needed during cycles of exacerbation. You
do not need to be on any of these drugs for long stretches of time.

In addition, there is **Neurontin®**, a unique medication that is used in
many people with neurological disorders and that also has been found to
be a potent pain medication. Blocking the GABA receptors in the brain,
it interferes with a totally different neurotransmitter, called gaba-
aminobutyric acid. It is given in doses up to 1800 mg per day. The dose is
accelerated slowly and weaned off slowly. It should be given by an experienced practitioner who will monitor you closely.

Finally, a medication has become available that is used to treat interstitial cystitis specifically. Called **Elmiron** (sodium pentosan polysulfate), it
is the only drug approved for the specific treatment of interstitial cystitis.
Elmiron is taken every day, three times a day, and is generally very well tolerated. It takes anywhere from 3 to 6 months to exert its effect. It works by

repaving the bladder lining to correct the defects in the wall of the bladder that lead to the pain. The results of studies on the use of this drug have come mostly from the manufacturer. Some reports have shown significant improvement in symptoms, while others show no change compared to placebo. Side effects are rare. The most common is hair loss, but this occurs in less than 2% of patients on the drug.

The bad news about all treatments is that no drugs are available to *cure* interstitial cystitis. The good news is that many medications are available to help you through the most difficult periods before the disease goes into remission. Nearly everyone will be able to find some medication or some combination of medications that will help you cope and gain some relief. Finding the right practitioner to help you work out a good program can be the most challenging part of treatment. Websites and organizations of inter-stitial cystitis sufferers are available to guide you. The Interstitial Cystitis Association is a patient advocacy group that offers support groups, a newsletter, and referrals to physicians for patients and their families. If you do an internet search for interstitial cystitis, the various website names will pop up.

Nerve Stimulators

Nerve stimulators have been used for years by pain management specialists to divert pain sensation away from the source. The target nerves are stim-ulated either directly or through the skin by an electrical current. This con-stant stimulation induces inhibitory nerve endings to be activated and shut down the overactive nerve that is causing the symptoms. The **TENS** (tran-scutaneous electrical nerve stimulator) unit delivers the current through the skin. Electrode pads are stuck to the skin with EKG leads and the wire is snapped onto the pad. At the other end, the wire is attached to a hand-held device that is set to fire at a rate you determine. You yourself, set the level as high as possible without inducing pain. It can be left on for a few minutes at a time for each treatment.

The **Interstim® neuromodulator** is an implantable device in which wires are inserted into the sacral spinal cord by a urologist or urogynecol-ogist. Similar in concept to a TENS unit, the nerves that supply the bladder are directly stimulated by a pacemaker that is inserted surgically under the skin of the buttock, similar to the implantation of a cardiac pacemaker. The nerves to the bladder are stimulated directly, as opposed to through the skin, the way the TENS unit works. The unit is set to fire regularly all of the time. The constant firing overrides the stimulatory effects of the native nerves to the bladder. The Interstim device has been very successful in treating the frequency and urgency associated with interstitial cystitis, but the pain component does not seem to respond as well. The drawbacks are obvious: a wire is inserted into the spinal cord. An operation is required. However, a test stimulation is done in the office first to see if the device will be effective. If it is not helpful during the test stimulation, then the permanent implant is not performed.

Surgery

Surgical management of interstitial cystitis should be reserved as a last-ditch effort at relief. Less than 2% of women with interstitial cystitis will even be candidates for anything more involved than hydrodistention. That means that 98% of you will respond to either behavioral therapy, intravesical instillations of agents, or medication. Women who consider surgery suffer from end-stage disease. The indications for surgical intervention include intractable symptoms, failure of nonsurgical treatment, and a bladder capacity of less than 400 cc under anesthesia. The surgical options include hydrodistention, bladder denervation procedures (separating the bladder from its nerve supply), and bladder removal.

Hydrodistention

Hydrodistention is the least-radical surgical procedure, and is used as both a diagnostic and a therapeutic tool. For diagnosis, it will help confirm the presence of the disease in those of you whose symptoms are not clear. The procedure is done under anesthesia in an operating room and it takes about 15 minutes to complete.

No standard method for hydrodistention is available, but the basic procedure is as follows. After you are asleep, a cystoscope is inserted into your bladder through the urethra. Water is drained into the bladder through the scope at a pressure of 80 cm of water until the bladder is full. Once the bladder is full, the water is left to dwell for a few minutes. It is then drained from the bladder into a container. The volume of water that the bladder holds is recorder and bloody output is observed. Some physicians will repeat the procedure a second time. The urethra can then be dilated or stretched to expand its diameter. You are then awakened and taken to the recovery room to come out of the anesthesia before discharge home an hour or so later.

Response can be experienced within hours of the procedure. Some women will go into remission from the disease for up to 12 months. Over 30% of you will experience some symptomatic relief as a direct result of the procedure. However, another 30% will have *worsening* of your symptoms.

Predicting who will gain therapeutic benefits and who will suffer is difficult. Some practitioners suggest that if the bladder can hold less than 600 cc of water under anesthesia, relief is more likely to be expected. A fairly harmless procedure, hydrodistention can be done multiple times if it is the only acceptable way that you can obtain relief. Rarely, a woman will request that it be done every six to eight months to keep the disease at bay. No evidence, as yet, supports its use or disproves its efficacy. The choice to do it is entirely in the hands of the patient and her caregiver.

Bladder Denervation: Cutting the Nerves to the Bladder

Bladder denervation procedures encompass a long list of surgeries with very disappointing results. Separating the bladder from its nerve supply was thought to help relieve women from the pain associated with the disease. Originally, in cases selective nerves were severed, so a woman would be able to urinate voluntarily, but she would not have a normal urge to go. However, with this selective removal of the nerves, the pain would come back. So, in an effort to alleviate the pain, all of the nerves to the bladder were severed. The loss of bladder function required intermittent catheterization in order to empty the bladder. Sadly, the pain would usually return anyway, but the function of the bladder would not. Fortunately, these procedures have been abandoned.

Botox® Injections

Botox injections (botulinum toxin is the generic name) into the bladder wall have recently come into favor as a way of temporarily deadening the nerves without causing any permanent damage. The use of botulinum toxin for all types of bladder disease is still under investigation, but the results look promising. At least whatever damage is being done, it is not permanent, which is important in a disease with such a dynamic course. Botox seems to be most useful in reducing the frequency and urgency associated with interstitial cystitis, more than with the pain component. It is very expensive and needs to be repeated at least every six months. It can be done in the office without anesthesia.

Bladder Removal

Finally, **bladder removal surgery** has had mixed results, similar to the denervation surgeries. It is generally not offered anymore. In women with bladder capacities under 2 ounces, the size of the bladder is increased by removing most of the diseased bladder and replacing it with a piece of intestine reshaped into a dome. The wall of the bladder and the corresponding nerves are removed with the hope that the disease will disappear with the removal of most of the diseased bladder. You can still urinate normally, but your bladder will not be made out of its original tissue and muscle. This procedure is called an *augmentation cystoplasty*. Good idea, bad results. Many, if not all of these women, had recurrence of their pain in spite of the removal of the bladder.

More drastic surgery was then proposed. Remove the bladder and the urethra entirely, reconstruct a new bladder out of intestine, and have the patient drain urine into a bag. This procedure is called *a complete cystectomy with urinary diversion*. In these women, again, the urgency and frequency were eliminated but the pelvic pain returned. Many women who received this operation felt that the surgery was somewhat successful because they could sleep throughout the night and function during day. Nowadays, very few patients undergo bladder removal surgeries of any kind as a treatment for interstitial cystitis.

Summary
Interstitial cystitis is a pelvic-floor disorder that presents with frequency, urgency, and pelvic pain. It is manageable in nearly every woman who is diagnosed correctly with the disorder, but it is not curable. Researchers have yet to identify the cause of the disease, so physicians are left with the responsibility of treating the symptoms as opposed to the disease itself. Many of you who suffer from interstitial cystitis are stigmatized as hysterical, problematic, and, often, even psychotic women and are sent to psychiatrists for treatment. Because urologists and gynecologists are not always familiar with the disease, it is important that you take an interest in your condition and *help the caregiver help you*. Knowledge about new treatments and support from other women is available on the internet and should be accessed by patients. Most importantly, remember that you may have to live with the disease, but you still must live. Help, relief, support, and understanding is out there. Take control, find it, and avail yourself of it.

IRRITABLE BOWEL SYNDROME

Irritable bowel syndrome is an intestinal disorder characterized by painful bloating, gas, diarrhea, and constipation. Its exact cause is unknown but it is suspected to result from spasms within the colon, also known as the large intestine. Many women with irritable bowel syndrome also suffer from urinary problems and vice versa. Because of the overlap, many physicians group irritable bowel syndrome and interstitial cystitis into one category, called pelvic pain syndrome. Like interstitial cystitis, the cause of irritable bowel syndrome is unknown, and no cure is available.

The bowel and the bladder share many of the same nerves, all of which interact with the nerves that supply the pelvic-floor muscles. If the bowel is off-kilter or the bladder is off-kilter or the pelvic muscles are in spasm, then symptoms will result in any or all of the pelvic organs. In interstitial cystitis, the bladder is clearly involved. In irritable bowel syndrome, the intestines are involved.

The large intestine, also called the colon, reabsorbs fluid and salt from the contents of the stool before it is evacuated. The stool is moved down the intestine through regular contractions that are mediated by a pacemaker in the wall of the gut. The right side of the colon does the work, the left side of the colon stores the stool until it is ready to be eliminated. In irritable bowel syndrome, the contractions that move the stool are irregular, which affects the movement of the stool as well as the absorptive ability of the colon. For this reason, you will have constipation, which is where the stool is too hard due to overabsorption of fluid and slow contractions. Others will have diarrhea, which is underabsorption of water from the stool due to fast contractions. In making a diagnosis, a colonscopy is done to be sure that no life-threatening disease is present, such as colon cancer, ulcerative colitis, or Crohn's disease. The intestines will look totally normal on examination, with no bleeding, no ulceration, and no inflammation.

The diagnosis is made when all other explanations are eliminated. We call this a diagnosis of exclusion. No blood is seen in the stool and colonoscopy is normal. If the history supports the diagnosis, you are told that you have irritable bowel syndrome.

Treatment involves dietary changes, exercise, physical therapy, and occasionally medication. Diet affects irritable bowel syndrome because eating stimulates bowel contractions. Foods that are particularly irritating include fatty foods, seeds, nuts, and dairy products. Reduction in the consumption of these foods may be enough to reduce the symptoms to tolerable. Exercise and stress reduction help everything, so they are included in the treatment of all incurable disorders. Physical therapy may be helpful in relaxing the resultant pelvic-floor spasms that result from the pain and discomfort of the syndrome.

Zelnorm® was recently approved for the treatment of irritable bowel syndrome. Fiber products can help regulate the water absorption in the colon to try to normalize the frequency and the texture of the bowel movements. Antispasmodics, such as oxybutynin (Ditropan®), may be helpful, but they can cause constipation which is not good if that is part of the presentation. Muscle relaxants, such as diazepam, may help reduce the muscle spasms induced by the problem. Antidepressants are also prescribed to help patients to cope with their symptoms. I am not sure this last intervention is necessary.

ENDOMETRIOSIS

Endometriosis is a more well-defined disease that presents with pelvic pain. It is caused by deposits of the uterine lining (called the endometrium) that, for some reason, escape the cavity of the uterus and attach to other pelvic organs. These deposits can sit in the pelvis, on the bladder, on the ovary, or inside any organ in the area. These deposits respond to estrogen stimulation just like the normally located uterine wall. With the increasing levels of hormones at the beginning of the cycle, the lining will enlarge. During the second half of the cycle it will remain dormant, and then shed and bleed during menstruation. The hallmark of endometriosis is that the symptoms change with the menstrual cycle. The blood will irritate the organ on which the lining is sitting and cause painful symptoms. Sometimes, the body will wall off the bloody lining and form a cyst. These cysts, called endometriomas, can sometimes be seen on x-rays or laparoscopy.

Any pelvic pain that is cyclic in nature can be caused by endometriosis. Because it is easily diagnosed and treated, you can be cured of this problem. Many of you will have both endometriosis and interstitial cystitis. Helping one problem can allow the second problem to be dealt with more effectively.

The diagnosis can be suspected on imaging studies. MRI and CT scan will show endometiomas if they are over 1 cm in size. The best screening tool for endometriosis is laparoscopy, which is a surgical procedure done in an outpatient setting. The gynecologist puts a scope into the abdominal cavity through a tiny incision at the bellybutton. Through the scope, she can identify any lesions and burn them. Destroying them with electrocautery will usually get rid of them completely. Generally, laparoscopy is reliable in making the diagnosis. Occasionally, a woman will have a normal laparoscopy but a very reliable history. In these cases, treatment should ensue despite the normal surgical findings.

Treatment of endometriosis involves hormonal manipulation if surgery does not ablate, or destroy, all of the abnormal tissue. Birth control pills can regulate the amount of estrogen that reaches the tissues and causes the lining to bleed. If pills do not work, then the body's supply of estrogen can be shut off completely by giving a gonadotropin-releasing-hormone inhibitor, such as Lupron®. Given by injection once every month, Lupron puts you into a menopausal state. You produce no estrogen, therefore, the tissue never bleeds. The symptoms are alleviated. Some women will experience menopausal symptoms, such as hot flashes and headaches as a result of the Lupron. In many cases, the side effects of the Lupron are far better than the pain of the endometriosis. Eventually, the endometriosis cells will become dormant and stop responding to estrogen. The Lupron can then be discontinued. Sometimes, the normal released of estrogen is suppressed long after the Lupron has been discontinued. It should be used with caution is women of child-bearing age. Although most drug plans will cover it, it is very expensive.

Like interstitial cystitis and irritable bowel syndrome, the symptoms of endometriosis can range from mild to severe. Unlike the other disorders, however, it is more easily diagnosed and treated. Many women, such as N., will suffer from two or even all three of these problems, which can make their management difficult, especially since different specialists treat all three problems: interstitial cystitis is treated by urologists, irritable bowel syndrome by gastroenterologists, and endometriosis by gynecologists.

SUMMARY

Pelvic pain syndromes are terrible for patients to live with and frustrating for physicians to treat. Little is understood about these diseases, so treatments can be elusive. The relationship between urethral syndrome, interstitial cystitis, irritable bowel syndrome, and endometriosis cannot be proven, but they seem interrelated in their symptoms and management. Researchers continue to pursue an understanding of all four syndromes, which should only lead to better treatments and, ultimately, to cure.

PART FIVE

RELATED ISSUES

CHAPTER 10

Menopause, Hormones, and the Development of Female Pelvic Problems

M.A. has just received an invitation to her best friend's 50th birthday party. She can't believe that the whole group is entering "middle age." Fifty used to seem really old, but now. . . . They still have nearly half of a lifetime to live, yet so many changes have begun to happen.

Although her menstrual cycle had been irregular for about six years, M. stopped getting her period about 18 months ago. Not that she misses all of the unpleasant stuff that goes with menstruation, but the adjustment to a new phase in life has been challenging. For one thing, she gets hot flashes, which are embarrassing and uncomfortable. Her gynecologist told her that they will subside in a few months, but she still gets them every now and then. Another thing is her moods. She feels cranky and irritable more than she used to. For no reason, she'll lash out at her friends or family. It makes her feel bad, but she doesn't feel like she has much control over it.

She and her friends are very open about their lives. They have all talked about their experiences with menopausal changes. One of her friends began taking hormones nearly immediately. As soon as she missed her period for three months in a row, she began to take medication. She says that she has had virtually no symptoms of menopausal changes. She feels healthy and strong. Her skin is smooth. She exercises regularly and has no problems with bone loss. She has no desire to stop taking the hormones because she feels so well, despite the bad press regarding hormone replacement therapy.

Another one of M.A.'s friends had breast cancer in her late 50s. She cannot take any estrogen-based medication because the breast cancer was estrogen-receptor positive. That means that the tumor may come back if she exposes her body to estrogen. She also feels fine. Ever since her diagnosis, she has been on a strict diet of fruits, vegetable, grains, and fish. She exercises regularly, and basically lives a healthy life. She has become an expert laywoman on the subject of women's health. She would not use hormones even if breast cancer were not part of her history.

M.A. is now at the point where she needs to figure out what she wants to do for herself. So many physical things with her body have changed that she isn't sure what is age-related and what is hormone-related. She is about 20 pounds heavier than she was in college. She walks a lot but doesn't go to the gym on a regular basis. She goes to the bathroom more often than before, and she gets up a few times at night to urinate. She gets fatigued more easily and, more often than not, would rather stay home than go out for a big fancy dinner. She was never that interested in sex, but lately, she has virtually no interest in sex. Her libido is basically nonexistent, which is fine, because she has no partner now anyway. When she thinks about it, M.A. is in a little bit of a slump. Maybe a shot of estrogen is just what she needs!

The gynecologist discussed the different ways in which hormones can be taken. There are pills, creams, and patches. The most recent research regarding oral estrogen replacement questions the safety of taking it regularly, but the doctor has many women on hormones for various reasons. Because M.A. has not had surgery to remove her uterus, she will need to take both estrogen and progesterone. The doctor explained that she won't bleed every month but she will take the progesterone only during certain days of the "cycle." The idea is to mimic the normal hormonal fluctuations in the body without producing a period.

M.A. wanted to know how hormone replacement therapy, as the gynecologist referred to it, would change her life. How would it make her better? She told the doctor about her two friends and their very different feelings about estrogen therapy. Which one was correct? M.A. heard that hormones would protect her against heart disease (her father died of a heart attack at the age of 76). She also read that it would protect against bone loss and the progression of osteoporosis. Some women claim that it makes them feel good. It stabilizes their moods and it keeps their skin supple. However, it may contribute to the development of breast cancer. What does the doctor think? What does the data show from all the studies that have looked at hormone replacement therapy in healthy women like M.A.?

> *Surprisingly, the doctor had very little hard evidence to offer M.A. regarding whether to start medication or not. The Women's Health Initiative is the biggest study that has been published on the subject of menopause and oral hormones. It suggests that oral estrogen does more harm than good. She could not say that hormones certainly will help with one condition or another. It was a matter of "personal preference." Personal preference! How should M.A. know what her "preference" is? Her preference is not to take any medication ever for anything. She just wants to make an educated decision before she embarks on taking a medication for the rest of her life.*

Menopause is defined as the time during which the ovaries stop functioning, resulting in the permanent loss of the menstrual period continuously for 12 months. The average age of menopause in the United States is 52. According to the 2000 Census, the life expectancy of the average American woman is 78 years, up from 51 years for the 19th century. Therefore, the average American woman will spend one-third of her life as a postmenopausal person. For the year 2000, the world population was 6.2 billion, and projections for the year 2020 put the world population at 7.9 billion. Eight point eight percent, or 796 million, of those people will be over age 65, and 124 million will be over 80. Since women live longer than men on average, we are talking about a huge population of postmenopausal women who will live many years with some of the symptoms of those changes. In the year 2000, over 50 million menopausal women were alive and well in the United States.

The issue of hormones and their impact on the various organ systems of the female body continues to baffle physicians and researchers, let alone women like M.A. Studies prove both sides of the argument: that hormones *do* help and that they *do not* help the symptoms that many women attribute to menopause. The use of hormone replacement therapy has become a religion: either you believe or you don't believe in their efficacy. Many women attribute hormone replacement with wonderful results: youthfulness, good sex, positive mood, and overall good health. Some women think that hormone replacement therapy has been sold to women as a fountain of youth that actually exposes users to an increased risk of cancer.

Fortunately, I am a urologist, so I can focus on a small, but major part of the female body that undergoes changes during menopause. Unfortunately, very little is really known about the effect that hormones and menopause have on the bladder and pelvic-floor muscles. I will try to clarify what *is* known about how estrogens and progesterones affect the urinary tract, what happens during menopause, and what treatment options are available. Perhaps, then, an educated decision can be made regarding the use of hormones for urinary tract problems.

THE PHASES OF MENOPAUSE

Menopause has been divided into three phases. Together, they are referred to as the "climacteric." The first phase is called **perimenopause**. It is defined as the beginning of diminished ovarian function and presents with irregular menstrual cycles. Just to review a few basic concepts about the life cycle of a woman: every girl baby is born with the number of eggs that she will have for the rest of her life. These eggs will not begin to mature until menarche, the age at which she begins to menstruate. At the beginning of each menstrual cycle, an egg matures within a follicle in the ovary, which ruptures at the time of ovulation and travels down the fallopian tube into the uterus. If it is fertilized by a sperm, the egg implants into the uterine wall, and the woman becomes pregnant. If it is not fertilized, 14 days later the egg and the uterine wall slough off during the menstrual period, while another follicle prepares for the next egg to mature. During the perimenopausal period, that original number of eggs that the woman was born with is dwindling, so the number of developing follicles diminishes.

Menopause occurs when no menstrual period occurs for 12 months. Hormonal levels can be measured to confirm the menopause. Estradiol-17β (the active estrogen produced by the ovary) levels are reduced and FSH (follicle-stimulating hormone, produced by the pituitary and a stimulator of the ovarian follicle) is elevated because it is not suppressed by the production of estrogen. No more follicles are able to mature, so menses stops.

Postmenopause is the state of being that spans for the next 30 years for the average woman. During this time, no eggs are maturing, but the body is still producing a small amount of estrogen, some of which is coming from the ovary.

ESTROGEN

Our bodies produce different types of estrogen, most of which comes from the ovary and the rest from the adrenal gland. In the premenopausal woman, the main form of estrogen that is produced is estradiol-17β. Eighty percent of the body's estrogen at this stage in life comes from the ovary. After menopause, estrone is the more prevalent hormone. It is mostly made in the adrenal gland and the fat cells, which convert cholesterol, testosterone, and other steroids into this type of estrogen. Interestingly enough, the postmenopausal ovary is not completely dormant; it makes about 20% of the body's total estrogen supply. Other hormones continue to be manufactured in the postmenopausal ovary, including testosterone, whose levels do not change at all throughout the climacteric, and androstenedione, a precursor hormone with strong estrogenic effects. Progesterone levels plummet to almost zero. So, postmenopausal woman have unopposed estrogen production, albeit at low levels.

Smoking causes menopause to occur 1.5 to 2 years earlier than would occur if a woman did not smoke. Smoking affects estrogen metabolism by promoting the breakdown of estradiol, one of the most active forms of estrogen in the menstruating female, into its less active metabolites. Yet another reason to stop smoking!

The Estrogen Receptor
Estrogen exerts its effects through binding to a receptor. First discovered in the 1960s, two receptors have been described. The way estrogen affects a certain target tissue such as the uterus or the breast depends, at least in part, on the type of receptor to which it binds. The receptor can change its shape, and thus its effect on a certain tissue, for no known reason. How the same estrogens affect target tissues differently is not understood. Nor do we understand how it is that different estrogens can interact with the same receptor and have a different effect. For instance, tamoxifen, a breast cancer treatment, binds to the same receptor on the breast and on the uterus; however, it has totally different effects on the two tissues.

When the importance of the receptor became clear, researchers began to look for receptors in different tissues in the female urogenital tract. So far, receptors have been found in the vulva (the opening of the vagina), the vagina, the cervix, the uterus, the fallopian tubes, the urethra, and the bladder. Some scientists have found that the urethra and the vagina are more sensitive to estrogen than the lining of the uterus. The sensitivity of these tissues is related to the increased estrogen-receptor activity that has been observed. Fewer estrogen receptors have been identified in the bladder than in the urethra. Estrogen receptors have been found in the supporting structures of the bladder as well. These structures include muscles, blood vessels, and connective tissue fibers.

PROGESTERONE

Progesterone is an even more mysterious hormone than estrogen. It works as a muscle relaxant and appears to account for many of the changes seen in the urinary tract during pregnancy. Like estrogen, it works through receptors, which have been found in the bladder and the urethra. Unlike estrogen, it is not produced by the postmenopausal ovary. As far as its impact on the urinary tract, nothing is known about progesterone. In general, it is not clear what progesterone does if given to the postmenopausal woman, except prevent the overgrowth of the uterine lining.

DEVELOPMENT OF THE UTERUS, VAGINA, AND URINARY TRACT IN THE FETUS

Why would a chapter on hormones be included on a book about urinary tract disorders in women? The simple answer is: because the urinary tract and the female organs are integrally involved with one another. As a matter of fact, the bladder, the urethra, and the vagina form from the same embryologic structure. During fetal development, all of the structures begin as the cloaca, which divides into the urogenital sinus and the hindgut. During the second trimester of fetal development, the hindgut becomes the intestine, and the urogenital sinus becomes the vagina, the bladder, and the urethra. Because of their common origin, the cell types are similar, as is the blood supply and the nerve supply.

The urethra is a very short structure in the female. It is 3.2 cm or 1.5 inches in length and only 6 mm or $\frac{1}{4}$ inch in diameter. This tiny organ can be divided into layers. The outer layer comes in contact with the urine. The next inner layer supports the blood supply that keeps the urethra nourished and healthy. It is believed that healthy, juicy blood vessels keep the urethra thick and elastic. As a woman ages, the blood vessels begin to shrink, making the urethra thinner and the walls stiffer. Studies in the laboratory proved that these blood vessels are sensitive to estrogen.

EFFECT OF ESTROGEN ON THE URINARY TRACT

Signs of ovarian failure, as menopause is referred to in the medical literature, occur up to 10 years before menopause actually sets in. Perimenopausal symptoms include urinary incontinence, sexual dysfunction,

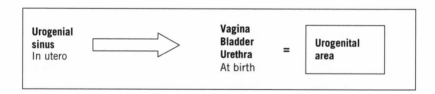

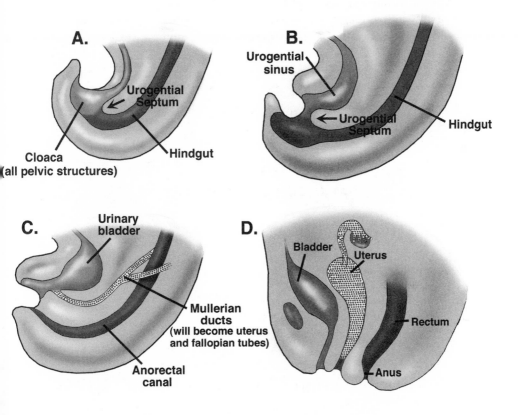

FIGURE 1. *Embryology of the Urogential System.*

increased risk of bone fractures, mood changes, hot flashes, and increased risk of cardiovascular disease. The most common urological problems that are encountered are narrowing and drying of the vagina, urinary leakage, with frequency and urgency, and recurrent urinary tract infections. Women with low estrogen levels can have changes seen in the bladder wall during cystoscopy, a procedure in which a scope is inserted into the bladder to visualize the lining.

Although less common than the other urological disorders, uterine and vaginal vault prolapse also occur much more often in postmenopausal women. With advancing age, the severity of the symptoms worsens. Approximately 9% of women over the age of 52 will develop pelvic-floor prolapse, in the form of a dropped bladder, rectum, or uterus. Bladder prolapse is the most common of the prolapse disorders. The urological disorders seen in postmenopausal women generally become symptomatic a few years after the onset of menopause, and tend to persist, and even worsen with age.

MOST COMMON CHANGES TO THE BLADDER AND VAGINA THAT OCCUR AFTER MENOPAUSE

Vaginal atrophy	Thinning of the walls of the vagina, with burning and itching
Urinary problems	Urgency and frequency of urination Difficulty reaching the toilet with an urge Leakage with activity
Urinary tract infections	Recurrent bladder infections
Sexual dysfunction	Pain with intercourse Reduced arousal/interest in sexual activity Decreased lubrication

---

Although we now feel confident that estrogen affects the urinary organs, we don't know what role it plays. Studies that actually look at these effects are few and far between. Observation and increased experience treating postmenopausal women has revealed the following impact that estrogen appears to have on urinary tract health. Estrogen maintains the acidity of the vaginal canal, which helps to maintain the proper balance of yeast and bacteria, thereby preventing urinary tract infections. When the estrogen levels in the vagina go down, the acidity diminishes and the balance of the flora changes. Bacteria can overgrow in the vagina, and then track up into the 1.5-inch urethra, and ultimately end up in the bladder. The result is recurrent infections.

The thickness of the vagina is increased by estrogens, which increase the blood flow to the tissues. This increased blood flow will also allow for better lubrication during sexual arousal. The thickened, juicy vaginal tissues of the premenopausal women are visibly different from the pale, thin-walled tissues of the postmenopausal woman. The lack of lubrication can cause burning, itching, and pain with sexual activity. Estrogen also increases the function of the urinary sphincter, the structure within the urethra that helps us maintain continence. The urethral muscle fibers are sensitive to estrogens, which help maintain pelvic-floor support and muscle tone. Therefore, sexual function and continence can both be altered as the estrogen levels in the bloodstream begin to diminish.

In summary, estrogen comes in many forms and exerts its effects through binding to receptors. Postmenopausal women produce estrogen, only it is in lower volume and with different predominate subtypes than in premenopausal women. The postmenopausal ovary is still productive, although its function is diminished. The actual impact that a particular type of estrogen has on a particular tissue depends on the receptor. Estrogen receptors have been found in the urethra and bladder, which originate from the same structure, embryologically, as the vagina. Progesterone is a complete mystery: its receptors have been found in the urinary tract, but how it affects these organs is not known.

WHAT HAPPENS TO THE URINARY TRACT AFTER MENOPAUSE

Approximately one-third of women over 50 will have some problems with their urogenital area, meaning the urethra, the bladder, and the vagina. Incontinence, urethra irritation and burning, frequency both day and night, recurrent urinary tract infections, and urgency of urination are the most common urinary problems that we experience. Vaginal complaints include dryness, painful intercourse, recurrent vaginal infections, foul odor, and discharge. The combination of urinary and vaginal disorders has been termed "senile urethral syndrome" by some, less-sensitive physicians who deal with these problems.

Estrogen deficiency seems to produce more problems with frequency of urination both day and night, as well as burning with urination, more than it causes leakage. In both men and women, urinating at night is more common with advancing age. The role of estrogen in promoting waking up at night because of an urge to urinate can only be assumed, not proven. The prevalence of incontinence in women living independently is anywhere from 30 to 50%, depending on the study that is quoted. Because incontinence is more common in older women and menopause occurs in older women, the speculation is that menopause contributes to the development of incontinence. However, not every postmenopausal woman has incontinence, which leads us to the conclusion that urinary control is a complex problem of which estrogen depletion is only one factor. Estrogen has some impact on incontinence and the urethra. We just don't know what impact that is.

In this section, I review the impact of low estrogen on the vagina and the urethra. Vaginal atrophy, voiding dysfunction, recurrent infections, and changes in sexual function are discussed.

Vaginal Atrophy

Vaginal atrophy is a description of the anatomical changes that can be seen in the vagina after menopause. The condition can be divided into symptomatic changes to the vagina and physical changes to the vagina. Symptomatic changes refer to the way the tissues *feel* when they are no longer estrogenized. Physical changes refer to the way the vaginal tissues *look* when they are no longer estrogenized. Symptomatic changes are experienced by you; physical changes are observed by your doctor.

SYMPTOMS OF VAGINAL ATROPHY

- Feeling of dryness
- Vaginal itching
- Vaginal burning
- Vaginal soreness
- Painful intercourse

PHYSICAL CHANGES SEEN WITH VAGINAL ATROPHY

- Narrowing of the vaginal opening
- Paleness of the tissue
- Vaginal shortening
- Pinpoint bleeding
- Retraction of the cervix
- Thinning of the pubic hair
- Thinning of the vaginal lips

Symptoms of vaginal atrophy include vaginal dryness, itching, burning without urination, soreness, vaginal discharge, and painful intercourse. These symptoms may occur before any physical changes are noted during examination. Usually, the *first* sensation is the feeling of dryness, which occurs as a result of reduced mucus production from the glands in the vaginal wall. The lack of lubrication that occurs during arousal results from the shrinking of the blood vessels under the vaginal wall. The *most common* complaint of vaginal atrophy is vaginal itching and burning. Some observers believe that the inflammation and irritation of the vaginal tissues contributes to symptoms of urgency and frequency of urination. Even the few of you who are still on oral estrogen replacement therapy may experience the symptoms of vaginal atrophy. It is estimated that between 10 and 25% of those of you will have at least some of the symptoms described above despite systemic estrogen use.

The physical changes to the vagina that can be seen in the postmenopausal woman include narrowing of the vaginal opening, which also becomes less elastic. Inside, the lining of the canal thins, becoming similar in texture to the tissue that coats the back of the hand. The canal also shortens, with loss of the vaginal folds. The vaginal lining becomes pale and bleeds easily. The thin vaginal tissue is susceptible to trauma and infection. Sometimes on exam, small paper-cut–like lesions can be seen along the outside of the vaginal canal. The cervix shrinks and retracts into the canal. It can be difficult for the gynecologist to locate the opening in order to perform a PAP test.

The vaginal lips, called the labia, decrease in size, with loss of fatty tissue and elasticity. The pubic hair tends to thin as well. The glands that line the vaginal wall shrink, producing less lubrication. The result is often dryness in the vaginal canal with itching and irritation, even without sexual activity.

Just because the physician may note physical changes during the examination does not mean that they need to be treated. The *symptoms* of vaginal atrophy are much more meaningful than any observations. Many women have no symptoms of vaginal atrophy, despite its physical presence. Any lumps, bumps, or isolated white spots that a physician sees in the canal should be biopsied, even if they are not causing pain. All postmenopausal vaginal bleeding also needs to be addressed, even if you have no associated symptoms. Aside from these two instances, physical changes do not need to be treated, but symptomatic changes do. You will not die from urogenital atrophy, like you can from heart disease, osteoporosis, or breast cancer, but you can be made uncomfortable from it.

Frequency, Urgency, and Getting up at Night to Urinate
Clearly, urinary changes occur in most of us as we get older. The relationship between hormonal changes and urinary symptoms remains elusive. The drive to urinate and the control of leakage are very complex phenomena that cannot be attributed to a single factor, such as estrogen. However, the changes that are noted to the bladder and the urethra are somewhat predictable. Physical changes to the structures are seen on exam, and symptomatic changes are experienced by you. Just because a woman has physical changes does not mean that she will experience symptoms. Only *symptoms* need to be treated.

You may experience urgency, frequency, nighttime awakening to urinate, burning with urination, and urinary leakage. Replacing estrogen either orally or directly to the urethra with creams generally will not reduce these symptoms. So the question remains: how are these symptoms related to estrogen depletion? So far, we only know what we have observed on physical exam in postmenopausal women in relation to what complaints they have regarding their voiding behavior. Observations that have been noted in postmenopausal women include reduced bladder capacity and slower flow during urination. Many of you do not empty your bladders completely during voiding. The residual urine will take up space in the bladder that cannot be used for new urine production. You also tend to feel full before your bladder is completely filled. In other words you sense a full bladder in spite of its only being at partial capacity. All of these observations together explain why older women urinate more often and get up at night to void. However, they do not explain the urgency to void and the increased incidence of leakage.

The urgency to void is related to vaginal atrophy and the sensitivity of the nerves in the urethra to stimulation. Estrogen creams that stimulate blood flow to the area may be helpful to treat this symptom of urgency, in particular. Providing a urinary tract infection has been ruled out, burning can be attributed to the same problem, and treated the same way.

Incontinence
Incontinence is a more complex problem. First of all, incontinence needs to be divided into two categories: stress incontinence and urge incontinence. Stress incontinence is leakage that results from coughing, laughing, sneezing, or activity. Urge incontinence is leakage that occurs with a strong desire to use the bathroom.

Stress incontinence results from weakening of the pelvic-floor muscles. Often, other pelvic floor defects are seen, such as a cystocele, rectocele, or uterine prolapse (see Chapter 7). Because the muscles are weak, they do not support the pelvic-floor structures well, resulting in leakage, and possibly, prolapse. In the older woman, another factor comes into play. The walls of the urethra thin out, resulting in a decreased sealing effect of the walls of the urethra. The decreased resistance will produce leakage. Estrogen creams can be used to bulk up the walls of the urethra through increasing the synthesis of collagen fibers and augmenting blood flow to the urethral lining. It also has been observed that vaginal estrogen will affect some of the receptors in the bladder and urethra that help maintain continence. Estrogen is often used in conjunction with other medications, such as pseudephedrine, that works on those receptors.

Urge incontinence is related to vaginal atrophy. Those of you with urge incontinence may not have an associated anatomical defect, such as a bladder prolapse, in addition to your leakage. Prolapse and urge incontinence are not as directly related as stress incontinence and prolapse are. Women with urge incontinence do not always have a history of childbirth or hysterectomy. As women age, the likelihood that they will develop urge incontinence increases. It is now considered one of the normal aspects of the aging bladder. Fortunately, urge incontinence is also responsive to local estrogen treatment. At present, other medications are available to treat urge incontinence more effectively, however, their effects can be boosted with estrogen cream.

Incontinence in the postmenopausal woman cannot be attributed solely to hormonal factors. In some cases, hormones may be helpful to supplement other treatments. Nonurological causes of incontinence must be evaluated and treated before estrogen supplementation is begun. These causes include dementia, urinary tract infections, fecal impaction, decreased mobility, confusion, medications (diuretics and sleeping pills, especially), hospitalization, and heart failure (see Chapter 6).

Pelvic-Floor Prolapse
Loss of pelvic-floor support is multifactorial as well. Genetics play an important role. Families will have multiple generations of women who have suffered from some degree of a dropped bladder. The history of a vaginal delivery is usually found in women who suffer from weakening of the muscles of the pelvic floor. Birth trauma certainly increases the risk of developing a problem. Estrogen depletion will not *cause* pelvic-floor prolapse, but it certainly contributes to its occurrence to some degree. An inciting event will occur, such as birth trauma or a hysterectomy, which will set the stage for the development of the muscle weakness. The actual manifesta-

tion of the problem will come after menopause. As the already weakened tissues shrink and lose their elasticity, the organs then begin to descend into the vaginal canal.

Urinary Tract Infections
Although urinary tract infections can plague women at any age, the cause of the infections changes throughout life. Approximately 15% of women over the age of 60 will suffer from frequent infections. The two reasons that women at this age are at an increased risk for developing a problem are 1) the presence of vaginal atrophy and 2) the loss of the vagina's acidity.

As mentioned earlier, vaginal atrophy is a term used to describe the physical changes that the vagina undergoes after estrogen levels drop. The tissues become thin and pale, which predisposes them to trauma and the introduction of bacteria. The bacteria can migrate up into the urethra and ultimately the bladder. The physical barriers that keep pathogenic bacteria out of the vaginal canal are altered by menopause. The vaginal lips shrink, with loss of the fatty bulk that covers the opening. The pubic hair thins out, eliminating another barrier to the introduction of bacteria.

The most popular theory regarding the cause of urinary tract infections lies with the change in the acidity of the vagina with age. The vaginal secretions are acidic in premenopausal women. The acidity maintains a balance of all of the different flora in the vagina, especially yeast and bacteria. The bacteria that are native to the vagina are called lactobacilli. Lactobacilli are healthy bacteria that maintain a balanced environment in the vagina. These organisms produce lactic acid which helps maintain the acidity of the vagina, thus inhibiting the growth of bad bacteria. Fragments of the lactobacillus cell walls can inhibit the attachment of *E.coli* to the walls of the vagina and the urethra.

With the change in hormone balance during menopause, the vaginal pH increases from a premenopausal level of 4.0 to a postmenopausal range of 6 or 7. The increase in the pH results in a disruption of the precarious balance that exists between the lactobacilli and other bacteria. Lactobacilli disappear from the vagina, allowing the vagina to become colonized by *E.coli* and other unhealthy bacteria.

Many of you who never suffered from urinary tract infections during your younger, more sexually active years may, all of the sudden, develop a problem with recurrent infections. The reasons are clear: hormonal changes to the vaginal tissues predispose you to infection. This problem is one of the few urological issues seen in postmenopausal women that can be directly attributed to hormonal changes.

Sexual Dysfunction

Female sexual function is a complex and poorly understood phenomenon. Some women experience changes in their sex life as they undergo menopause. In many cases, sexual activity remains stable with little change in the desire to have sex and the physical response to arousal. However, it is not unusual for postmenopausal women to experience postcoital bleeding and irritation, lack of lubrication, pain with sexual intercourse, difficulty reaching an orgasm, vaginal spasms upon penetration, lack of libido, and vaginal infections.

One of the earliest signs of low estrogen is lack of lubrication during arousal. Investigators speculate that the sensory nerves to the vagina become less responsive, leading to decreased sensation with stimulation. Less sensation leads to a reduction in the secretion of fluid from the vaginal glands, which normally are under neural control. Fewer sensory nerve endings also decrease the blood flow to the vagina, which is normally increased during arousal. The vagina does not respond with expansion and relaxation, which help to accommodate the penis during intercourse. These *physical* changes that occur due to low estrogen production make the woman think that she is less responsive *mentally*. If she is not lubricated, then she and her partner think that she must not be aroused.

Changes in the desire to have sex have also been reported by women going through menopause. The libido, or the desire to have sex, is a complex emotion that is under both hormonal and endocrine control. Interpersonal relationships, self-image, physical well-being, and psychological stability must all be factored into a women's interest in sex. It seems illogical to think that a single hormonal change, such as a reduction in estrogen production, would be wholly responsible for this complex disorder. Clinical studies have been unable to substantiate the use of estrogen, either orally or vaginally, to treat problems related to low desire. Oral estrogen therapy may help with hot flashes and sleep disturbances, which, when treated, may help indirectly with sexual desire.

TREATMENT

Treatment of urological disorders that may be attributable to estrogen depletion comes in the form of oral medication, skin patches, vaginal creams, and vaginal rings. The correct choice is individual and depends on the other symptoms from which you may be suffering. Most physicians will try one method or one product and see how you do—a trial and error approach to treatment. A little patience on the part of both parties can result in finding an acceptable solution. In my experience, estrogen therapy of any kind is usually accompanied by other treatments that address the urinary problem in particular, such as medication for overactive bladder or physical therapy for pelvic-floor spasms. Single-line treatment with estrogen alone will usually not manage any urological problem in the postmenopausal woman completely.

The goal of estrogen therapy is to provide the greatest relief of symptoms with the fewest side effects. Formal FDA approval for the use of estrogen has been obtained only for hot flashes and vaginal atrophy, the symptom complex of vaginal irritation, dryness, and shrinkage that can be seen in estrogen-depleted vaginal tissues. Progestins can be included in the regimen, but even less is known regarding its contribution to urological changes after menopause. Because the side effects of progestin can be quite bothersone, urologists do not usually include progestin treatment in an attempt to combat the changes seen in the vaginal and urethral tissues. Gynecologists add progesterone to prevent the overgrowth of endometrial tissue that can ensue with unopposed estrogen therapy.

TYPES OF ESTROGEN REPLACEMENT FOR UROLOGICAL DISORDERS IN THE POSTMENOPAUSAL PATIENT

> Pills taken by mouth
> Cream applied vaginally
> A ring inserted vaginally every 3 months
> A patch placed on the skin
> An injection given into the skin

Oral Treatment

Since the publication of the Women's Health Initiative report on the risks and benefits of oral Premarin® use, the recommendations regarding the use of oral estrogens has changed dramatically. The concern over the risk of breast cancer development has scared many women and physicians away from pills. However, there are many of you still taking oral estrogens and women in the future may choose to begin them despite the risk. For these women, I am going to review the hormone replacement therapies that are available and how they affect the urinary tract.

Oral estrogen comes in three forms: 1) *natural estrogen* that is extracted from plant products, 2) *equine estrogen* that comes from horse urine, and 3) *synthetic estrogen*, that is produced in a laboratory. The most common names for natural estrogens include *micronized estradiol* and *piperazine estrone sulfate*. The most commonly used equine estrogen is called *conjugated equine estrogen*. The most common synthetic estrogens are called *ethinyl estradiol* and *diethylstilbestrol*.

EXAMPLES OF NATURAL AND SYNTHETIC ESTROGENS

Generic name	Trade name
estradiol-17β	Estrace/Estring
Piperazine estrone	Ogen
Estrone sulfate ⎫	
Equilin ⎬	Estratab
Estradiol valerate ⎭	
Equilenin	
Estradiol cypionate	
17α-ethinyl estradiol	Estinyl
Δ⁸-estrone	
Mestranol	
Tamoxifen	
Reloxifen hydrochloride	Evista

The most common estrogen used for postmenopausal estrogen replacement is conjugated equine estrogen (Premarin®). The Women's Health Initiative used conjugated equine estrogen for their study. All the results are based on this form of estrogen. Containing 10 different estrogens, the agent is extracted from the urine of pregnant mares. It is a natural product, in that the estrogen has not been chemically modified. The "natural" estrogens come from plants, such as soy or the Mexican Yam. Natural estrogens include ethinyl estadiol, diethystilbestrol, and norethindrone acetate. These estrogens have to be chemically modified before the human body can use them. Therefore, "natural" estrogens have to undergo some processing in order to be functional.

No matter what form they begin in, all oral estrogens pass through the liver on their way to the distant tissues of the vagina and the urethra. As they pass through the liver, they are broken down into smaller parts, called metabolites. In many cases, those metabolites are less potent than the form that is ingested. Because of this breakdown, higher doses of oral agents may be required to combat the urological symptoms for which you are seeking treatment.

It takes about three months of therapy before you will know whether the treatment is effective in addressing the urological issues. Approximately 10 to 25% of patients on oral estrogen therapy will still experience the symptoms of urogenital atrophy. In other words, the tissue levels of estrogen in the vagina and the urethra do not reach a therapeutic level. The most effective use of oral estrogens lies with treatment of mood disorders, hot flashes, and sleep disturbances, not with urinary problems. **I do not advocate the use of oral estrogens to treat the urological disorders of menopause.**

Many physicians will include progesterone in the treatment of estrogen deficiency in the postmenopausal woman. Progesterone prevents the overgrowth of the uterine lining (endometrium) that can occur with estrogen therapy alone. If you have had a hysterectomy, progesterone is not necessary to include in the regimen. The actual benefits of progesterone are not known. It does not appear to improve symptoms in any noticeable way. It is solely used to prevent endometrial overgrowth.

Many different progestins are available for use. Like estrogen, progestins come from natural materials or can be produced in the laboratory. The advantages and disadvantages of synthetic versus natural progestins are not known. When progestin is added to estrogen, the combination therapy is called *hormone replacement therapy*. If estrogen is used alone, it is called *estrogen replacement therapy*.

PROGESTINS AVAILABLE FOR HORMONE REPLACEMENT THERAPY

Progesterone
Medroxyprogesterone acetate
Norethindrone
Norgestrel
Norethindrone acetate
Norgestimate
Desogestrel
Gestodene

Estrogen Creams

Estrogen creams, applied directly into the vagina, have become more popular for the treatment of the urogenital symptoms of menopause than oral treatment. Estrogen cream applied to the vagina does not get absorbed into the bloodstream. Therefore, the cream does not present the same potential risks that oral estrogens do. However, the creams will induce significant changes to the tissues of the vagina, The risks of use are low and the benefits are high. In addition, the estrogen that is present in the cream attaches to the vaginal tissues in the form in which it is packaged. It does not get broken down by the liver before it gets to the target organ, as do the oral estrogens. Estrogen creams are so safe that they are sold over the counter in Sweden. Women with a history of estrogen-receptor–positive breast cancer can usually use estrogen creams, rings, or tablets, even if they are also on tamoxifen. Always discuss this with your oncologist before using creams.

The cream is inserted into the vagina either with an applicator or with your finger. The initial dose is applied daily five days per week for two weeks, and then maintained with applications two to three times per week thereafter. Estrace and Premarin are the two most commonly used creams in the United States. Estrace is synthesized in the laboratory, while Premarin comes from the urine of pregnant mares. They are equally effective. The main difference lies within the agent in which the estrogen is suspended. Some women will react to the "cream" part of the estrogen cream with itching or burning. If that happens, you can switch to the other cream. Occasionally, a woman will experience transient breast tenderness or nipple sensitivity during the initial daily application. This response will diminish with continued use of the cream.

Other vaginal applications of estrogen come in the form of a ring and a tablet. The Estring is a plastic ring impregnated with the estradiol form of estrogen. You insert the ring yourself or your doctor can do it. The ring releases a low dose of estrogen into the vaginal tissues on a continuous basis for three months before it needs to be changed. Vagifem is estradiol-17β in a tablet. The pill is inserted into the vagina with the same regimen as the cream. Some women find it less messy than the cream. It is a natural estrogen which many women like more than the synthetic estradiol, but it does not come from horses. Generally, all of the vaginal estrogen products are safe, effective, and easy to use.

The "vasomotor symptoms," which include hot flashes, are not treated with vaginal estrogen. Those symptoms require oral hormones or the estrogen patch, which release estrogen into the blood stream. Now, many gynecologists are using other treatments for the symptoms of menopause and staying away from the oral estrogens and the patches. Vaginal estrogen, however, is safe.

VAGINAL ESTROGEN PRODUCTS

Estrace cream
Premarin cream
Vagifem vaginal tablet
Estring

Estrogen Cream for Vaginal Atrophy

Vaginal estrogen therapy is very successful in treating the local symptoms of menopause, especially vaginal atrophy and senile urethral syndrome. Vaginal atrophy describes the changes to the vagina that occur with decreased estrogen. They include itching, burning, and shrinkage of the vagina, accompanied by paleness and easy tearing of the thinned vaginal skin. Senile urethral syndrome describes the symptoms of frequency, urgency, and urination at night that is seen in postmenopausal women. Local treatments deliver relatively high doses of medication without causing the side effects in the rest of the body that can be seen with oral therapy, the most notable being endometrial proliferation that needs to be treated by adding progesterone.

Because vaginal estrogen is delivered pretty much unaltered to the local tissues, the results are good. The vaginal tissues become moister, pinker, and more elastic after four to eight weeks of use. Many of you will experience resolution of symptoms such as itching, vaginal spotting, dryness, and irritation. Reduction in frequency of urination is a less likely change, but some of you may also see changes in your urinary symptoms while using vaginal estrogen. The treatments need to continue on a regular basis of twice per week in order for the benefits to be continued. In other words, vaginal estrogen therapy will not cure vaginal atrophy and senile urethral syndrome, but it will manage the symptoms.

Estrogen Creams for the Prevention of Urinary Tract Infections

One of the more direct benefits of vaginal estrogen cream that is not seen with oral therapy is in the prevention of urinary tract infections. Estrogens are helpful in replenishing the supply of lactobacilli in the vagina. Good bacteria, lactobacilli, balance the vaginal flora and prevent bladder infections. Postmenopausal women have a paucity of lactobacilli in their vaginas because the vaginal pH is too high to maintain them. Vaginal estrogen will lower the vaginal pH, making the vagina more acidic, allowing the lactobacilli to grow. Continued use of vaginal estrogen on a twice-weekly basis is all that is needed to continue to foster lactobacilli growth. Any active urinary tract infection needs to be treated with antibiotics. But for prevention, vaginal estrogen can be effective.

The Use of Hormones in the Treatment of Urinary Incontinence

Urge Urinary Incontinence

Estrogen replacement alone, of any kind—vaginal, oral, or the patch—is not going to manage or cure urinary incontinence. No placebo-controlled trials have been done to look at the relationship between incontinence and estrogen therapy; however, the studies that have been done do not support the use of estrogen alone for the treatment or control of any type of incontinence. The logic behind the use of estrogen as *part* of the management of incontinence lies with the observation that incontinence clearly worsens with age and occurs in postmenopausal women at a higher rate than in premenopausal women. Because incontinence occurs more frequently in older women, and older women have considerably lower levels of estrogen, then there must be a relationship between estrogen production and incontinence. I would agree that a relationship exists; I just don't know how direct it is. Other treatments for incontinence are better than estrogen replacement alone. Therefore, I never prescribe estrogen alone for the treatment of incontinence, especially in light of the new information we have on the risks of estrogen replacement.

Urge incontinence is the loss of urine that is accompanied by a strong desire to urinate. This type of incontinence is treated with medications that relax the bladder and allow it to hold higher volumes of urine before expulsion. Urge incontinence is seen in postmenopausal women. It is part the effect that aging has on the bladder. Local estrogen applied vaginally can be used in combination with bladder medications to help control the leakage. Many of you with urge incontinence suffer from vaginal atrophy in addition to urgency and urge incontinence. The supplemental estrogen can help with the vaginal changes as well.

Stress Urinary Incontinence

Local estrogen may cause changes to the anatomy of the urethra and the bladder that some physicians think may indicate their usage in the treatment of stress urinary incontinence. Estrogen replacement may induce scar formation in the tissues around the bladder and the urethra. The scarring will strengthen the ligaments around the urethra, preventing the mobility that leads to stress incontinence (the leakage associated with movement and coughing). Estrogen may also increase the blood supply to the tissues below the urethra. The increased blood supply should bulk up the tissues and allow the walls to close better during movement. Progesterone receptors have not been identified in the bladder or the urethra; therefore, progesterone is not used to treat or augment treatment of urinary incontinence. Although the theories sound good, using estrogen, orally or as a cream, will not improve stress incontinence to any noticeable degree. I don't advocate its use for this problem.

In summary, estrogen therapy alone of any kind will not manage urinary symptoms in the postmenopausal woman. If local estrogen therapy is used, it must be accompanied with another medication to control the symptoms of urinary frequency, urgency, and incontinence. Many women with urinary incontinence also suffer from vaginal atrophy. Local estrogen therapy will treat vaginal atrophy and may augment the medication that is being used to treat the bladder symptoms.

Contraindications to the Use of Estrogen

There are a number of reasons why a woman cannot take oral estrogen tablets. Advanced breast or uterine cancer, recurrent blood clots in the legs, unevaluated uterine bleeding, and a history of severe liver disease are the absolute reasons why a woman cannot take oral estrogen. Other disorders that may be aggravated by the use of estrogen by mouth include uterine fibroids, endometriosis, history of gallstones, history of migraine headaches, high triglycerides in the blood (related to cholesterol), and a history of blood clotting during pregnancy. Before starting estrogen, if you have of these conditions, you must discuss this with your doctor. Estrogen can be used if any of these disorders are present as long as the physician is monitoring you carefully.

Women who have been diagnosed with breast cancer should not take estrogen of any kind without consulting with a physician. Many breast cancer survivors can take vaginally applied estrogen; however, this must be done under a physician's supervision. Although vaginal estrogens are safe, there are cases in which physicians do not want their patients on any sort of hormone replacement.

Progestins can also produce side effects. If you are put on an oral estrogen and progesterone combination pill, you may experience side effects from the progestin component of the tablet. These side effects include headaches, fatigue, depression, bloating, menstrual cramps, and bleeding.

SUMMARY

The role of hormones in urinary tract disorders remains confusing, even for those of us in the business of providing care and counsel to patients. The Women's Health Initiative Study made it clear that oral estrogen has risks and should not be prescribed without a clear reason. On an individual basis, educated decisions can be made between you and your doctor, depending on what menopausal symptoms you need to treat. Hormone depletion causes changes in the urinary tract, especially the urethra. Visible changes to the vaginal canal correspond to the symptoms that many of you may experience from low estrogen, including dryness, itching, and burning in the vagina and the urethral area. Vaginal applications of estrogen will help these symptoms while causing very few side effects. Systemic estrogen has a less clearly defined role in the treatment of urinary tract disorders in the postmenopausal woman. In terms of urinary leakage, estrogen therapy alone will not treat the problem. However, combination therapy of vaginal estrogen and a bladder medication may alleviate symptoms more than either would alone.

CHAPTER 11

Anesthesia for Surgery and a Crash Course in Pain Medications

J. knows that she needs surgery to correct her pelvic-floor prolapse and incontinence problem. We have been discussing it for months. Surprisingly, she has little anxiety about the operation. She feels confident in the surgery, but she is very nervous about the anesthesia. She has had other surgeries, but they were when she was much younger. After her last operation, she awoke nauseated and feeling terrible. She developed a rash from one of the medications that was administered. It took her weeks to recover. Now she is 30 years older, so her fears are even greater.

During our discussions about the operation, I had mentioned that she could opt for either total anesthesia or an epidural. Total anesthesia means that she would go to sleep using gases and intravenous medications. Spinal or epidural would numb her body from the waist down. She would be in a twilight state during the surgery. She had no idea which was better. These were not decisions that she was interested in making. I told her that she would have the opportunity to discuss the options with the anesthesiologist on the day of the operation. Although the day of the operation did not seem to be the optimal time to make such an important decision, I reassured her that I would be present during the discussion to give her some help. She was relieved.

One week before the operation, her family doctor did blood work and took an EKG and a chest x-ray. This medical clearance is done to be sure that she does not have any abnormalities that could interfere with the anesthesia. She received a clean bill of health and was all ready to go. J. asked her family doctor what he recommended in terms of anes-

thesia, but he suggested that she discuss that with the professionals who know the most about it. She was cleared for either a general anesthetic or a spinal/epidural.

On the day of the operation, J. and her husband arrived two hours before the scheduled start time. She changed into a hospital gown and answered innumerable questions about her health history, her allergies, and when she last ate or drank anything. Finally, she went to the bathroom, her glasses were removed and put with her clothes, and she was wheeled into the preoperative holding area. Now, she would meet the anesthesiologist, the person who was going to keep her alive during the surgery!

A pleasant, young doctor, dressed in operating room regalia, introduced herself. While she reviewed the chart, she asked the same questions that the nurses had asked her upon her arrival. Then, she began to discuss the anesthesia options for the type of surgery that J. was about to have. Basically, she said that both were safe and effective. J. and I both thought the spinal approach would be better for her. It involved less medication injected into her system, so the risk of nausea was lower. Plus with the spinal, she would have some numbness after the surgery which would help with pain control. J. did not want to be in pain. She signed the consent with the knowledge that if the anesthesiologist was unable to deliver a spinal anesthetic, then general anesthesia can be induced. As long as J. was unaware of the operation, she was happy with that choice.

The spinal anesthesia was administered without any difficulty. After numbing her legs within seconds, J. was sedated and fell asleep. The surgery transpired uneventfully. When she awoke, she was in the recovery room and had no recollection of having ever entered the operating room. Her legs were numb, which was a strange but welcome sensation under the circumstances. A catheter was in her bladder draining urine, so she did not need to use the bathroom. Since she could not walk, that would have been a serious problem!

Over the course of the next few hours, J.'s legs began to come back to life. She felt hot and cold, and finally pinprick sensation. By dinnertime, she was sitting in a chair and eating. She could walk with assistance, mostly because of the soreness from the surgery, and not from the weakness in her legs. That was pretty much gone.

By the next morning, the pain in her pelvis was present, but not horrible. Clearly, the spinal anesthesia has worn off completely. The nurses gave her pain medication by mouth, which nearly bowled her

over. She felt drunk, her mouth was dry, and she was terribly consti-
pated. She slept most of the day and tried to stay off of the painkillers,
but she needed something to relieve her discomfort. Tylenol was not
doing the trick, but she hated the sensation that the other pills brought
on.

She called me from the hospital to ask me to change her
medication, if I could. I ordered a different injection, Toradol®, that
would take the edge off without making her feel so sick. It could only
be taken for three days because it can affect the kidneys. Great—if
its not one thing, it's another. I reassured her that her pain would be
greatly diminished by then and the medication issues will not be a
problem.

After the catheter was removed, J. urinated and went home. She
took a prescription for a milder narcotic pain medication home with her
just in case she needed it. Although the side effects of the medication are
unpleasant, being in pain is worse. Fortunately, she only needed one pill
before bedtime, and that was only necessary for the first few days at
home.

Overall, J. was very pleased with her experience. She is dry, her
prolapse is repaired, and she did not have any bad reactions to the
anesthesia. It did take a few weeks to recover completely from the
operation. She thought that she would bounce back more quickly, but
her body just doesn't have the reserve that it used to have. Now, she
wonders why it took her so long to do this in the first place!

Most people make the decision to undergo elective surgery with trepida-
tion. Confidence in the surgeon helps allay one's fears, while successful outcomes in friends and relatives confirm the choice. However, the risks of
anesthesia rarely come into play when the options are discussed. With media
awareness of the potential problems from anesthesia, people are becoming
more and more cognizant of how critical this part of the surgical procedure
actually is. This chapter is essential for inclusion in any book that discusses
surgery. The two disciplines, surgery and anesthesia, cannot be separated. If
one is to have surgery, anesthesia will be required. The following discussion
is not exhaustive. It is only meant to guide you through the various aspects
of anesthesia and help sort out the choices that will be offered. Pain management follows any surgery. Educated decisions regarding both anesthesia
and postoperative pain management can help turn a frightening experience
into a rewarding outcome.

GOALS OF ANESTHESIA DURING SURGERY

Anesthesia: Sleepiness
Analgesia: Painlessness
Amnesia: Forgetfulness

Anesthesiology is the general term that is used to refer to the discipline of managing the patient during the operation so that the surgeon can attend to his work. It did not evolve into a separate medical specialty until the 1930s. Today, it is regarded as one of the most complicated and important areas of expertise. The anesthesiologist is responsible for getting the patient comfortable, keeping her comfortable, and maintaining proper organ function during the operation. He is also expected to keep the patient from moving under all circumstances so that the operative field sits like a canvas for the surgeon to do his work. Postoperative pain management has now fallen under the domain of anesthesia, with specialized training incorporated into most residency programs.

Three main aspects to intraoperative care fall under the domain of the anesthesiologist. They include anesthesia, analgesia, and amnesia. Anesthesia refers to the art of putting the patient to sleep, either with gases or intravenous medications. Analgesia refers to the avoidance of pain during the surgery. Amnesia refers to the lack of memory regarding the events surrounding the operation. Successful anesthesia involves sleepiness, lack of pain, and little memory of the operating room. The following discussion encompasses how the anesthesiologist is able to accomplish these goals. Intravenous medications for the induction of anesthesia, muscle relaxation, and pain control are discussed. Then, the gases that are employed to maintain anesthesia are reviewed. Spinal and epidural methods of operative management are mentioned. Finally, a discussion of the postoperative pain management completes the chapter.

Adequate preparation for surgery, both psychological and physical, will help ensure a positive outcome. Even the most common and minimally invasive surgery will induce a stress response in your body. The incision, itself, will cause the body to release stress hormones that will increase the heart rate, raise the blood pressure, reduce intestinal motility, and fatigue you. Surgeries that involve vital organs, like the bladder, or that involve large incisions, like in the vagina, produce greater reactions in your body. Even if the incisions cannot be seen, as is the case in vaginal surgery, the body "knows" that something has violated it, and the stress hormones will flood the system. On top of this response, immobility, semi-starvation for a day or two, sleep disturbances, and pain will all weaken the system and tax the heartiest of people. No surgery is small, especially if it is being done on your body.

For these reasons, optimization of all organ systems should precede the operation. Each hospital has its own set of rules regarding surgical clearance. Each patient has her own medical profile that will dictate what testing is required. If the surgeon or the anesthesiologist asks you to see a specialist for any reason, or to get a lab test for any reason, it is in your best interest to do as you are advised. Being overcautious never hurt anyone. The more information that the surgeon and the anesthesiologist have, the more prepared they will be for the unexpected, should the unexpected occur. That is not to say that every woman needs an exhaustive workup. It just means that recommended testing should be followed up.

Once it is determined that you are in a safe condition for surgery, you are instructed not to eat or drink any fluids from midnight the night before the operation. That means no water, no coffee, not anything. If medications are taken on a regular basis, instructions will be given regarding how and when those medications can be taken on the morning of the operation. When in doubt, ask your doctor or don't take the medication. Forgotten medications can always be taken at the hospital, especially if the pills are brought with you. If a mistake is made and you ingest some water or toast or something, let the nurses or the anesthesiologist know. They must make special provisions in the anesthesia to account for food in the stomach. No aspirin or ibuprofen should be taken one week prior to surgery.

Special holding areas are designated in most hospitals where patients go immediately before the operation. The anesthesiologist will introduce himself at this time and discuss the options for anesthesia. Unlike surgeons, anesthesiologists do not have separate offices away from the hospital. They come attached to the hospital or the surgical center. Many surgeons work with specific anesthesiologists whom they have gotten to know through experience. In other situations, the surgeon will work with which ever anesthesiologist is assigned to his room that day. Because the anesthesiologist does not know whom he will be caring for on a given day, he meets his patients in the holding area before the surgery.

Not all anesthesia caregivers are physicians. Nurses can deliver anesthesia if they get special training beyond their four-year registered nurse degree. Nurses who deliver anesthesia are called nurse anesthetists. They work under the direction of a physician, but they function independently during the operation. Most nurse anesthetists are excellent at what they do. Experience, good training, and adequate supervision ensure that equally good care comes from a nurse anesthetist as from a physician.

Finally, it is time to enter the operating room. Some anesthesiologists will give you a sedative before you go into surgery, especially if you are particularly anxious. That is an individual choice. Regardless, once everything is over, very few of you will actually remember entering the operating room. The medications that are given to induce sleep also induce forgetfulness for the short time immediately before surgery and immediately after. Most people only remember being wheeled into the operating room and waking up in recovery. So, what goes on in between? Read on.

INTRAVENOUS MEDICATIONS: DRIFTING OFF TO SLEEP

INTRAVENOUS MEDICATIONS

- Begin anesthesia
- Maintain relaxation
- Pain control

As soon as you enter the operating room, you are placed on the operating room table, which is narrow and hard. Warm blankets are supplied because the room is cool for maintenance of the machinery and the comfort of the surgeons who are draped in layers of sterile clothing. All of the operating room staff is covered in hats, shoe covers, and masks to prevent the spread of infection. Monitors are placed on your chest for measuring vital signs. An oxygen monitor is clipped to your finger, and a blood pressure cuff is placed around your upper arm.

An intravenous line is placed in your opposite arm or hand. The reason for this direct access into the bloodstream is to inject medications for many different functions. Intravenous fluids can be given this way, as well, in order to replace the liquid and the electrolytes that have been lost from not eating or drinking prior to surgery.

If general anesthesia is going to be induced, intravenous sedatives are used to begin the anesthesia. The gases that are breathed in are extremely irritating, smell bad, and can cause agitation. In response, the blood pressure and heart rate can rise, leading to risks to the cardiovascular system. You will not experience any of these sensations because you are first sedated heavily with one of numerous agents that will dampen the effect of the gas. These intravenous sedating medications are called induction agents. They prepare you for the inhalation of the gas which will ultimately maintain sleep.

In 1872 the first induction agent was introduced for use in the operating room. It was chloral hydrate, which has a quick onset and is still used in pediatric surgery. In 1903 barbiturates were found to depress the vital functions through depressing the brainstem. They have a quick onset and short duration of action, so they can be controlled easily. Thiopental, a barbiturate, is one of the common induction agents still used today.

BEGINNING ANESTHESIA: INDUCTION AGENTS

- Chloral hydrate
- Barbiturates
  Phenobarbital
- Opioids/narcotics
  Morphine
  Fentanyl
- Benzodiazepines
  Diazepam (Valium)
  Lorazepam (Ativan)
  Midazolam (Versed)
- Ketamine
- Etomidate
- Propofol

First isolated from the opium poppy in 1805, morphine was not used medically until 1916 when it was found to be useful in both sedation and pain relief during surgery. The first synthetic form of morphine, meperidine, was developed in 1939. Fentanyl, sufentanyl, and alfentayl are the newer synthetic opioids that are used today. They are inexpensive to produce, have a short onset of action, and provide excellent pain relief. They block pain activity in the brain, the spinal cord, and in the distant organs. However, they do not provide strong sedative action. Benzodiazepines, which include diazepam, lorazepam, and midazolam, offer greater sedative qualities with less pain relief than the opioids. They suppress the function of the cerebral cortex, which controls conscious awareness. The combination of an opioid and a benzodiazepine offers enough sedation and pain relief to perform many procedures, such as colonoscopy. For major operations, they are not powerful enough to insure immobility and proper control of the vital organs, so gases are used to maintain anesthesia. These two medications are very useful in helping you to relax and allowing you to enter general anesthesia with good control.

Ketamine was synthesized in 1962 specifically for help in inducing anesthesia. The patient would become unaware of her surroundings, but would still be breathing, swallowing, and moving as if she were awake. This dissociative state would allow for protection of the patient's breathing until the gas could be administered and a tube could be inserted into the windpipe. It is no longer used because it causes people to hallucinate. It is sold on the black market as PCP or angel dust.

Synthesized in 1972, etomidate suppresses the stress response to anesthesia. It causes problems with the adrenal glands, so it is not used very often any more. Propofol is a newer agent that has become one of the main sedating medications for use today. It is unclear exactly how it works, but it has a quick onset, causes a sleep-like state, and does not have the postoperative hangover-like effect that opioid narcotics do. Short procedures can be done with propofol alone. The major drawback is the burning it produces as it goes into the vein.

The point of mentioning all of these medications is to reinforce the complexity of the anesthesia. Many different medications will be given, so allergies, reactions to medications, and bad prior experiences with anesthesia or pain medications need to be shared with your physicians. If someone has some idea of what the categories of medications that will be given are, perhaps she will be able to remember adverse reactions better. Once you are asleep, you now have be paralyzed so that you can be positioned and absolutely still for the surgeon to work.

Paralysis during surgery strikes most people as a terrifying reality. "What if I am aware of everything that is going on, but I cannot move and I cannot communicate?" This is a fear that I hear from a lot of women. Fortunately, this fear is not a reality because the stress induced by such a situation would result in elevation of blood pressure and heart rate, which are picked up by the monitors. The first sign that the sedation is wearing off is an elevation of the vital signs. Buzzers go off and the anesthesiologist is alerted. Either the gas is turned up or more sedation is given. You will not wake up and become conscious during surgery.

MAINTAIN RELAXATION: MUSCLE RELAXANTS

Curare
Succinylcholine
Vecuronium
Pancuronium

Paralytic agents offer two benefits. If general anesthesia using a breathing tube is indicated, the muscle relaxant will allow the anesthesiologist to insert the tube without traumatizing your windpipe. The second function is for relaxation during surgery. The sedatives and gases may offer some relaxation, but if more is needed, other agents are available. Vaginal surgery usually does not require muscle relaxants in order to perform the operation, but, if necessary, they can be used.

In 1942, curare, a poison found in nature, was noted to provide relaxation during intubation and abdominal surgery. Lower doses of gas and sedatives could be given if a muscle relaxant was included in the cocktail. In 1949, succinylcholine was synthesized and is still the standard agent used today. It takes effect within 30 to 60 seconds and provides profound muscle relaxation. Approximately 10 other paralytic agents are available for use today.

Pain control during anesthesia is done using morphine and its derivatives. No other medications has been developed that controls pain better than narcotics. Morphine is a natural product whose active ingredient can now be synthesized. The manufactured formulations aim to reduce the side effects of morphine while capturing its benefits. The section on postoperative pain control addresses the options that are available. Intraoperatively, morphine, Demerol®, and fentanyl are still the most common intravenous agents that are used.

Finally, most surgeons request that the anesthesiologist inject intravenous antibiotics before the incision is made. Infections can be prevented by giving a single dose of a broad-spectrum agent 20 minutes before the surgery is to begin. If synthetic materials are used in vaginal surgery, this step is particularly important in minimizing postoperative complications.

INHALATION AGENTS: MAINTENANCE OF SLEEP WITH GAS

General anesthesia refers to the use of gas to keep you asleep. Breathing can be done on your own with the gas delivered through a mask, or a tube can be inserted down the windpipe and the gas inspired through a machine that delivers it at a given pressure. Gases diffuse into the bloodstream directly through the lungs. The body does not change the gas before the agent circulates into the brain and affects the conscious state. The anesthesiologist has tight control over of the amount of material getting into the system, so that limited doses can be given. Adjusting the dose of the inhalation agent will allow the anesthesiologist to give the surgeon the proper balance of relaxation and responsiveness.

Applied in the operating room in 1842, the first gases to be used in general anesthesia were ether, nitrous oxide, and chloroform. Highly combustible, ether and chloroform are not longer used. They have been replaced with newer agents that cause fewer side effects, are less irritating to the lungs, and are easily stored in the hospital. The gases that are used today include halothane (FDA approved in 1956), methoxyflurane (approved in 1960), enflurane (approved in 1973), isoflurane (approved in 1981), desflurane, and sevoflurane. Nitrous oxide is a colorless, odorless, natural gas. It causes relaxation and anesthesia and is totally eliminated through the lungs and the skin. It will not cause liver or kidney damage. The problems with nitrous oxide are that it is highly combustible and it causes bowel distention. Its explosive nature makes it difficult to store, and the bowel distention precludes its use in intestinal surgeries. It is still widely used.

Unlike nitrous oxide, halothane gas is not explosive. A synthetically produced air, it is broken down by the liver. Halothane is no longer used because of its potential toxic effects on the liver. Also a noncombustible, synthetic gas, methoxyflurane is cleared through the kidneys, where active metabolites are released. The sweet, fruity odor makes it more pleasant for you to inhale. Enflurane and isoflurane are safe agents that are well tolerated. The newest agents available, desflurane and sevoflurane, have a very quick awakening time. They are more potent than nitrous oxide, but less potent than the others. Deep anesthesia can be achieved effectively with awakening that takes half the time of the others.

Complications from general anesthesia are rare. The most common problem is pneumonia, which is usually only seen in people with risk factors preoperatively. Fever, cough, or difficulty breathing before the operation usually requires delaying the procedure until these symptoms pass because they can lead to postoperative pneumonia. Intense reactions to the gases can happen, but generally, people are not allergic to the agents that are commonly used. Blood pressure elevation indicates sensitivity to the gas, but this can be controlled with medication. The beauty of anesthesia is that the anesthesiologist has control over the cardiovascular system, so he can adjust the gases to respond to your vital signs: your heart rate and blood pressure.

If he cannot balance proper anesthesia with blood pressure and heart rate, he can always inject medications to protect the heart and brain.

Post-awakening nausea and vomiting are common. Temporary disorientation and loss of bowel and bladder function occasionally happen. Sore throat from the tubes that are used to protect the windpipe may be annoying for a few days. Seldom, the vocal cords can be injured, causing temporary paralysis. This is manifested by hoarseness. Sometimes evaluation and treatment by an ear, nose, and throat doctor will need to be sought. As with all medical situations, elderly people do not tolerate anesthesia as well as younger ones. Temporary brain injury from the toxic effects of the gases and intravenous medications may take days or weeks from which to recover. Great advances have been made in reducing the amount of medication that needs to be given and the duration of their actions, so that elderly people recover more quickly. Surgery has never been safer than it is now, thanks to progress with anesthesia.

SPINAL AND EPIDURAL ANESTHESIA

Regional anesthesia refers to the numbing of the area on which the surgery is being done while the rest of the body remains sensate. Spinal and epidural anesthesia fall under this definition, as do topical agents that go on the skin, and local nerve blocks that only affect a very small part of the anatomy, such as the finger or the groin. The first regional anesthetic to be used was cocaine in 1884, approximately 30 years after being isolated from the cocoa plant. The hypodermic needle came into use in 1855, and the first spinal block is attributed to August Bier in 1898. We now have over nine medications that can be injected into the spinal cord for use during surgical procedures, including procaine, tetracaine, lidocaine, bupivicaine, and narcotics. Advances in technique and instrumentation as well as more tightly controlled medications have broadened the appeal of spinal and epidural anesthesia, especially in pelvic and vaginal surgery.

Spinal and epidural anesthesia are very similar. The differences have more to do with where the medication is injected and how it is infused than with how you are affected. Spinal anesthesia means that the medication is injected into the spinal canal, which houses the nerves that supply the torso and limbs. Epidural anesthesia involves placing the drug outside of the spinal canal and its coverings but inside the bony vertebrae. This tiny space can hold a thin tube through which medication can be delivered continuously. The medication will then diffuse across the dura, or the covering of the spinal cord, and into the nerves beneath it, numbing them. *Epi-* means

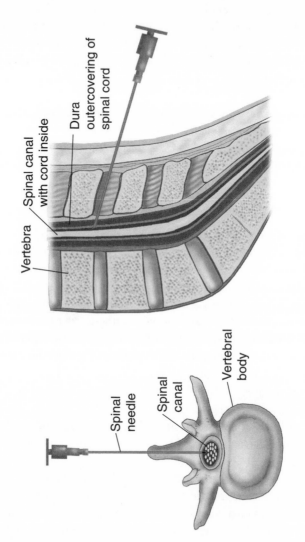

FIGURE 1. *Spinal Anesthesia.*

outside, and *dura* refers to the covering over the spinal cord. That is where the name *epidural* comes from.

The same medications can be used for both types of regional pain control. Spinal anesthesia usually involves a single injection that will last a given period of time. The time depends on how long- or short-acting the injected drug works. Once the spinal anesthetic wears off, either the operation should be over, or general anesthesia will need to be induced. Epidural anesthesia can continue long-term because the medication can be delivered through a catheter continuously. It can even be infused after surgery for postoperative pain control.

Prolapse repairs and incontinence surgery are usually done under spinal as opposed to epidural. These operations last for a predictable period of time and postoperative pain control with strong local drugs is not usually necessary. Pelvic surgery is particularly amenable to spinal anesthesia because the operative area is very low on the body. The nerves that control breathing and other vital functions are not near the site of injection, so you can be numb and still be breathing on your own. A sedative is given at the time of the spinal anesthesia so that you are not aware of what is going on, but no breathing apparatus needs to be used. Less medication enters the system, so drug reactions, nausea, and disorientation are minimized. Elderly women do very well with spinal anesthesia as long as they do not have severe spine problems. Prior surgery and bad bones in the back will make inserting the spinal needle very difficult, if not impossible.

Not everyone is a candidate for spinal anesthesia. Absolute contraindications for spinal or epidural anesthesia include problems with blood clotting, infection in the skin over the site of the injection, and lack of consent on your part. Women with chronic low back pain, history of spinal surgery, severe anxiety, or nerve disorders in their feet should discuss these problems with the anesthesiologist before consenting to spinal pain control. Age does not preclude its use.

Spinal anesthesia has a bad reputation as potentially causing paralysis. This event has not been documented in and medical journals. However, complications from spinal anesthesia can occur. Most of them are minor, and they go away within a few days, at most. The most common complication is pain at the injection site on the lower back, which will go away by itself over time. Backaches can occur if the muscles surrounding the injection site go into spasm. Sometimes requiring physical therapy, this usually resolves within 10 to 14 days.

Spinal headache results if some of the fluid that bathes the spinal cord and brain seeps out of the injection site. You will notice the headache 6 to

12 hours after the spinal needle is inserted, feeling it when you first sit up after the operation. Young women are at the highest risk for the development of a spinal headache. It is treated with intravenous fluids and pain medication, such as acetomenophen (Tylenol) or narcotics. If that does not work, blood can be drawn from your arm and injected at the site. The blood clot will plug the hole and stop the leakage. Newer treatments include intravenous infusions of caffeine and other medication. Spinal headaches are uncommon since the size of the needles that are used are so tiny. Other problems from spinal anesthesia are very rare.

In order to have surgery, anesthesia is necessary. Obviously, if we could avoid exposing you to all of these medications, we would choose to. However, that is not the case. Poor anesthesia will result in cardiovascular compromise due to an overwhelming stress response, inadequate surgery due to movement on your part, and an unsatisfactory overall outcome. It is better to have good anesthesia and a good outcome, than no anesthesia and a poor outcome. Because so many elderly women are having operations, anesthesiologists are familiar with their fragile constitution. Fortunately, science and technology have allowed them to develop their craft with the growing elderly population.

POSTOPERATIVE PAIN MANAGEMENT

After surgery, the return to a normal activity level requires pain relief, adequate nutrition, and mobilization. Postoperative fatigue inhibits mobility and delays recovery. This fatigue is caused by the surgical injury itself, the lack of food around the time of the operation, and the loss of muscle tone. Unfortunately, pain medication will only help deal with the pain, not with the other aspects of recovery. People don't realize the degree to which surgery can upset one's biorhythms. Efforts to eat well, even if in small quantities, and to get out of bed, even if it is to sit in a chair, will help speed up recovery and also reduce the risk of embolisms or blood clots. Adequate pain management will help achieve a smooth postoperative course and promote healing.

The type of medication ingested is one aspect of pain management, which will be discussed in detail in this section. The other aspect is the method through which it is delivered. While still in the hospital, acute pain can be managed with intravenous injections, intramuscular injections, patient-controlled pain pumps, and epidural infusions. Intravenous injections directly enter the bloodstream through an access that is placed during the surgery. The nurse on the floor or in the recovery room gives the injection based on your needs. Although it is an effective method of relieving pain, intravenous injections require busy, skilled nurses to deliver the medication, which can delay relief. Intramuscular injections do not require an intravenous line because the needle is inserted into the arm, the leg, or the buttock muscle. The medication diffuses into the bloodstream slowly, delaying pain relief but delivering a slow steady dose of the drug. Again, skilled staff must administer the injection.

First proposed over 25 years ago, patient-controlled anesthesia (PCA) allows you to give yourself intravenous infusions of pain medication when you need it, as opposed to waiting for the nurse to inject it. The pump is attached to a bag of a liquid narcotic which is connected to the intravenous line. A low dose of medication is steadily infused to give a baseline level of pain control. For extra relief, you can push the button and an extra dose of the drug will be delivered. The machine is set to limit the amount of medication that is delivered each time and to pause for five or eight minutes or so between injections. You will receive less medication using a patient-controlled anesthesia pump because you feel more secure. If you are worried about getting the medication from a health-care worker, you will tend to ask sooner, more often, and for more each time. If you can control the dosing, you will use only the absolute limited amount that you need.

Epidural infusions of pain medication are effective because narcotics can be avoided. Local anesthetics, like lidocaine, can be continuously infused through a pump to relieve pain. The problem with epidural pain relief is that you are not very mobile because you need to lie down regularly in order to get an adequate level of relief. Short-term use of epidurals can be helpful, especially if epidural anesthesia is used during the surgery. Once discharged from the hospital, most women are prescribed oral pain relievers.

Besides the route of administration, the type of medication must be determined. The mainstay of postoperative pain control is narcotic medication. Morphine was the first narcotic to be identified, and it is still a commonly used and highly effective pain reliever. Many different formulations of narcotics based on the morphine molecule are now available, some of which are mixed with acetaminophen, aspirin, or ibuprofen. The combination of drugs can act synergistically, helping one another to work better while reducing the side effects of each one. Regardless of the route of administration (intravenous, intramuscular, epidural, or oral), narcotics can cause nausea, vomiting, constipation, urinary retention, itching, and sedation.

In response to the difficulties produced by narcotic painkillers, a new category of pain medication has been developed that offers an alternative to narcotics. Called cox-2 inhibitors, these medicines fall into the category of nonsteroidal antiinflammatory drugs (NSAIDS). These agents inhibit the inflammatory pathway that is set off by an enzyme called cyclo-oxygenase 2 (cox-2). Cyclo-oxygenase 1 is a similar enzyme that protects the stomach lining and kidney function. The cox-2 inhibitors do not interfere with cyclo-oxygenase 1. Cox-2 inhibitors reduce inflammation, relieve pain, and lower fevers. They do not cause nausea, vomiting, constipation, sedation, or itching. However, they do not relieve pain nearly as effectively as narcotics. For this reason, they are not used for acute postoperative pain. They are better off being used for outpatient oral pain relief. There is one NSAID that is used intravenously in the hospital for acute pain. It is called ketoralac (Toradol). It can only be used for three days because it can cause kidney failure. It is used for intravenous, intramuscular, and oral pain relief in the acute postoperative period.

The market is now flooded with different pills to help manage pain. No magic bullet has yet been discovered, but with all of the choices out there, something will help you get through those first few days of surgery when you need relief. Most of the time, a few days of oral pain pills will suffice. Some women take longer to heal. Some of you may still be using the medications for a few weeks postoperatively, especially at night. Good pain management will certainly help speed up the return to your activities of daily living.

The accompanying tables list the most commonly used postoperative pain medications and the routes through which they can be administered. Except for a few drugs, pain medications fall into two main categories: narcotics (also called opioids) and nonsteroidal antiinflammatory drugs (NSAID). Both groups have formulations that can be given intravenously, intramuscularly, through an epidural catheter, and orally.

Narcotic Pain Medications

Generic Name	Trade Name	Route of Administration
Codeine		Oral, intramuscular
Codeine + acetomenophen	Tylenol #3	Oral
Fentanyl	Duragesic	Patch
Fentanyl citrate	Actiq	Oral
Hydrocodone + ibuprofen	Vicoprofen	Oral
Hydrocodone + acetomenophen	Lortab	Oral
	Maxidone	Oral
	Vicodin	Oral

Narcotic Pain Medications—continued

Generic Name	Trade Name	Route of Administration
Hydromorphone	Dilaudid	Oral, intramuscular, intravenous
Levophenol	Levo-Dromoran	Oral, intramuscular, intravenous
Meperidine	Demerol	Oral, intramuscular, intravenous
Meperidine + promethazine	Mepergan	Intramuscular, intravenous
	Mepergan Fortis	Oral
Methadone	Dolophine	Oral, intramuscular
Morphine	Astramorph	Intravenous, epidural
	Duramorph	Intravenous, epidural
	Avinza	Oral
	Kadian	Oral
	MS Contin	Oral
	Oramorph	Oral
Morphine sulfate	MSIR	Oral, intramuscular, intravenous
Oxycodone	Oxycontin	Oral
	Oxyfast	Oral
	Roxycodone	Oral
	OxyIR	Oral
Oxycodone + acetomenophen	Percocet	Oral
	Roxicet	Oral
	Tylox	Oral
Oxycodone + aspirin	Percodan	Oral
	Endodan	Oral
Pentazocine + aspirin	Talwin	Oral
Pentazocine + naloxone	Talwin NX	Oral
Propoxyphene napsylate	Darvon	Oral
Propoxyphene + aspirin	Darvocet N	Oral

Nonnarcotic Pain Medications

Generic Name	Trade Name	Route of Administration
Celecoxib	Celebrex	Oral
Diclofenac	Cataflam	Oral
	Voltaren	Oral
Diclofenac + misoprostol	Arthrotec	Oral
Diflusinal	Dolobid	Oral
Etodolac	Lodine	Oral

Nonnarcotic Pain Medications—continued

Generic Name	Trade Name	Route of Administration
Fenoprofen	Nalfon	Oral
Flurbiprofen	Ansaid	Oral
Ibuprofen	Motrin	Oral
Indomethacin	Indocin	Oral
Ketoprofen	Orudis	Oral
	Oruvail	Oral
Ketorolac	Toredol	Oral, intramuscular, intravenous
Meclofenamate		Oral
Mefenamic acid	Ponstel	Oral
Meloxicam	Mobic	Oral
Nabumeone	Relafen	Oral
Naproxen	Naprosyn	Oral
	Anaprox	Oral
	Nalrelan	Oral
Oxaprozin	Daypro	Oral
Piroxicam	Feldene	Oral
Tolmetin	Tolectin	Oral
Valdecoxib	Bextra	Oral

Miscellaneous Pain Medications

Generic Name	Trade Name	Route of Administration
Acetomenophen	Tylenol	Oral
Gabapentin	Neurontin	Oral
Tramadol	Ultram	Oral
Tramadol + acetomenophen	Ultracet	Oral

Surgery has never been safer than it is today. In many respects, this fact is due to the advances in anesthesia. The medications are safer, the monitoring devices are more sensitive, and the anesthesiologists are more highly trained. Only recognized as a medical specialty since 1939, anesthesia has grown into a discipline with six areas of specialization, including cardiac anesthesia, critical care, neuroanesthesia, obstretics, pediatric anesthesia, and pain management. People are becoming more and more aware of the importance of anesthesia in the overall success of the operative experience. Safe anesthesia includes careful preoperative preparation, open disclosure of foods and medications ingested by you before surgery, and the selection of appropriate agents in the operating room.

Adequate postoperative pain management follows successful intraoperative anesthesia. The balance between effective pain control and reduced side-effects from the medications can be tricky. Trial and error will finally tease out the best choice. Because so many options are available, everyone should be able to find something that will relieve their discomfort without too many problems. Under the best circumstances, surgery is difficult; and the recovery trying. Patience, realistic expectations, and positive thinking always help expedite a speedy recovery. Confidence in the team that performs the surgery and the support staff that manages the perioperative course will ensure the best possible environment for a positive experience.

CHAPTER 12

A Visit to the Urologist's Office

Definitions and Explanations of the Diagnostic Procedures

L. has had recurrent urinary tract infections for a few months now. Mostly consulting with her gynecologist, her doctor has suggested that she see a urologist to get a handle on the problem. L. always thought that urologists treated men. She had never heard of women going to the urologist until her mother told L. about her own experience with a urologist many years ago.

L.'s mother, M., had a problem with infections when she was in her early 20s; just about the same age as her daughter is now. She went to a urologist who prescribed sulfa antibiotics on many different occasions. Eventually, the antibiotics stopped relieving her symptoms of frequency, urgency, and pain. He inserted catheters in an effort to get sterile urine specimens for culture and he put a scope into her bladder to evaluate the lining for abnormalities. The cultures were often negative. He told M. that her bladder wall was red, which was consistent with cystitis, or infections. She took more courses of antibiotics, without resolution of her problem.

Finally, the urologist suggested that she have her urethra dilated. Out of desperation, she consented to the office procedure. Metal rods were inserted into her urethra in gradually increasing sizes. Although it was painful, the dilatation seems to have worked. M. had no more infections for years. She agreed with the gynecologist: that L. should see a urologist, even though that would mean being poked and prodded. At least, she would get some answers, and perhaps, some respite from this chronic problem.

The idea of seeing a doctor who was going to insert metal devices into her bladder terrified L. She would rather get infections than go through what her mother described. Maybe she could go and talk to the doctor before he does anything invasive. Getting information about the treatment, perhaps with some medication to alleviate her anxiety before anything is done, would suffice for the first visit. L. had no idea what to expect. Should she call the urologist and ask what he is planning to do on the first visit? That seems silly since he doesn't even know her problem, so how could he tell her what he would do for her?

Urologists certainly have earned out reputation for inflicting pain on people. Not that a great deal of good does not come out of the procedures that we do, but the anxiety that both men and women suffer in anticipation of a urological exam cannot be understated. The purpose of this chapter is to take you through a routine office visit with a urologist to alleviate your apprehension and prepare you for what may lie ahead.

Before any discussion ensues, it must be emphasized that nothing should transpire between you and your physician without an explanation and some form of consent either written or verbal, from you. If the intentions of the doctor are not clear, then you or your family member should ask for clarification. There are very few things that we do in the office that cannot be described in plain English. If you do not speak English, then a translator may need to be present to be sure that the procedures to be done are clearly understood.

Nothing that we do now is that painful. In the past, the instruments that we used were much larger and more cumbersome. Technology has allowed for greater visual resolution with smaller scopes. Topical numbing agents offer local anesthesia to ease the pain and discomfort of many of our procedures. Some offices even employ anesthesiologists a few days per week to come in and help sedate people during more invasive procedures. In the area of female urology and urogynecology, I don't see a need for sedation during any of our tests. In most cases, you will need to cooperate during the test and that means you must be conscious, so sedation cannot be used.

In most urology and gynecology offices, you will be asked to give a urine specimen when you check in at the front desk. Because people who visit a urologist's office have urinary problems, the container is given immediately so that you can empty your bladder as soon as you get to the office, and you don't have to hold it. Sometimes, a wipe will be provided to insure a clean specimen. I do not use these in my office. You can urinate directly into the cup and we can make determinations based on those findings.

THE OFFICE VISIT

When you meet your doctor for the first time, the most comfortable environment is usually in a consultation room, sitting in a chair, and fully clothed. Not all physicians have their practices set up this way. If you prefer to meet the practitioner sitting up with your clothes on, let him or his staff know that when they ask you to undress and put on a gown before meeting him.

The first thing that happens is a lot of talk. He will want to hear what the problem is in your own words. Reports from other doctors may be helpful, but the real problem needs to be described by the person experiencing it, not a third party. Description of the pain, the frequency, the leakage, the getting up at night, the whatever, needs to be as accurately recorded as possible. Most doctors will prompt you with pointed questions to help get a clear picture of the problem. The better you can describe your symptoms, the more likely the doctor will be able to hone in on the problem. If it is an abnormal lab test that brings you to the doctor, a copy of the abnormal data should be brought to the visit in case the doctor's office did not receive a copy.

A list of medications that you are taking, as well as your allergies, can be provided to the practitioner. Past medical and surgical history will be discussed. Family history and social habits will round out the discussion.

Following a thorough history, the physician will bring you into an examination room. It is appropriate to ask what will transpire from this point. Usually, you will be asked to remove your clothes and cover yourself with a gown. When the examiner enters the room, he will wash his hands, don a pair of gloves, and begin the physical exam. A thorough urological exam includes evaluation of the abdomen and the pelvis. A pelvic exam is not only appropriate for a urologist to perform, but necessary, given that the urethra lies above the vagina. Masses, discharge, irritation, and weakening of the muscles can all be assessed through a simple examination. No instruments are needed. Rectal examination may be necessary as well. Generally, the doctor will warn you before he inserts his finger.

Some physicians will use a speculum to examine the vagina. Others will not. If there is a question regarding what is being done, just ask the doctor. He will explain why he is performing whatever is being done. Some urologists and gynecologists like to obtain catheterized specimens of urine in certain women. If there is a problem with urinary tract infections, or if the physician wants to measure the residual urine in the bladder *and* get a sterile sample, he will need to obtain a catheterized specimen. A small plastic tube is gently inserted into the urethra just far enough into the opening to drain the urine. That means it will only enter about 2 inches. A dab of anesthesia jelly can be placed on the tip of the catheter to ease the discomfort. The procedure is not painful if it is done with care. At most, it will smart for a second. Again, if the practitioner wants to do anything invasive, he should let you know before he does it. Warning you will take away 90% of the unpleasant sensation.

The urine sample that was given earlier will be analyzed on the spot. Blood, white blood cells, protein, and sugar can be detected if they are spilled into the urine. The pH and the presence of bacteria or bacterial byproducts may also be recorded. This evaluation is called the *urine analysis*. The urine analysis (also called urinalysis and u/a) is a quick way of getting information during the visit. The results can vary from day to day based on diet, fluid consumption, activity level, and medication use. Definitive testing follows all abnormal findings on the urine analysis, but clues to the source of a problem can be found in this two-minute office test.

After the examination is done, most doctors will have you get dressed and meet them in the consultation room to go over their findings so far. He will summarize the main complaint, review the findings on physical exam, and report on the urine analysis results. Further testing may be discussed at this point, or therapeutic intervention may be offered immediately.

OFFICE-BASED TESTS

If further testing is recommended, an explanation of the procedures that are needed should be offered. Any maneuver that involves inserting an instrument into the body is considered an invasive test. Invasive testing requires your understanding of the test and why it is being done. Before a test is started, ask the physician or his associate what information will be gained from the test that cannot be gained in some other way. The less manipulation of the body that is required, the better it is for you.

Most urology and urogynecology offices these days are equipped to do procedures. In the past, hospital admission and an overnight stay were required for many of the tests that now take less than a half an hour in the office. Some of the procedures that may be recommended are uncomfortable, but none of them are actually painful. If anything that is done is painful, a topical anesthetic should be offered before a procedure is undertaken.

PROCEDURES THAT CAN BE DONE IN THE OFFICE

Sonogram = ultrasound
Cystoscopy
Urethral catheterization
Urethral dilation
Bladder instillations
Clean intermittent catherization
X-rays
Urodynamics

Sonogram = Ultrasound

Sonograms (also known as ultrasound) can be done in the office. A sonogram is a radiological procedure in which a small wand is rubbed on the skin overlying the organ that needs to be studied. Seen on a monitor, an image of the organ in question can be analyzed by the trained eye. Used to define the picture, sound waves rely on the changes in the density of tissues in order to increase the resolution of the image. No radiation is used, so it is a safe medium under nearly all circumstances, including pregnancy.

In urology, ultrasound technology has been revolutionary. Fluid in the bladder and the kidneys can be seen easily. If a urologist wants to know if any fluid is sitting in the bladder, all he has to do is put the probe on the lower abdomen. No catheterization is required. Fluid, masses, and cysts in the kidneys can also be visualized. Ultrasound is a noninvasive method of getting information about internal organs without any danger, discomfort, or pain to you.

USE OF ULTRASOUND IN UROLOGY

Evaluate for post-void residual urine
Check the kidneys for stones and tumors

Ultrasound is used in women to check the **post-void residual** urine in the bladder. After you go to the bathroom and empty as much as you can, you are brought into the sonogram room and the probe is placed immediately above the pubic bone, underneath which sits the bladder. The amount of urine left over in the bladder after completing urination is called the post-void urine ("void" means to urinate) residual ("residual" means leftover). A circle is drawn over the oval shape that the bladder takes on when it is full of urine and the machine will calculate the volume in the oval. Some offices use a handheld ultrasound machine that can only be used for this purpose. Other offices have large free-standing machines that have different probes for other uses.

The kidneys can also be seen on ultrasound. Trained technicians will place a different probe over the upper back just below the ribs. A grainy image will appear on the monitor that is difficult to interpret without experience. Cysts, solid tumors, and blockages in the kidney can be visualized. Stones are sometimes difficult to identify because so many things look like stones. A large stone, one that is over half an inch in diameter, will be visualized fairly easily. Smaller stones are not so obvious.

Cystoscopy

Cystoscopy is the dreaded office procedure that so many people fear. Granted, it is not a pleasant experience, but it is tolerable, and can be made more so by a patient physician and staff. Cystoscopy is the process in which a long tube with a light at the tip is inserted into the bladder through the urethra in order to visualize the bladder lining. It would be comparable to looking at the inside of a balloon through the mouthpiece. The inside of the urethra and the urinary sphincter can be seen as well.

There are two main types of office cystoscope. One is a rigid scope; the other is a flexible scope. Most urologists now use flexible scopes because they are less traumatic and can be manipulated to see around corners and into pockets. The flexible scopes are the same diameter as the rigid scopes, but they seem to be more forgiving, and therefore, more comfortable for you. The optics of all of these instruments has improved dramatically. Because of fiberoptic technology, smaller-caliber sheaths allow for even better visual resolution than the larger ones of years ago. The brightness of the light will not fade as it travels down the long instrument, so even tiny lesions can be seen.

You lie on the examination table with your legs in stirrups. Some physicians will insert anesthesia-impregnated gel into the urethra and let it sit for a few minutes. The area through which the scope is to be inserted is wiped with cleaning solution on a cotton swab or a piece of gauze. The cystoscope is then connected to a light source, and tubing, through which water can be infused. The cystoscope is then inserted through the urethra which sits immediately above the vagina and below the clitoris. The urethra is 2 to 3 inches in length in women, but the scope looks like it is 3 feet long (it is about 18 inches long). That is because we use the same scopes for men and women. Men have longer urethras which can be made even longer by enlarged prostates and distended bladders. Women, sometimes get a little upset when they see this long instrument primed to be inserted into such a small area. But I reassure you, it only goes in a very short distance.

Once the scope is inserted, 3 to 4 ounces of water is drained into the bladder through the scope while the physician is looking around. The water will separate the folds in the walls behind which tumors can lurk. He can see the walls of the bladder as well as the ureteral orifices. These are the openings in the bladder that connect to the tubes that bring urine from each kidney into the bladder. These little openings (or orifices) squirt urine every 20 seconds or so from each kidney. If blood is coming from one kidney, it can sometimes be seen as that ureter drains urine. The scope needs to be manipulated to see all of the nooks and crannies in the bladder. Sometimes uncomfortable, this movement can put pressure on the muscles surrounding the urethra. The entire procedure takes about two minutes to complete.

You do not need to prepare for a cystoscopy. You come to the office as if you were coming for a routine visit, and you can go back to work or resume any usual activities. Unlike colonscopy, no sedation is administered. However, you should ask your physician at the time that you schedule the appointment whether or not he uses any sedation or anesthesia. Some offices do. Occasionally someone will ask me if they should take valium before coming in for the procedure. I do not encourage this because the effects of the valium far outlast the discomfort of the procedure. If a woman has tremendous anxiety, it will not detract from the performance of the test,

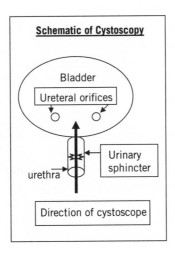

so she can take something without interfering with the procedure. If any sedating medication is going to be taken, you need to be accompanied by another adult who will be able to take you home. Under no circumstances should you drive a car while sedated.

After the cystoscopy, many physicians will give antibiotics to prevent infection. It is not absolutely necessary, and the length of treatment is not set in stone. Usually, anywhere for one tablet to three days of treatment is prescribed. Pyridium can be taken immediately after the scope is removed to help with the burning that may last for an hour or so afterward. A small clot may be seen in the toilet at the first urination after the procedure. Sometimes, a spot of blood can be seen on the toilet paper as well. This small amount of blood should not alarm you. If bleeding or burning persists, the physician should be notified. Most women feel normal by the time they leave the office after a cystoscopy.

INDICATIONS FOR CYSTOSCOPY

Blood in the urine
History of bladder tumor
Physician's discretion

Microscopic Blood in the Urine

Not every woman who sees a urologist will have an office cystoscopy, but many will. The only absolute indications for cystoscopy are a history of bladder tumor that is being followed for recurrence, and blood in the urine, either microscopic or obvious. That is not to say that every woman with blood in her urine will have a cystoscopy, but if it is persistent and does not go away with antibiotics, a urologist will do a cystoscopy. The need to see a urologist for blood in the urine will be determined by your internist. Once you get to the urologist, he will most likely want to look into your bladder at some point to evaluate for the blood in the urine.

Other reasons for cystoscopy depend on the physician doing the evaluation. Some doctors do cystoscopy routinely. They feel that the more information that they can get regarding the patient's anatomy, the more informed their recommendations for treatment will be. Other physicians only perform cystoscopy for specific reasons. Once the physician recommends a cystoscopy and explains why he is doing it, if it seems reasonable, there is no reason not to consent to it.

Urethral Catheterization

Compared with cystoscopy, urethral catheterization is a cake-walk. Urethral catheterization is when a small, pliable tube is inserted into the urethra to drain the bladder. "Catheter" is another word for a tube, implying a soft, plastic device. Although it is not usually painful, urethral catheterization should only be done if it is necessary since it is an invasive procedure. In other words, if the information can be obtained *without* inserting anything into the body, then the alternative should be done.

Urethral catheterization is performed for a number of reasons. The most common indication is to obtain a sterile sample of urine to test for infection. Contamination by vaginal flora can interfere with an accurate reading. Most of the time, the clean sample that you collect into a sterile cup is good enough, but, on rare occasions, a catheterized specimen will be needed. Another reason would be to get a fresh sample if blood is seen in the urine. Sometimes it is hard to tell if the microscopic blood is coming from the vagina or the bladder. Some urologists like to take a sample of urine directly from the bladder to see if the blood is still present. Finally, catheterized specimens can be done to measure the leftover urine after you urinate. If a fresh sample is needed, or not enough urine is obtained spontaneously to run various tests, the urologist can catheterize you and obtain the desired sample as well as measure the residual urine. Although the test is invasive, it accomplishes a number of things at one time.

INDICATIONS FOR URETHRAL CATHETERIZATION

Sterile sample for culture
Bladder sample for blood
Patient is unable to provide sample
Check for post-void residual
Urethral dilitation
Instillation of medication into the bladder
Self-catheterization for incomplete emptying

Inserting a catheter into the urethra is a simple, painless procedure if it is done carefully, using sterile technique. The vaginal area is swabbed with cleaning solution before a small, plastic tube with a hole on either end is inserted into the opening above the vagina. Tapered on one end, the tube slides easily into the opening. Lubrication helps. The urine drains into a container until the bladder empties. At the end, a small pinch may result as the bladder collapses around the end of the tube. The entire process takes less than a minute. If the practitioner prepares you for the procedure by alerting you to the steps as they are being done, the surprise factor is eliminated and very little discomfort will result.

Urethral Dilatation
Urethral dilatation involves inserting larger and larger caliber catheters into the urethra to stretch the opening. Metal rods are used that range from very small to very large. The idea is to improve the drainage of the bladder by widening the opening through which the urine drains. It is used in women who suffer from recurrent urinary tract infections and in women who urinate very frequently. They are told that their urethras are small and scarred. Women in both of these groups have small urethras that prevent the urine from draining efficiently when they go to the bathroom. Widening the opening will result in better drainage, fewer infections, and fewer visits to the bathroom.

Although the theory may sound good, there is no proof that it is true. First of all, women with recurrent bladder infections do not necessarily have elevated residual urine volumes after emptying their bladders. As a matter of fact, most women who get bladder infections have perfectly normal bladder function. Secondly, dilating the urethra does not improve emptying. If it helps, the effect lasts for a few days only. Most women who undergo urethral dilatation have the procedure repeated every three months because the results are so transient.

INDICATIONS FOR URETHRAL DILATATION

Recurrent urinary tract infections
Poor bladder emptying
Interstitial cystitis

A painful procedure that does not result in any noticeable improvement in a woman's condition should not be done. I do not think that there is a place for urethral dilatation at this time. Regardless of the size a woman's urethra on exam, every urethra can be stretched to accommodate an instrument. That does not mean that the urethra is too small for a woman's bladder. Perhaps someone will do a controlled study proving that it actually helps in some objective way. Until then, I do not advocate the use of urethral dilatation in the office.

Having said that, there are women who swear by its effectiveness. They are convinced that the dilatations have cured their urinary tract infections. My response to that is that the infections had run their course already by the time you got to the urologist. Had nothing been done, the results would have been the same. I am not necessarily right in refuting the efficacy of urethral dilatation, but I would like to see proof of its effectiveness before I will subject anyone to this painful procedure

Bladder Instillations

Bladder instillations refer to inserting medications into the bladder directly through a catheter. Different diseases can be treated by bathing the bladder wall with chemicals. The benefit of this method of directly delivering the treatment is that it prevents exposure of the entire system to the drugs, and it allows the drug to reach the bladder without being altered or diluted by the liver or the kidneys. After a small plastic tube is inserted into the urethra, the medication is pushed into the bladder with a syringe that is attached to the end of the tube. The medication will then sit in the bladder until you urinate.

The procedure is only as painful as the catheterization. Sometimes the medication will sting a little bit as it is infused, but usually you notice a sensation. Bladder instillations are used to treat certain types of bladder cancer as well as interstitial cystitis. Rarely, antibiotics are inserted directly into the bladder to treat difficult urinary tract infections. Trials infusing different medications are underway for a variety of different diseases, including overactive bladder.

INDICATIONS FOR BLADDER INSTILLATIONS

Interstitial cystitis
Bladder cancer
Urinary tract infections—rarely

Clean Intermittent Catheterization

Women can be taught to catheterize themselves. Once you understand your anatomy, nearly everyone can learn how to insert the catheter into your urethra. When a woman is told that she can be taught to catheterize herself, the response is nearly always, "no way." I tell women that it is analogous to putting contact lenses in your eyes. The idea of touching your eyeballs with your bare hands sounds unmanageable. But once the skill is mastered, the lenses can be popped in nearly anywhere. Catheterizing is similar in that once you master the skill you can do it in a public bathroom.

Self-catheterizing is done for poor bladder emptying. If a woman cannot empty her bladder well on her own, she may need to learn to drain the residual by inserting the catheter at regular intervals. High volumes of residual urine left in the bladder can cause urinary tract infections, worsening of bladder function, and, in long-standing cases, kidney compromise. Self-catheterization can prevent all of these problems.

INDICATIONS FOR CLEAN INTERMITTENT CATHETERIZATION

Incomplete emptying
Instillation of medication directly into the bladder

Many women are concerned that inserting a catheter regularly can cause recurrent bladder infections. On the contrary, regular bladder drainage will prevent the buildup of stagnant urine. Clean, not sterile, technique is all that is needed to ensure safe drainage. The catheter gets rinsed off in warm water and inserted into urethra with clean hands. No gloves are needed. Some women boil the catheters or use new sterile ones each time. These safeguards are not necessary. Every woman who learns to catheterize herself will introduce bacteria no matter how careful she is. Colonization is not the same as infection. Infection implies pain, burning, leakage, foul odor, and fever. Colonization just means that the bladder has bacteria in it but no inflammatory reaction has ensued.

Bladder catheterization for drainage and instillation of medications can be done fairly painlessly by a caring, patient practitioner. For the proper indication and with the right attitude on the part of the physician and the patient, inserting a tube into the bladder can be one of the most effective interventions that we as urologists can offer.

X-rays

A number of urology and urogynecology offices have the equipment to perform x-rays, radiographic tests that require exposure to radiation. A technician is trained to maintain the machinery and take the pictures. The newer equipment is digitalized, so actual films may not be produced. The images are transferred directly to a computer disc or stored in the x-ray machine at the office. Ultrasound does not use radiation; it is done with sound waves. Therefore, an ultrasound is not an x-ray. CT scans do involve radiation exposure, but they are done with special devices and software, so they are generally not referred to as x-rays. Like ultrasound, MRI does not involve radiation exposure.

Urological x-rays all have acronyms that stand for the part of the body being studied. The most common urological x-ray is an IVP. The other less well-known studies include KUB, VCUG, RUG, and a cystogram. **IVP** stands for intravenous pyelogram. The procedure requires that you lie down on the x-ray table for a plain film of the abdomen, which includes the location of the kidneys and the bladder. Those organs cannot be visualized on plain x-ray, which is why an injection of intravenous dye needs to be given. The dye will drain into the kidneys, turning them bright white. As the dye continues down the urinary tract, it will outline the ureters and the bladder. You empty your bladder about 45 minutes into the study, and a drainage film of the bladder is taken to see if the bladder empties.

RADIOGRAPHIC TESTS AVAILABLE IN SOME OFFICES

IVP

KUB

VCUG

RUG

Cystogram

Kidney stones, masses, anatomical abnormalities, and blockages can be visualized. The function of the kidneys can be extrapolated from the pictures as well. A nonfunctioning or poorly functioning kidney on IVP will need to be followed up by other studies to find out why the kidney is not draining the dye well. The dye is made of hypoallergenic material that used to be iodine-based, but is not anymore. Allergies to shellfish no longer interfere in the administration of the dye. Diabetics have the hardest time tolerating the dye, as do people who have had allergic reactions to any intravenous contrast materials in the past. Steroids can be given the day before the test to suppress the reaction to the dye if the test is absolutely necessary.

The IVP has a number of advantages and disadvantages. The main advantage is that it is both an anatomical look at the urinary tract as well as a functional test. It provides a view of the inside drainage of the entire urinary tract in a single picture that is repeated exactly the same way as the dye travels through the system. Comparisons between the films will allow the trained eye to pick up small abnormalities. It has been the standard test for urologists to perform in everyone with microscopic blood in the urine. However, other tests have been introduced that provide similar information with less radiation exposure, which leads us to the disadvantages.

An IVP requires a fair amount of radiation exposure for the limited information that is gained. Although a comprehensive evaluation of the urinary tract is done, no other organ system is visualized on IVP. If the diagnosis is uncertain, then only urological problems can be eliminated. Other tests will need to be done to look at the gynecological, gastroenterological, and musculoskeletal systems. The other problem with the IVP is that the findings can be very subtle. An experienced urologist and radiologist may see a finding that a less-experienced practitioner may miss. Newer tests have become available that allow for more readily accessible information with less radiation exposure. Finally, the intravenous contrast dye can cause problems in some people. Although dye reactions are unusual, they do occur. If the dye can be avoided, it is better to choose a noninvasive test if possible.

In spite of its drawbacks, IVPs are still used by many urologists to evaluate the urinary tract. It is an excellent, comprehensive evaluation of both the anatomy and the function of the kidneys, ureters, and bladder. An IVP should not be done in a woman who is pregnant or thinks that she may be pregnant. Radiation exposure during pregnancy should be limited, especially in the first trimester. If a woman has a kidney stone during pregnancy, there may be a need to perform a shortened two- or three-film IVP. That indication can be discussed with the urologist if the occasion arises.

A **KUB** (kidneys, ureter, bladder) is a single x-ray of the abdomen that includes the outline of the kidneys. The kidneys, the ureters, and the bladder cannot be seen on plain x-rays, where no dye has been injected. If a kidney stone is suspected, a KUB will show a white circle wherever the kidney stone is sitting. Most kidney stones can be seen this way because the calcium in the stone will appear white on the gray background. Approximately 20% of stones do not have calcium in them and cannot be seen on a KUB. These stones are made of uric acid and they can be seen on CT scan.

Besides kidney stones, KUBs can be done to look at a recently instrumented system after surgery. They can be done after an IVP or a CT scan to look at the passage of the dye through the system. A plain, single-shot x-ray of the abdomen can be useful in very specific situations, and little radiation exposure is required.

A **VCUG** is a voiding cystourethrogram, which is complicated name for a complicated test. The test involves radiation exposure. A catheter is inserted into your bladder through which dye is instilled. Once the dye enters the bladder, x-rays are taken that show the contour of the bladder. Stones, tumors, pockets, and abnormal shadows and shapes within the bladder can be visualized. Once the bladder is filled to capacity, the catheter is removed and you urinate into a receptacle as x-rays are taken. The dye will flow through the urethra, displaying the walls of the tube that would otherwise not be seen.

Narrowed areas, called strictures, can be seen along the urethra. Women rarely develop urethral stictures. Because the urethra in men is so much longer than in women, men are more likely to develop urethral strictures than women. However, women are prone to urethral diverticula, which are infected pockets of tissue that lie under the urethra on the top wall of the vagina near the opening. These pockets form when glands that become infected eat their way into the urethra and drain through the opening. Symptoms include burning and pain while sitting and during sex. You can feel a small ball of tissue in the vagina, which is seen by an examiner as pelvic exam, On a VCUG, the pocket will fill with fluid as you urinate. Nowadays, we have other tests, like CT scans and MRIs, that can make the diagnosis without catheterization. Some practitioners still like to do VCUGs to diagnose urethral diverticula. These pockets can be removed vaginally by a skilled vaginal surgeon.

The other indication for a VCUG is recurrent urinary tract infections that began in childhood. Children with bladder infections may have a

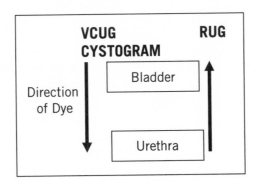

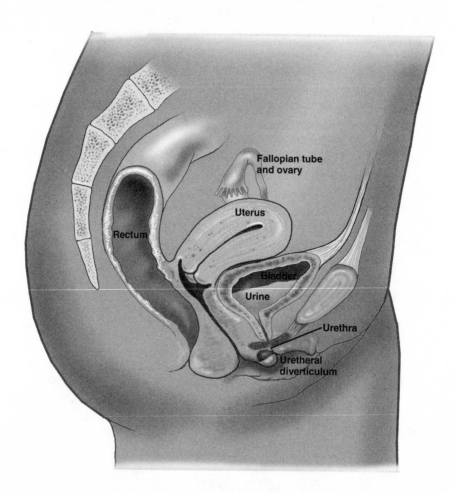

FIGURE 1. *Urethral Diverticulum.*

problem with reflux, a condition is which the urine travels up the ureter as well as out of the urethra during urination. Urine should never enter the ureter from the bladder. If it does, an abnormal condition is present that may need to be treated. There are instances in which reflux is diagnosed in adults. If it is suspected, then a VCUG will show the dye entering the ureter from the bladder during urination. Treatment of reflux includes antibiotic therapy, injection therapy, and surgery.

A **RUG** is a test in which the lining of the urethra is studied from the tip of the opening in towards the bladder, not going from the bladder to the opening. RUG stands for retrograde urethrogram. "Retrograde" means backwards, so the dye is injected in the opposite direction of the flow of urine. Again, x-ray exposure is required since regular films are taken of the pelvic area. The indications for a RUG overlap those of a VCUG. Women who are suspected of having diverticula or strictures may be asked to have a RUG performed. A RUG will not help in diagnosing any bladder conditions since the bladder is not filled during a RUG. Only the urethra is seen.

A **cystogram** is similar to a VCUG, except there is no voiding part. The bladder is accessed with a catheter after which it is filled with dye. The dye will outline the walls of the bladder. If there is a hole in the bladder, or a large outpouching, called a diverticulum (similar to a urethral diverticulum, but in a different place), it will be seen on a cystogram. Trauma in which the bladder may be involved is the most common indication for a cystogram. Blunt or sharp injury can damage the bladder, such as in a car accident or in the operating room. A cystocele, where the bladder falls into the vagina, can be seen on a standing cystogram. A cystogram will not diagnose a bladder tumor or polyp. For these conditions, a cystoscopy will need to be done. Cystograms require radiation exposure. For cystograms, VCUGs, and RUGs, the dye is not injected; it is instilled into the bladder throughh a catheter, so dye allergies are not an issue.

Finally, **urodynamics** can be done by many urologists and urogynecologists in their offices. This test evaluates the function of the bladder. It cannot determine whether or not a patient has cancer. Urodynamic studies are indicated in women who have problems urinating, either too much or too little. In women with incontinence, it can help define the type of incontinence. The study has two parts: the first part involves bladder filling, the second, bladder emptying. A catheter is introduced into the bladder to instill water and read pressures as the bladder fills. Another catheter is inserted into the rectum. This catheter does not involve any filling. It sits there and records pressures external to the bladder.

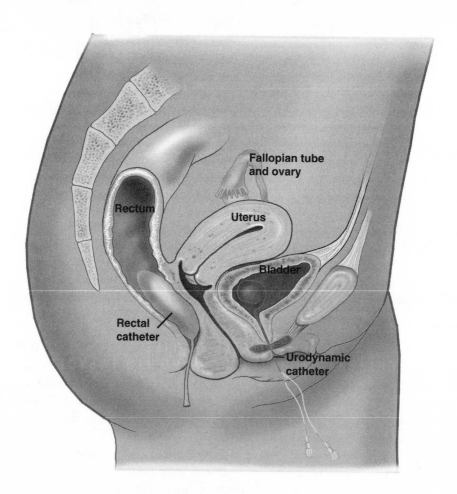

FIGURE 2. *Catheters for urodynamic testing.*

Water is slowly infused into the bladder as you sit on a special commode or table. Some practitioners use x-rays to visualize the filling in addition to viewing the pressure recordings that can be seen on a computer screen. You participate in the test by responding to cues from the technician regarding urges to urinate, sensation of leakage, and discomfort. When you feel that your bladder is full, you empty it spontaneously around the catheter which is still in place. The velocity of the urination and the residual water left in the bladder after you empty are recorded. No special preparation for a urodynamics tests is required. It is not painful, and with a skilled calming technician, it is not even unpleasant. The amount of information that we can glean from this test is enormous.

INDICATIONS FOR URODYNAMICS

Symptoms of stress and urge incontinence
Incontinence that does not respond to medication
Urinary problems in diabetics or women with neurological problems
Incomplete emptying
Difficulty after incontinence surgery

Not all urology offices are equipped to do all of the tests mentioned. If a doctor recommends that a study be done, it should be explained in detail. Most insurance companies require that diagnostic work be done at a different visit from the original consultation so that both the patient and the examiner have time to consider its necessity. Whether or not this is the most efficient approach, it gives you time to digest the information that is presented to you. If a catheter is to be inserted, you need to be prepared for that event so that you do not feel violated, surprised, or hurt. A simple, easy, painless procedure can turn into a disaster if you are not adequately warned of its occurrence.

OUTPATIENT DIAGNOSTIC STUDIES

More sophisticated tests may need to be done in order to make a diagnosis. CT scan, MRI, and renal scan evaluate the anatomy and the function of the organs being studied. These radiological tests are done in a hospital or a free-standing specialty office in which radiologists are present to read the results.

Radiologists are medical doctors who specialize in diagnostic testing of the entire body. They complete a residency in radiology before sitting for their own board exams. Specialties within radiology include neuroradiology (studies of the brain and spinal cord), body imaging (evaluation of the torso), pediatric radiology, bone imaging, interventional radiology (using radiographic images to guide in accessing the body internally), uroradiology (imaging of the urinary tract), and mammography.

Different methods of evaluation are used for different parts of the body. For example, the brain is not studied in the same way as the kidneys. Over the last couple of years, technological advances have exploded in the area of radiological imaging. In many cases, the diagnostic testing has surpassed our knowledge of the illnesses being identified. This leaves many physicians and patients in a quandary regarding how to manage lesions found incidentally on film. Many of these findings would have no impact on your life, but once we know that they are there, we have trouble ignoring them.

RADIOLOGIC TESTS DONE OUTSIDE OF THE UROLOGY OFFICE

CT scan

MRI

Renal scan

CT scanning has become one of the most commonly ordered radiographs, especially among urologists. The "CT" stands for *computerized tomography*, which is a fancy way of saying digital photographic slices of the body that are taken and stored in a computer. Radiation is used to produce the pictures. You are placed on a table in a cold room that has a large donut-shaped machine in the middle of it. The table slowly rolls through the donut as cross-sectional images of the body parts of interest are taken. Your head is always exposed, so there is no danger of claustrophobia. A single set of films takes about 20 minutes to produce.

INDICATIONS FOR A CT SCAN IN UROLOGY

Suspected kidney stones

Blood in the urine

Suspected kidney tumor

Undiagnosed flank, abdominal, or groin pain

The images that are produced by CT scan are all shades of gray, unless dye is used to produce contrasting colors. The dye or contrast can be ingested orally to outline the bowels. It can be inserted rectally to highlight the lower colon. Finally, it can be given intravenously, where it will coat the larger blood vessels of the body and drain through the kidneys and the bladder. The timing of the actual photography with the dye consumption is important because different things can be seen at different intervals. For example, early pictures after intravenous injection will show the kidneys, while later images will show the bladder. Earlier films after drinking the dye will show the stomach and duodenum, whereas later films will show the small intestine and colon. In some cases, you may be asked to drink the dye and wait one or two hours before the scan is performed. Although this can be tedious, it will produce the most comprehensive results.

The dyes that are used nowadays have special qualities that are hypoallergenic. Iodine-based materials were used in the past, which put people with seafood allergies at risk. There are still people who may react to the dye, but the reactions are much less severe than were experienced with the previous agents. The scheduling person at the CT scan office will ask you a number of questions whose answers may alert her to a possible risk of allergy. If there is concern but the scan is necessary, premedication with oral steroids can be arranged without difficulty or danger to you.

A CT scan of the abdomen and pelvis with and without intravenous contrast (dye) and with oral contrast is the most comprehensive single test of the urinary tract that you can have. Not only will the anatomy of the entire system be visualized, but the function can be inferred by the passage of the contrast through the whole tract. The part that is done before the dye is given will identify kidney stones nearly 100% if the time. After the dye is injected, tumors, cysts, infections, and blockages can be seen. The downside to having a CT scan is the time factor (it can take up to two hours to complete), the radiation exposure, and the possible dye allergy. Women with poor kidney function cannot get a CT scan done with dye because the dye can injure the kidneys. Pregnant women should only have a CT scan done if no other radiological test can determine the problem being investigated.

MRI stands for *magnetic resonant imaging*. MRI uses completely novel technology to visualize the internal organs. Magnets are used to pull the hydrogen atoms in the body in certain orientations that result in the formation of images. Hydrogen atoms are targeted because they are found in water, which is copious in the human body. No radiation is used. MRI can be done on anyone for any condition, unless you have metal anywhere inside your system. Because magnets are used, the metal can be dislodged and cause injury. Claustrophobia used to be a problem for some people because the machine is like a coffin, but open machines are now more plentiful to help ease this problem.

MRI visualizes the pelvic organs very well. Because hydrogen atoms are targeted by the machine, water-filled organs appear well-defined on the images. The bladder appears either bright white, or jet black, depending on the sequence being used. The ovaries, the uterus, the urethra, and the kidneys can be studied as well. The dye that is used to color the urine for visualization through the system is called gadolimium. Gadolimium can be given to people with kidney problems, unlike the contrast that is used for CT scans which is toxic to the kidneys.

INDICATIONS OF FOR MRI IN UROLOGY

Cannot tolerate CT scan dye
Urethral diverticulum
Suspected kidney tumor
Clarification of prolapse

MRI is done as an outpatient procedure, just like CT and ultrasound. Radiologists read the scans after they are done and pass the results on to the ordering doctor. Generally, the only preparation that is needed is a clear liquid diet for four to six hours before the test is done. The reason for this is to keep the bowels and stomach free of food, which can make the study difficult to interpret. Sometimes special instructions will be given if a specific diagnosis is being entertained. All directions should be followed closely so that the best information can be obtained from the study.

Nuclear medicine is a field within radiology in which different cells within the body are labeled with materials. The labeled cells are followed through the body as pictures are taken by a special machine. Information regarding the transit time, the amount of material that passes through each organ, and the location of the labeled cells will give information to the physician interpreting the results. Renal scan, indium scan, HIDA scans, and PET scans all fall under the purview of nuclear medicine.

In urology, **renal scans** can be very helpful in determining the function of each individual kidney without having to perform any invasive testing. After radioactive material is injected into your veins, a large machine is lowered over your body while you lie flat on your back. The machine records the passage of the material as it moves through each kidney into the bladder. If the material sits in the kidney and does not drain, the kidney is blocked. The degree of blockage and the function of the blocked and the unblocked kidneys can be calculated.

INDICATIONS FOR A RENAL SCAN

Kidneys are different sizes on X-ray
One kidney needs to be removed
Kidney blockage is suspected

Nuclear medicine uses radiation for diagnostic purposes, while radiation oncology uses radiation to treat illness. The ways in which the radiation is used are very different, as are the doses. If a physician feels that a nuclear test is helpful, the degree of radiation exposure should not deter you from having it done. The radiation washes out of the system in a few days at the most, and none of its effects are lasting.

HOSPITAL-BASED PROCEDURES

Besides surgery, very few procedures in urology are solely hospital-based. Most diagnostic work can be performed comfortably and safely in the office. The efficiency of office-based care for both women and their physicians has driven most of our work out of the hospital. The only strictly hospital-based procedure that is left, aside from surgery requiring anesthesia, is the placement of a temporary drainage tube into the kidney to relieve a blockage. Called a *percutaneous nephrostomy tube*, a drainage tube placed into the kidney is done if a ureter is blocked and cannot be unblocked from below. A radiologist with special training in interventional techniques (he is called an *interventional radiologist*) puts the tube in using x-ray equipment to direct the tube into the kidney.

Causes of kidney blockage include kidney stones, blood clots, tumors, and surgical mishaps. Occasionally, a severe pelvic-floor prolapse can cause both of the ureters to be kinked. If the kidneys begin to fail, tubes may need to be inserted into the kidneys until the prolapse can be repaired.

Slow onset of kidney obstruction is not usually painful. Sudden onset is. Blockage due to prolapse is usually a slow process involving both kidneys. The woman suffering from the condition may only notice that her urine output has diminished. She may feel no pain. If a kidney stone or blood clot falls into the ureter, that event will result in terrible pain. Women wind up in the emergency room on a morphine drip until a diagnosis is made and the blockage is alleviated. The need to insert a tube from outside into the kidney versus from inside through the bladder into the ureter depends on many factors. The urologist decides on the method of alleviating the blockage after reviewing all of the data and speaking to the patient and her family.

Surgical mishaps that result in tying off one or both ureters or kinking of the ureters can occur. When consenting to any pelvic surgery, this complication should be included in a discussion regarding possible problems. It is a rare event, but when it happens it needs to be addressed quickly. If rapid onset of back pain results after an operation for incontinence or prolapse, blockage of a kidney should be considered in the differential diagnosis. An ultrasound will make the diagnosis, and a percutaneous nephrostomy tube may need to be inserted until repairs can be made. The tube will allow the kidney to drain, which does two things. First, the pain will be alleviated, and second, the function of the kidney will continue unimpaired. Not only is the continued blockage painful, but it can jeopardize the kidney. Four weeks of continued blockage results in loss of kidney function.

INDICATIONS FOR A PERCUTANEOUS NEPHROSTOMY TUBE

A blocked kidney due to
- **Stone**
- **Tumor**
- **Surgery**

Interestingly, blockage of one kidney will not result in loss of urine output. Only one kidney needs to work in order to maintain normal urine production and blood tests. If both kidneys are blocked, the urine output will cease entirely.

Percutaneous Nephrostomy Tube
The insertion of the tube is done under local anesthesia with sedation. If the kidney is dilated, the procedure does not usually take very long because the distance between the skin and the drainage system in the kidney is short. The tube is put in over a wire, which is then removed. The tube is connected to a bag that collects the urine. The bag can be attached to your leg. The

whole apparatus is hidden under your clothing and no odor is produced. Although it may be uncomfortable at times, a percutaneous nephrostomy tube can be worn for many weeks without danger. It will protect the kidney effectively until definitive treatment can be undertaken.

Besides precutaneous nephrostomy tube insertion, surgical procedures are the only other treatments that are done in the hospital. Surgery for incontinence and pelvic-floor prolapse are discussed elsewhere in the book. In general, any procedure involving heavy sedation or anesthesia should be performed in a monitored setting, either in a surgical center or a hospital. Local anesthetics can be given in the office safely, allowing us to perform many of our tests in the office for the convenience and cost-saving benefit of both patient and physician.

SUMMARY

The point of this chapter is to alleviate one's fears about visiting a urologists's office. Although we are a procedure-oriented field, none of the tests that are performed in the office need to be painful or unpleasant. A competent staff and a compassionate practitioner can make any test tolerable. Urinating in front of an audience is surely an anxiety-producing concept, but when it is done with a professional technician in a private, relaxing environment, even the most inhibited person will feel at ease. The information that is gleaned from these tests can be invaluable. Effective treatment comes out of careful history taking, thorough examination, and comprehensive testing. In order to remain collaborative with your doctor, you need to know the reason for the tests being done, the results that are obtained, and the outcomes of treatment that are chosen.

CHAPTER 13

Safety in Numbers

The Epidemiology of Urinary Incontinence

Here is a typical scenario that will be reported to me by patients and their families. S. has recently developed leakage of urine when she coughs, laughs, sneezes, and exercises. Her gynecologist told her that she has something called stress urinary incontinence, a condition common in women who have delivered babies vaginally. Because the accidents have become bothersome to her, S. wants to do something to reduce them. She has heard that medications are available but she is reluctant to go on something that she may need to take for the rest of her life. Surgery is also an option, but that seems so drastic for a problem that she would describe more as an inconvenience than anything else.

Lately, the problem of urinary incontinence in women has been getting a lot more attention that ever before. S. has seen advertisements on television for pills that will delay the urge to go to the bathroom. The number of different pads that are available to people in the pharmacies seems to have multiplied over the years. The internet is loaded with information on bladder problems in women. The evening news has even had a few special reports on urinary incontinence.

S. discussed the problem with her gynecologist when she went for her routine physical examination. He was very knowledgeable on the subject, and discussed all of the options for both evaluation and treatment. She asked how common her problem was, and why she developed this, when many of her friends had not. Unfortunately, not nearly as much information was available regarding the prevalence of urinary incontinence in her age group as she would have liked. Either more people are willing to discuss this problem now, or more people actually suffer from it. The result is that more and more treatment options are available than ever before.

The statistics regarding the number of women who suffer from urinary incontinence are difficult to get a handle on because so many variables play into the picture. Incontinence can be caused by bladder problems, muscle problems, and problems unrelated to the urinary tract altogether. Factors such as mobility, medications, mental status, and neurological problems can all cause incontinence, but have nothing to do with bladder function at all. So even if we do know how many people suffer from urinary incontinence, it may not help any individual patient understand her own condition because each situation is so complex. However, some studies have attempted to get an idea of the number of Americans who have some degree of urinary leakage or urinary disorder.

For the sake of surveys, incontinence is described as the involuntary loss of urine that occurs in sufficient volume to be considered a problem. Frequency of urination is defined as the need to urinate more than eight times per day and more than two times per night. The Agency for Health care Policy and Research Public Health Service (AHCPR), a branch of the U.S. Department of Health and Human Services, defined these terms to help standardize the information that different epidemiologists obtain. These definitions have been applied to research in drug efficacy as well, and help us establish reasonable goals for therapy with patients. So, if a woman is placed on a medication because she gets up to urinate four times per night, her goal on the medication should be getting up only twice per night, as opposed to sleeping through the night which is not a reasonable goal for a middle-aged woman.

According to this definition, 10 to 35% of all American adults are incontinent. Fifty percent of institutionalized adults are incontinent and over 50% of the homebound elderly are incontinent, regardless of age. In 1999, 30.6 million women in the United States were over the age of 55, and 12% of the population was over 65 years old. This means that over 13 million Americans in both the community and the institutional setting are incontinent of urine. These numbers include older women with children, young women without children, and men.

The accuracy of these statistics cannot be confirmed because most people will not talk to their physicians about incontinence, unless the physician brings it up first. Only one quarter of the women who suffer from urinary leakage will seek out formal advice from a health-care provider. Studies show that variable identification of incontinence on the part of health care providers also underestimates the true incidence of this problem. Many doctors do not ask about it, do not examine patients for it, and do not know what treatments are available. What we do know, however, is that the annual incidence of people who become incontinent while they are in the hospital or nursing home is approximately 27% per year. In 1998, 121,000 operations were preformed for stress urinary incontinence and 247,000 operations were performed for pelvic-floor prolapse, not including hysterectomy (National Center for Health Statistics). Although these numbers give us some idea of the degree to which the problem affects people, it only reveals the tip of the iceberg. I know from my practice, very few people actually come to surgery for either problem. At least two-thirds of the patients either manage their urine loss on their own, or seek non-surgical treatments.

The other complicating factors regarding statistics lie in the unpredictable natural history of incontinence and the varying degrees of leakage with which people present. Incontinence is not a progressive disease. Although rare, it can get better on its own. Usually, it remains stable or, it gets better and worse intermittently. Women with severe incontinence of any type tend to be the ones who complain about the problem most openly. Women with intermittent problems tend not to bring it up to their doctors. Older people are less likely to bring it up with a doctor. Many of you think that leaking urine a natural part of aging or that nothing can be done about it, so there is no reason to discuss it. However, when asked, this population also reports that incontinence is severely limiting to their social and physical activity, and they feel that it seriously inhibits their lives and well-being.

COST OF INCONTINENCE

The direct costs associated with caring for people with urinary incontinence of all ages are estimated to be between 11 to 15 billion dollars annually. This figure includes expenses attributed to supplies; illnesses due to leakage, including bedsores and skin breakdown; loss of work; and the costs of institutionalization. Urinary incontinence is one of the leading causes of institutionalization among the homebound elderly. The cost to society will only increase with time because more those people are getting older.

PREVALENCE AND INCIDENCE OF URINARY INCONTINENCE

Prevalence is defined as the probability of a person *being* incontinent within a defined population. *Incidence* is defined as the probability of *becoming* incontinent during a defined period of time. Prevalence data is obtained by determining the number of people who are incontinent over the total number of people in the population being studied. It is useful for understanding incontinence information at a particular point in time. From this information, health and medical needs can be projected for the community being studied. Prevalence data cannot clarify the onset and course of the problem within a woman or a group of people. The few studies looking at the prevalence of incontinence have been done in Europe. Those results have been extrapolated for use in the United States.

The prevalence of urinary incontinence in all people over the age of 65 is anywhere from 8 to 34%, depending on the study. The range of results is so broad because the definition of incontinence is not consistent from study to study, the types of populations that are studied are variable, and the age range of the sample is not consistent. The three main definitions that were used in the studies cited are 1) any uncontrolled loss of urine in the prior 12 months without regard to amount (a very broad definition), 2) more than two incontinence episodes in one month (very narrow), or 3) urinary leakage that results in hygiene problems or incontinence that is objectively demonstrated (very esoteric). If definition 1 is used, the prevalence is 34%. If definition 2 is used, the prevalence is 8 to 18%. If definition 3 is used, the prevalence is 24%.

The prevalence of stress incontinence versus urge incontinence has not been well characterized either. Approximately one-third of all incontinent people have a component of stress incontinence. The prevalence of stress incontinence averages around 20% for postmenopausal women. The prevalence of urge incontinence cannot be deduced from these numbers because there is a great deal of overlap between the two major causes of incontinence in women.

PREVALENCE AND INCIDENCE OF URINARY INCONTINENCE

Prevalence 8–34%
The likelihood of being incontinent at a given time

Incidence 10–20%
The likelihood of becoming incontinent over a one-year period

---

Incidence data helps to understand the onset and course of a disease. It is defined as the probability of becoming incontinent during a defined period of time, such as one year, two years, or five years. As difficult as prevalence studies are to conduct and reproduce, incidence studies are even more challenging because the same information is obtained over different time periods. Participants are asked to report on symptoms at day one and, let's say, day 30. Leakage can be variable, so if you have leakage on day one, but none on day 30, the study would report cure of the problem, which is not accurate. Just because the participant has no leakage on a particular day does not mean that she no longer has leakage. Incidence numbers that look at severe incontinence are the most reliable because the presence of leakage is indisputable and consistent. One-year incidence rate for incontinence in women is 20%, and in men, 10%. In other words, the likelihood that a woman at the age of 65 will become incontinent is 20%.

Few epidemiological studies look at pelvic-floor prolapse alone. Urinary incontinence and pelvic-floor prolapse occur frequently in the same women, so significant overlap occurs. The lifetime risk of needing to undergo prolapse surgery is 11%. The re-operation rate for prolapse surgery is the same: 11%.

URINARY INCONTINENCE AND ITS IMPACT ON QUALITY OF LIFE

The negative impact of urinary incontinence on women's self-esteem has been well determined. Severe incontinence, in particular, causes psychological decline leading to depression and lower life satisfaction. Incontinent women are more likely to have low self-esteem and feel shame and guilt, which keeps them from working and partaking in social activities. Independence is compromised due to a reduction in physical activity, increasing isolation, and dependence on care givers.

Forty-two percent of severely incontinent women responded "yes" to a questionnaire that asked, "Do you feel that your leakage has affected your mental well-being?" Anxiety, depression, and loss of interpersonal relationships all worsen in the incontinent woman.

The degree to which the decline in mental health can be directly attributed to incontinence is not clear. Many of these women suffer from other debilitating illnesses that curtail their activity. However, women have reported that it is the urinary leakage that is the most limiting physical ailment from which they suffer. Urinary incontinence leads to bed sores, skin breakdown, falls secondary to frequent trips to the bathroom, and ultimately, institutionalization. Urgency and urge incontinence negatively affect a woman's lifestyle more than stress incontinence because it is unpredictable.

RISK FACTORS LEADING TO URINARY INCONTINENCE

At some point during the initial visit, nearly every woman asks me, "Why did this happen to me?" The answer is not clear, as are so many things in the area of bladder disorders in women. We just do not know why some women suffer from leakage problems and some women do not. A few risk factors have been proven to lead to problems, and other presumed risk factors have never been clearly causally related to the development of urinary leakage.

RISK FACTORS LEADING TO THE DEVELOPMENT OF URINARY INCONTINENCE

Risk Factor	Related to Incontinence
Gender	YES: women more than men
Age	YES: older more than younger
Vaginal births	YES: all you need is one!
Family history	YES: like mother, like daughter
Immobility	YES: the quicker you get there, the less likely you'll leak
Neurological problem	YES: strokes, spinal cord injury, multiple sclerosis, back problems
Obesity	NO: not proven
Race	YES: see family history

Being a woman clearly puts a person at a higher risk of developing some form of incontinence over her lifetime. Starting at the age of 65, women are one and a half to two times more likely to develop incontinence than a man of the same age. Younger men have even less problems with incontinence than women their age. Pure stress incontinence is much more common in women than men of any age, unless the man has had prostate surgery. Prostate surgery predisposes men to the development of stress incontinence.

URINARY INCONTINENCE IN PEOPLE 15–64 YEARS OLD

MEN	1.5–5%
WOMEN	10–30%

URINARY INCONTINENCE IN PEOPLE OVER 65 YEARS OLD

MEN and WOMEN   20–50%
Variation depends on the history of the patient and the other conditions
from which they suffer.

Age as a "risk factor" for the onset of incontinence is difficult to analyze. Incontinence is more common in the elderly, however, many other illnesses are also more common in the elderly. So, is age the cause or are the other co-morbid conditions the cause? Menopause and hormonal changes may contribute to the development of incontinence. Menopause occurs in women in their 50s, with incontinence usually beginning about that time. Is age the problem, or are the hormonal changes?

Although the bladder undergoes changes over time, urinary incontinence is not considered a normal part of the aging process. Frequent urination and increased getting up at night to go to the bathroom naturally worsen with age. These changes are not considered abnormal if a woman or a man in their 70s or 80s complains of them. But, *leakage* is not an acceptable condition that we are expected to live with even if you are over the age of 65. So, incontinence is more likely to occur in older people, but it is not considered a natural part of aging.

A woman's history of having delivered a baby vaginally, as opposed to through a C-section, increases her risk of developing stress incontinence during her lifetime. A single vaginal delivery is all that is needed to increase the risk. The need for an episiotomy, use of forceps, or a vacuum-assisted delivery can traumatize the muscles of the pelvic floor, which alters the support of the urethra and bladder. The number of vaginal deliveries does not matter; one, alone, puts a woman at risk. Not every woman who delivers a child vaginally develops incontinence, and many women with no children, or who delivered by C-section do develop incontinence. Therefore, an obstetrician cannot recommend against vaginal delivery in order to prevent incontinence.

Prolapse occurs more often in women who have delivered children vaginally, as well. Stretching of the vaginal muscles and the muscles of the pelvic floor results in weakness of the support structures of the bladder, the urethra, and the rectum. Over time, these muscles continue to weaken, and, in some women, result in prolapse.

Family history seems to play a fairly large role in the risk of developing urinary leakage. No studies have looked at this directly, but women often report that their mothers had the same problem, but never talked about it. Studies looking at mother/daughter incidence of disease seems simple enough to do, but are not in the case of conditions like urinary incontinence or pelvic-floor prolapse. First of all, many women in previous generations would not discuss these problems with their physicians. Second of all, women would not discuss these conditions with their families. If anything were done, they would not tell their children what condition they were having treated. Finally, women did not live as long as they do now. Longevity contributes to the increasing incidence of both of these problems.

Inability to move clearly affects the occurrence of urinary incontinence, certainly more than pelvic-floor prolapse. As anyone who has experience running to the toilet after putting the key in the door knows, the quicker you get to the bathroom, the less likely you are to have an accident. If a woman is confined to the bed, getting someone to help her to a bathroom may take more time than she has, once the urge has hit. In many nursing homes, the personnel are not available to move people from the bed to the commode, so they are left in diapers. They are incontinent only because they never get to a bathroom, let alone get there in time. Of course the issue also may be the underlying condition. Again, immobile patients are usually immobile because they have pretty serious medical conditions that leave them bedbound. Those underlying conditions may be contributing to the urinary problems as well.

Neurological conditions predispose women to urgency and urge incontinence. Brain injuries, such as tumors, strokes, Parkinson's disease, and dementia, can all cause incontinence, alone. No other risk factors need to be present to explain the presence of the incontinence. Age, gender, history of childbearing, and family history may all contribute to the degree, but the neurological condition alone can explain the presence of the leakage. Spinal cord disorders, like disc herniation, spinal stenosis, and arthritis, can cause swelling of the nerves to the bladder, especially if the condition is in the lumbar spine. Studies should be done by a urologist to correlate the injury to the bladder problems before any conclusions are drawn. Although these disorders can cause incontinence, the two conditions can coexist as well.

Obesity has not been proven to be a risk factor. Many of you have reported to me that their physician told them to lose 30 or 40 pounds and see if their problem gets better. Not only is that impractical, but it may not help. You are in a catch-22. You cannot exercise because of the leakage, but you can't cure the leakage without losing weight. In addition, many thin women with low body mass indices suffer from urinary leakage.

Finally, women of all races and ethnicities suffer from urinary leakage. In the United States, studies suggest that Caucasian and Hispanic women have a higher incidence than African-American or Asian women. The protein make-up of the skin and soft tissues found in Caucasian women may play a role. It is possible that the statistic is more related to the fact that Caucasian women discuss the problem with doctors more often or seek medical treatment more readily. Race and family history are closely related, which may explain some of the racial differences that we see.

SUMMARY

The epidemiology of urinary incontinence is complex. Clearly, older women suffer from the condition more than any other group of patients. However, other conditions can contribute to its presence, and certain behaviors can make it worse. Regardless of the cause of urinary incontinence and pelvic-floor prolapse, we do know that both conditions are on the rise, they are costing people and society a fortune in supplies, and they can be treated successfully by an interested health-care professional.

Glossary

ABDOMEN: Body cavity in which the intestines are located. The kidneys sit behind the abdomen.

ANTERIOR REPAIR: Surgical repair of a cystocele, which is done through the vagina, either with or without supporting material. It is synonymous with cystocele repair.

ANTIBIOTICS: Medication that kills bacteria.

BACTERIA: Foreign organisms that can cause infections, responsive to antibiotics.

BLADDER: Pelvic organ that holds and empties urine.

BOARD CERTIFICATION: Credential within a particular area in medicine. It implies that a doctor has met certain educational and training criteria established by the medical profession and examinations have been successfully passed.

BURCH PROCEDURE: Similar to the MMK for the treatment of stress incontinence. An abdominal (bikini) incision is made and the tissue next to the urethra is tacked near the pubic bone.

CATHETER: A tube that can be inserted into the bladder to drain urine. It comes in different sizes and is made of plastic, rubber, silicone, or metal.

COLONIZATION: Bacteria live in the bladder but do not cause symptoms of an infection.

CT SCAN: (computerized tomography) A radiographic test in which the internal organs are visualized. Radiation is used. Sometimes dye is injected intravenously. Not claustrophobic.

CYSTITIS: Bladder inflammation, usually but not always caused by bacteria.

CYSTOCELE: A bladder that has slipped into the vaginal canal.

CYSTOGRAM: X-ray of the bladder after it is filled with dye, a fluid that allows the bladder to be seen on a plain film.

CYSTOSCOPY: Office procedure in which the inner lining of the bladder is visualized with a scope inserted through the urethra.

CYSTOMETRICS: Part of a urodynamic study in which the bladder pressures are measured as water is infused into the bladder.

DILATION: Stretching open.

FECAL INCONTINENCE: Leakage of stool.

ENTEROCELE: Descent of the small bowel into the vaginal canal, an unnatural state.

EPIDURAL ANESTHESIA: Numbness of the lower half of the body that is induced to allow for surgery to ensue without pain or movement. The medication is inserted into the space between the layers covering the spinal cord. It can be given continuously, as opposed to a spinal which is of a finite duration.

ESTROGEN: One of the many hormones in women that is produced by the ovaries and the adrenal glands.

FISTULA: An abnormal communication between two organs, such as a hole between the bladder and the vagina.

FOLEY CATHETER: The most commonly used catheter, which is made of rubber and stays in the bladder with an inflated balloon.

GENERAL ANESTHESIA: Method of inducing sleep with pain management in which gas is inhaled in a controlled setting.

GYNECOLOGY: Specialty that focuses on medical and surgical problems of the female reproductive organs.

HYSTERECTOMY: Surgical removal of the uterus, either through the vagina or the abdomen. When the ovaries are also removed, the term oophorectomy is added.

INCONTINENCE: Leakage of either urine or stool.

INTERMITTENT CATHETERIZATION: A small tube is inserted into the bladder to drain urine in people who cannot empty on their own. The catheter is removed after drainage, and reinserted at the next urge or time interval. Clean, not sterile, technique is required.

INTRAVENOUS PYELOGRAM: X-ray in which the kidneys, ureters, and bladder are visualized using an injection of dye into the veins.

INTERSTITIAL CYSTITIS: A bladder condition in which pain, frequency, urgency, and night time urination plague the sufferer.

KEGEL EXERCISES: Used to strengthen the pelvic-floor muscles. The way to identify the muscles is to try to stop the flow of urine while you are going to the bathroom. Once you feel the contraction, finish urinating, and contract those muscles at times that you are not going to the bathroom. Do 10 contractions while waiting for a traffic light or during the commercials while watching TV.

KIDNEY: Two organs, one on each side of the body, located under the lower ribs in the back that function to drain toxins, make red blood cells, and metabolize calcium, among other things.

KUB: Plain x-ray of the abdomen.

LAPAROSCOPY: Method of doing surgery in which carbon dioxide is infused into the abdomen and instruments are placed into ports. It is considered minimally invasive.

MEDICAL HISTORY: The patient's current and past medical problems, including medications and surgeries. All relevant information should be available to the practitioner at the initial visit.

MENOPAUSE: Stage of life in which a woman's estrogen production is decreasing. It takes approximately 10 years to occur. The average age of onset is between 42 and 52 years old.

MESH: Netting that is used to reinforce muscle repairs. It can be made of many different materials.

MICROSCOPIC BLOOD IN THE URINE: Blood cells that are detected in a urine analysis but not seen with the naked eye. This finding should be reviewed by a urologist.

MMK: Similar to the Burch. Stress incontinence surgery in which an abdominal incision is made and the tissues around the urethra are affixed to the pubic bone.

MRI: (magnetic resonance imaging). Radiological test in which magnets are used to visualize the internal organs. No ionizing radiation is used. The dye is not toxic to the kidneys. May be claustrophobic, but open machines are available. It is contraindicated if metal materials are in the body.

NARCOTICS: Pain medication with highly addictive qualities, but excellent effect. They usually cause constipation and some nausea.

OVERFLOW INCONTINENCE: Uncontrollable loss of urine due to a full bladder.

PELVIC EXAMINATION: examination of the pelvic organs in a woman while her legs are in stirrups. It is part of any gynecologic or urologic evaluation of a female patient.

PELVIC-FLOOR REHABILITATION: A specialty of physical therapy that uses exercise, massage, biofeedback, electrical stimulation, and weights to strengthen and relax the pelvic muscles.

PELVIC-FLOOR SPASMS: Uncontrollable, and often painful, contractions of the muscles of pelvic floor. It presents with frequency, urgency, and burning without urination.

PELVIS: Body cavity in which the bladder, uterus, ovaries, and small intestine sit.

PERCUTANEOUS NEPHROSTOMY TUBE: A plastic device that drains urine from the kidney out through the skin and into a collection bag.

PERINEUM: The space between the back wall of the vagina and the anus.

PERSISTENT URINARY TRACT INFECTION: An infection that will not go away. This problem implies that something in the urinary tract is preventing the resolution of the infection, such as a stone or a foreign body.

PESSARY: Silicone ring used to support organs that have prolapsed into the vagina.

PHYSICAL EXAMINATION: The examination of the patient's body by a licensed physician. It should include a pelvic examination in a woman.

POST-COITAL PILL: Antibiotic that is taken within 24 hours of intercourse to prevent infections related to sexual activity.

POSTERIOR REPAIR: Surgical repair of the back wall of the vagina overlying the rectum. Synonymous with rectocele repair and suggests the vaginal approach.

POST-VOID RESIDUAL: The amount of urine remaining in the bladder after a person urinates.

PROLAPSE: Descent of the pelvic organs into the vaginal canal.

PROLINE: A type of nylon used to make mesh for hernias and prolapse repairs.

PROPHYLACTIC MEDICATION (same as suppression): Treatment that is used to prevent a problem. It is especially effective when used to help manage difficult recurrent urinary tract infections. One low-dose antibiotic tablet is taken daily.

PUBIC BONE: Bone that sits in front of the bladder and under which the urethra passes.

PUBOVAGINAL SLING: Surgery in which a support is placed under the urethra in order to prevent stress incontinence.

PYELONEPHRITIS: Kidney infection. Much more serious than a bladder infection. Presents with fever over 101.5°F, elevated white blood cell count in the blood, and back pain.

RECTOCELE: Prolapse in which the rectum pushes up into the vaginal canal, causing a bulge.

RECURRENT URINARY TRACT INFECTION: New bacteria colonize the bladder after a recent infection has just been treated. This implies that the last infection has resolved before the new one began.

REFLUX: Abnormal condition in which urine goes from the bladder into the kidney instead of out the urethra.

RESIDENT: A physician who is training within a medical or surgical specialty. They cannot work independently yet.

SONOGRAM: Same as an ultrasound. A radiological test in which the organs are visualized using sound waves. No radiation is used.

SPINAL ANESTHESIA: Numbness is induced from the waist down by inserting medication into the fluid that bathes the spinal cord.

STENT: a plastic tube that is inserted into the urinary tract to divert the urine around a blockage.

STRESS INCONTINENCE: leakage of urine with couging, laughing, sneezing, or activity.

SUPPRESSION (same as prophylactic): Medication that is taken to prevent an infection in women who get recurrent urinary tract infections.

SUPRAPUBIC TUBE: A plastic or rubber tube that is inserted into the bladder through the skin overlying the pubic bone. The tube can be plugged and drained intermittently, or attached to a bag and left to drain continuously.

SUTURE: Surgical thread used to sew tissue together.

TOTAL INCONTINENCE: Uncontrollable loss of urine due to a hole in the bladder, called a fistula.

ULTRASOUND: Same as a sonogram. A radiological test in which the organs are visualized using sound waves. No radiation is used.

URETER: The two tubes that drain urine from the kidneys to the bladder. In normal anatomy, each kidney has its own ureter.

URETHRA: Tube that empties urine from the bladder to the outside. In women it is very short. In men, it is long.

URETHRAL CARUNCLE: A dilated vein that is seen on the urethra, especially in women who push to empty. It is similar to a hemorrhoid on the anus.

URETHRAL DIVERTICULUM: A growth under the urethra and on top of the vagina that may or may not be painful. It needs to be surgically removed.

URGE INCONTINENCE: Urinary incontinence that is induced by the urge to go to the bathroom.

URINARY RETENTION: The inability to urinate or incomplete urination.

URINARY TRACT INFECTION/ UTI (same as cystitis): A bladder infection that is usually caused by bacteria.

URINE ANALYSIS/URINALYSIS: Test on a urine sample that can be done in the office. It can suggest infection, but it is not a definitive test. Protein, blood, and urine pH can be assessed as well.

URINE CULTURE: Test in which bacteria can be detected in the urine. It takes at least 24 hours to get the result. Antibiotic sensitivities can be determined as well.

URODYNAMICS: Test that assesses bladder function. It involves inserting a catheter into the bladder and into the rectum. The bladder is slowly filled with water as the pressures and volumes in the bladder are being recorded on a computer screen. After filling is complete you empty your bladder into a receptacle that measures flow and volume. Although uncomfortable, it is not painful.

UROGYNECOLOGY: Specialty of gynecology that involves additional training after residency focusing on urinary problems in women.

UROLOGY: Area of surgery that focuses on the management of the urinary tract (kidneys, ureters, bladder, and urethra) as well as the male genital organs (prostate, testicles, and penis).

VAGINAL ATROPHY: Dryness, itching, pallor, and thinning of the vaginal tissues that results from low hormone levels.

VCUG: (voiding cystourethrogram) X-ray in which the bladder is filled with dye through a catheter and films are taken as the patient urinates.

Index

A

Abdominal examination
in evaluating incontinence in the
elderly, 151–152
in evaluating urge incontinence, 115
Abdominal surgery, for stress
incontinence, 88
Acetylcholine
bladder contraction, control by, 109. *See
also* Anticholinergic medications
Acidity, of the vaginal environment
and bacterial growth, 241
effect of vaginal estrogen on, 330–331
role of estrogen in maintaining,
318–319
and urinary tract infections, 324
Adherence of bacteria to tissues, 239–240
figure, 241
Adherence theory, of interstitial cystitis,
282
Age
and incontinence, 131–173
and pelvic-floor prolapse, 184
and sleep cycle changes, 111
and stress incontinence, 32–33, 70,
386–387
and urinary tract infections, 228
in elderly women, 268–269
urological infections during childhood,
18
Alfentanyl, use in surgery, 341
Allergies
to collagen, checking for, 85
interstitial cystitis associated with, 285

to penicillins, 260
to sulfa-based antibiotics, 257
Alpha agonists, for stress incontinence,
82–83
American Board of Obstetrics and
Gynecology, fellowship for female
pelvic disorders certification, 52
American Board of Urology, fellowship
for female pelvic disorders
certification, 52
American Medical Association (AMA),
list of practicing physicians in the
United States, 47
Amitriptyline, for treating interstitial
cystitis, 298–299
Amnesia, after surgery, defined, 338
Analgesia, defined, 338
Anaphylactic shock, from penicillin, 260
Anaprox, antiinflammatory agent for
treating interstitial cystitis, 300
Anatomic incontinence, defined, 30–31
Anatomy
abnormalities of, and urinary tract
infections, 242–245
of the bladder, normal, 135
embryology of the urogenital system,
317
of the female pelvis, 3–13, 40, 190
from below, 230
after hysterectomy, 205
side view, 12, 229
of the male pelvis, 8, 181, 232
of the perineum, 231
in uterine prolapse, 190

Androstenedione, production of, in menopause, 315
Anesthesia
  defined, 338
  for prolapse surgery, 203–204
    complications of, 221
  for surgery, 335–353
Animal tissue, for pubovaginal slings, 95
Antibiotics
  for infections of the urinary tract, 18, 215, 250–251, 254–266
    prophylactic treatment with, 252
  intravenous prior to surgery, 343
Anticholinergic medications
  for treating incontinence in the elderly, specificity of, 146
  for treating urge incontinence, 121–129
Antidepressants, for treating interstitial cystitis, 298–299
Antidiuretic hormone, change in production, with age, 111
Antihistamines, for treating interstitial cystitis, 298
Antiinflammatory drugs
  effect in urethral syndrome, 278
  for treating interstitial cystitis, 300
Antispasmodics, for treating interstitial cystitis, 298
Aspirin, avoiding prior to surgery, 339
Asymptomatic bacteriuria, in the elderly, 144, 156
Atrophic vaginitis, in the elderly, 144–145
Attending physicians, qualifications of, 48
Augmentation cystoplasty, 304
Aumentin, for treating urinary tract infections, 260
Autoimmune disease
  cystitis as, 25
  interstitial cystitis as, 282–284

B
Bacille Calmette-Guérin (BCG), for treating interstitial cystitis, 297
Background checks, in selecting a physician, 55

Bacteria
  resistance of
    to antibiotics, 263–265
    to penicillin, 260–261
  in the urine, evaluating, 116, 156, 289
Bacterial persistence, in urinary tract infections, 236
Bacteriuria, defined, 233
Barbiturates, historic use for induction in surgery, 341
Behavior modification
  goals in urge incontinence, 118–121
  for leakage, 164–165
  for managing stress incontinence, 79–82
  for treating interstitial cystitis, 293–296
Benzodiazepines, use in surgery, 341–342
Bextra, antiinflammatory agent, treating interstitial cystitis, 300
Biofeedback
  to manage interstitial cystitis, 296
  to manage stress incontinence, 81
Birth trauma, and pelvic-floor prolapse, 323–324. See also Vaginal delivery
Bladder, 5–7
  aging, and normal changes, 134–138
  complications of prolapse surgery related to, 213–217
  denervation of, to manage interstitial cystitis, 303
  descent into the vagina, 15–16
  detrusor muscle, 5–7
  failure to empty, 137, 157
    evaluating in a physical examination, 152–153
  failure to fill, 136
  flaccid, defined, 35
  function of, postoperatively, 210
  injury to, in pubovaginal sling surgery, 98
  instillation of, to treat interstitial cystitis, 296–297
  lining of, in interstitial cystitis, 283
  location relative to the uterus, 10
  muscles of
    contractions and age, 137–138

effect of potassium on, 282
loss of function of, and age, 158
spasms of, and urge incontinence, 153
normal functioning process, 108–110
reduced capacity of, with age, 136–137
removal of, to treat interstitial cystitis, 303–304
training of, to manage urge incontinence, 120–121
wall of, in interstitial cystitis, 290–291
Bladder-emptying studies, in evaluating prolapse, 195–196
Bladder instillations, in the office, 365
Bladder prolapse (cystocele), 38–41
case example, 15–16
figure, 39, 187
symptoms of, 186–188
Bladder surgery
overflow incontinence following, 35
Bladder training, in interstitial cystitis, 295
Bleeding, after prolapse repair, 217–218
Blockage
of the ureter, 3–5
to urine flow, 137, 157–158
α-Blocker, for treating men with outlet obstruction, 82–83
Blood
filtration of, by the kidneys, 3
in a urine specimen
as an indication for cystoscopy, 362
significance of, 77, 289
Blood flow, in tissues, effect of estrogens on, 319, 325
Blurry vision, side effect, of anti-cholinergenic medications, 128
Board certification, of doctors, 47–48
Botulinum toxin (Botox)
injections of, to manage interstitial cystitis, 303
to prevent involuntary bladder contractions, 127, 168
Bowel
functioning after surgery, in the elderly, 172

injury to
in prolapse surgery, 220
in pubovaginal sling surgery, 98
Brain, the bladder control center of, 110
Breast cancer, estrogen-receptor-positive, and use of estrogen creams, 329, 332
Bubble baths, infections caused by, 238
Burch colpopexy, 88
figure, 89

C
Cadaveric materials, for pubovaginal slings, 94–95
Calcium, metabolism of, by the kidneys, 3
Calcium channel blockers, effect of, on urination at night, 149
Caruncle, on the urethra, 157, 178
Catheterization
indications for, 158–161, 172, 363–364
infections related to, 269
Catheters, figure, 372
Causes
of incontinence in the elderly, reversible, 153–155
of interstitial cystitis, 281–288
of overflow incontinence, 34–36
of pelvic-floor prolapse, 183–185
of stress incontinence, 66–70
of urge incontinence, 106–107
of urinary incontinence, 142–150
of urinary tract infections, 237–245
Celebrex, antiinflammatory agent for treating interstitial cystitis, 300
Cephalosporins, for treating urinary tract infections, 261–262
Chemotherapy, urinary tract infections associated with, 245
Chlamydia, pelvic inflammatory disease due to, 28
Chloral hydrate, historic use of for induction in surgery, 341
Chloroform, historic use for general anesthesia, 344
Clean-catch specimen, defined, 246

Clean intermittent catheterization, 365–366

Clorpactin (oxychlorosene), instillation of, to treat interstitial cystitis, 296–297

Clostridium difficile, colitis due to, 265

Cocaine, historic use for regional anesthesia, 345–348

Collagen
injection of, figure, 86
for treating stress incontinence, 85–87

Colonoscopy, to diagnose irritable bowel syndrome, 305

Colony forming units (CFU), in clean-catch urine, 247

Complications
of anesthesia
general, 344–345
during prolapse surgery, 221
spinal, 346–347
of indwelling catheters, 162
of prolapse surgery, 212–221
of pubovaginal sling surgery, 97–99

Computed tomography scans, 374–375
for evaluating kidney infections, 266–268
for evaluating prolapse, 197
for evaluating urinary tract infections, 249

Congestive heart failure, 148–149

Conjugated equine estrogen (Premarin), use in the Women's Health Initiative, 327

Constipation
and pelvic-floor prolapse, 185
rectocele causing, 41
as a side effect of anticholinergenic medications, 128

Contigen (collagen), for treating stress incontinence, 85–87

Contractions, involuntary, of the bladder, 136

Contraindications
to anticholinergenic medications, glaucoma, 128
to estrogen therapy, 332
to spinal or epidural anesthesia, 346

Controlled substances, state laws covering prescription of, 299–300

Cost
of antibiotics for urinary tract infection, 255
of incontinence
for direct care, 383
management of urge incontinence, 105
managing in nursing homes, 133
of prolapse surgery, 212

Cox-2 inhibitors for pain control, 350

Cranberry juice for preventing urinary tract infection, 253–254

Creatinine measurement, to check kidney function, 294

Curare, as a relaxant, 343

Cystectomy, complete, with urinary diversion, 304

Cystitis
autoimmune, 25
defined, 233
hemorrhagic, 24–25
interstitial, 23–24, 271–304
nonbacterial, 25, 269–270
symptoms of, 17–20
viral, 25

Cystocele, 38–41, 178
defined, 183
pessary for managing, 171
surgical repair of, 204–208
figure, 206

Cystogram, in the office, 371

Cystometrics. *See* Urodynamic testing

Cystoscopy
for evaluating interstitial cystitis, 290
for evaluating prolapse, 196
for evaluating urinary tract infection, 250
identifying misplaced mesh during surgery, 208
as an office procedure, 360–362

D

Darafenacin (Enablex) for treating urge incontinence, 125

DDAVP (artificial hormone), for treating urge incontinence, 127
Delirium, causes of, in the elderly, 144
Demerol for pain control during anesthesia, 343
Detrusor muscle of the bladder, 5–7
Diabetes mellitus
    excessive urine output in, 148
    incontinence accompanying, in the elderly, 152
    overflow incontinence in, 33–34, 141
    urinary tract infections in, 245
Diagnosis
    of urinary tract infections, 245–250
    of interstitial cystitis, 275–276
Diaphragm, contraceptive, and urinary tract infections, 242
Diarrhea, antibiotic-induced, 265
Diazepam (Valium) for managing pelvic-floor spasms
    in interstitial cystitis, 298
    in irritable bowel syndrome, 306
Diet, modification of
    to manage interstitial cystitis, 294
    to manage irritable bowel syndrome, 305
Dimethyl sulfoxide (DMSO), for treating interstitial cystitis, 297
Diphtheroids, in the rectum, 228
Dipslide culture (Uricult), for identifying urinary infections, 248
Dipstick method, of urinalysis, 246–248
Disinhibition, in bladder functioning, defined, 109–110
Ditropan XL, for treating urge incontinence, 124
Doctor
    referring urge incontinence patients to a specialist, 117
    selecting an individual, 51–55
    selecting a specialist, 45–59
Douching, recommendation on, 238
Duloxetine for treating stress incontinence, 84–85
Durasphere for treating stress incontinence, 85–87
Dyes, for computed tomography scans, 375

E
E. coli
    resistance of, to fluoroquinolones, 264
    urinary tract infections caused by, 237–245
        effect of lactobacillus on, 324
        sulfamethoxazole for treating, 257
Education, of a doctor, 46–51
Effexor for treating interstitial cystitis, 298–299
Elderly, defined, 132
Electrical stimulation for physical therapy in the elderly, 166
Elmiron (sodium pentosan polysulfate), for treating interstitial cystitis, 274–275, 300–301
Endocrine imbalances, interstitial cystitis associated with, 285
Endometrial overgrowth, prevention of, with progesterone added to estrogen therapy, 328
Endometriosis, 26, 306–307
Enterocele, 41–44
    defined, 183
    figure, 191
    repair of, 208–210
Enterococcus faecalis, urinary tract infections caused by, 237
Epidemiology
    of interstitial cystitis, 279–281
    of urinary incontinence, 381–389
Epidural anesthesia, 345–348
Epidural infusion of pain medication, 349
Episiotomy, closing after childbirth, 208
Erosion, of mesh materials used in surgery, 96–97
Estring, for vaginal application of estrogen, 329
Estrogen
    and breast cancer, 311–312
    effect of, on the urinary tract, 316–319
    and elasticity of the vaginal canal, 31
    local, for urge incontinence treatment, 323
    production of, during menopause, 314
    for treating atrophic vaginitis, 144–145

Estrogen (*cont.*)
for treating stress incontinence, 83–85
and types of urinary tract infections,
240–242
for urinary tract infection prevention,
253
Estrogen creams, for treating urogenital
symptoms of menopause, 329
Estrogen receptors, 315
Estrogen replacement therapy
and urological disorders,
postmenopausal, 326–328
and vaginal atrophy, 321
See also Hormone replacement
therapy
Estrogens, 314–315
contraindications to the use of, 332
natural and synthetic, list, 327
See also Hormones; Women's Health
Initiative
Estrone, production of, 314–315
Ether, historic use for general anesthesia,
344
Etomidate for sedation in surgery, 342
Evaluation
for incontinence in elderly women,
150–154
for interstitial cystitis, 288–291
for pelvic-floor prolapse, 193–198
for stress urinary incontinence,
71–79
for urge incontinence, frequency, and
urgency, 112–117
for urinary tract infections, 245–250
Examination, in an office visit, 357–358
Exercise, for elderly women, 165–166

F
Fallopian tubes, 10
Family history. See History, family
Fatigue, after surgery, 348
Fellowship, in specialty training, 47–48,
52
Fentanyl
for pain control during anesthesia,
343
use in surgery, 341

Fetal development of the uterus, vagina,
and urinary tract, 316
Fistulas, between the bladder and vagina
after prolapse surgery, 216–217
in total incontinence, 36–37
Flaccid bladder, defined, 35
Flexeril, in interstitial cystitis, 298
Fluid restriction
to manage incontinence
from congestive heart failure, 149
in the elderly, 156
to manage urge incontinence, 119,
133–134
to manage stress incontinence, 79–80
Fluid shifts, during sleep, 111
Fluoroquinolones, for treating urinary
tract infections, 258–259
resistance of E. coli to, 264
Foley catheter, indwelling, 159–162
Follicle-stimulating hormone,
production of, during
menopause, 314
Follow-up, in urinary tract infections,
indications for, 248–249
Foreign bodies, in the bladder, infection
due to, 243
Frequency of urination
defined, 382
at night, 110–112
Functional incontinence, in the elderly,
141–142

G
Gantrocin (sulfa-based antibiotic), 257
Gardinerella, vaginitis caused by, 242
Gases, for general anesthesia, 340–341,
343–345
Gender
and urinary incontinence, 386–387
and urinary tract infection, 230
Genetic factors, in pelvic-floor prolapse,
184–185
Genital organs, structure of, in relation
to the urinary tract, 10–13
Glomerulations, post-distention, in
interstitial cystitis, 291
Glossary, 391–396

Glycosaminoglycan layer of the bladder, role in defense against bacteria, 239

Gonadotropin-releasing hormone inhibitor, for treating endometriosis, 306–307

Gonorrhea, pelvic inflammatory disease due to, 28

Grading, of a prolapse, 194

Group practices, types of, 58

Gynecological disorders, painful, 26–28

Gynecological examination, for evaluation of incontinence, 151–152

Gynecological surgery, total incontinence following, 36–37

Gynecology, compared with urology, 48–49

H

Halothane, for general anesthesia, 344

Headache, in spinal anesthesia, 347–348

Helicobacter pylori, peptic ulcer disease caused by, 282

Hemorrhagic cystitis, 24

Heparin, for treating interstitial cystitis, 297

Hernia. *See* Prolapse

Hippurate, for preventing urinary tract infection, 252–253

History
for evaluating incontinence, 151
for evaluating stress incontinence, 71–75
family
of incontinence, 387–388
of stress incontinence, 70, 75
taking, in an office visit, 357

Hormone replacement therapy, 312–314
defined, 328

Hormones, 311–333
effect on fluid accumulation in the bladder, 111
manipulation of, to treat endometriosis, 306–307
oral, for vasomotor symptoms of menopause, 329
See also Estrogens

Hospital-based practice, comparison with private practice, 58

Hospital-based procedures, 377–379

Hospitals
information about, 55–59
types of, 56–57

Hunner's ulcer, 290–291

Hydrodistention
cystoscopy with, under anesthesia, 290
to treat interstitial cystitis, 302–303

Hydroxyzine (Vistaril or Atarax), for treating interstitial cystitis, 298

Hypercalcemia, in the elderly, excessive urine output in, 149

Hysterectomy
and pelvic-floor prolapse, 185
small intestine location after, 13
small intestine prolapse after, 41–42, 210
stress urinary incontinence, 70, 75
stress urinary incontinence after, 30
for treating uterine prolapse, 204

I

Ibuprofen
avoiding prior to surgery, 339
for treating interstitial cystitis, 300

Imipenem-cilistatin, for treating urinary tract infections, 260–261

Imipramine
for treating stress incontinence, 83
for treating urge incontinence, 126–127

Immunosuppression, effect of, on urinary tract infections, 245

Incidence, of urinary incontinence, 383–384

Incontinence
defined, 382
difference between men and women resulting in, 7
after menopause, 322–323
role of estrogen in, 320
total, 36–37

Incontinence (*cont.*)
See also Stress incontinence; Urge
    incontinence
Indications
  for bladder instillations, 365
  for clean intermittent catheterization,
    366
  for cystoscopy, 362–363
  for a percutaneous nephrostomy tube,
    378
  for surgery for incontinence
    for interstitial cystitis, 302
    for prolapse, 202–203
  for urethral catheterization, 363–364
  for urodynamic tests, 373
Induction agents, before general
    anesthesia, 341
Indwelling catheter, 172–173
Infections
  in catheterized patients, 162, 172–173
  interstitial cystitis following, 282
  of the kidneys, 3
  of a mesh hammock used to repair a
    cystocele, 207
  after prolapse surgery, 215
  recurrent, cultures for diagnosing,
    248
  of the urinary tract, 17–20
    in the elderly, 144
    finding on urinalysis, 77
    after menopause, 324–325
    pelvic-floor spasms due to, 22
Inhalation agents, for general surgery,
    343–345
Injection therapy, for stress incontinence,
    85–87
Integrated theory, of interstitial cystitis,
    287–288
International Continence Society, 103,
    108
Interstitial cystitis, 23–24, 271–304
  defined, 275–278
Interstitial Cystitis Association, 301
Intramuscular injections, of pain
    medication after surgery, 349
Intravenous medications for anesthesia,
    340–343

Intravenous pyelogram (IVP)
  for evaluating urinary tract infection,
    249
  as an office procedure, 367–368
Irritable bowel syndrome, 304–306

K
Kegel exercises
  for elderly women, 165
  to manage stress incontinence,
    80–81
Ketamine (PCP), historic use for
    sedation, 342
Ketoralac (Toradol)
  for pain relief after surgery, 337
  for treating acute pain, 350
Kidneys
  blockage of, in pelvic-floor prolapse,
    137
  evaluating
    renal scans for, 376–377
    x-rays for, 367
  path of infection to, from the bladder,
    267
  structure and function of, 3–4
  ultrasound examination of, 359
  urinary tract infection involving, 254,
    266–268
Kidney stones, infection in, 19, 243
Klebsiella pneumoniae, urinary tract
    infections caused by, 237
KUB (kidneys, ureter, bladder) x-rays,
    368–369

L
Labia, changes in, after menopause,
    321
Laboratory tests, to evaluate stress
    incontinence, 76–78
Lactobacilli, in the vagina, 228, 238,
    324
Laparoscopic surgery, for stress
    incontinence, 88–91
  figure, 90–91
Laparoscopy, for screening for
    endometriosis, 306–307
Leakage, night time, evaluating, 114

Leukocyte esterase (LE), in urine, as an indication of infection, 247

Lidocaine, for treating interstitial cystitis, 297

Lifestyle changes, limiting water intake, 74

Long-term (persistent) incontinence, 143
  in the elderly, 150
    treatment of, 164

Low back pain, pelvic muscle spasms due to, 22

Lubrication, lack of, as a symptom of estrogen deficiency, 325

Lupron, for treating endometriosis, 306–307

M

Magnetic resonance imaging (MRI), 375–376
  for evaluating prolapse, 196–197
  for evaluating urinary tract infections, 249

Male pelvis. See Anatomy, of the male pelvis

Marcaine, for treating interstitial cystitis, 297

Massage, in physical therapy in the elderly, 166

Masses, evaluation of, during physical examination for stress incontinence, 76

Mast cells, in interstitial cystitis, 284, 291
  antihistamines for stabilizing, 298

Medical conditions, urinary tract infections associated with, 245

Medical specialties, list, 48

Medical treatment, of urge incontinence, 121–129

Medications
  effects of, on urinary emptying, 133
  in the elderly, incontinence related to, 145–147
  for frequency, urgency, and urge incontinence, list, 121
  goals of, in treating urge incontinence, 118–119

oral, for managing interstitial cystitis, 293, 298–301
  for postsurgical pain, list, 350–352
  for stress incontinence, 82–87
  for urge incontinence
    case, 101–103
    in the elderly, 167

Menopause, 311–333
  change in urinary tract bacteria during, 240–242
  defined, 313
  as a phase of the climacteric, 314
  See also Age

Mental health
  effect of incontinence on, 383
  and interstitial cystitis, 285

Meperidine, use in surgery, 341

Mesh, synthetic
  for cystocele repair, 207
  erosion of, 215–216
  evaluation for reduced recurrence in prolapse surgery, 220
  for incontinence repairs, 96–97

Methenamine mandelate (Mendelamine), for preventing urinary tract infection, 252–253

Methoxyflurane, use for general anesthesia, 344

Microscopic analysis, for urinary tract infection, 246–248

Mittelschmerz, defined, 27

Mixed incontinence, defined, 71, 78

Mobic, antiinflammatory agent for treating interstitial cystitis, 300

Mobility
  restricted, in the elderly, 149
  urinary incontinence due to lack of, 388

Morphine
  for postoperative pain control, 349
  in surgery, 341

Motivation to continue physical therapy, 165

Mucosa, of the urinary bladder, 5–6

Muscle relaxants, in surgery, 343

Muscles
  effect of potassium on, 282
  pubococcygeus, strengthening to
    manage stress incontinence,
    80–81
  See also Bladder, muscles of; Pelvic-
    floor muscles
Mutation, bacterial resistance to
  antibiotics due to, 263–264

N

Narcotics
  for treating interstitial cystitis, 299–300
  for treating postoperative pain,
    349–351
National Center for Health Statistics,
  information about incontinence
  and surgery for incontinence, 383
National Institutes of Diabetes and
  Digestive and Kidney Diseases
  (NIDDK), criteria for diagnosing
  interstitial cystitis, 275–276
National Institutes of Health, U.S., 108
Native tissues, for surgical treatment of
  stress incontinence, 91–94
Nausea, from anesthetics, 345
Nerve damage, interstitial cystitis related
  to, 284–285
Nerve stimulators, to treat interstitial
  cystitis, 301–302
Nerve supply, shared, between the
  bladder and the uterus, 10
Neurological disorders
  incontinence related to, 388
  interaction with urge incontinence,
    32–33
  interstitial cystitis associated with,
    figure, 286
  overflow incontinence caused by, 34–35
Neurological examination of the genital
  area, in evaluating urge
  incontinence, 115
Neuromodulation
  for treating interstitial cystitis, with
    Interstim, 301–302
  for treating urge incontinence,
    129–130

Neurontin, for treating interstitial
  cystitis, 300
Neurotransmitters, of the bladder system,
  108–110
Nighttime urination, changes in, with
  menopause, 322
Nitrates, in urine, as an indication of
  infection, 247
Nitrofurantoins
  natural resistance of *Proteus* to, 264
  for treating urinary tract infection,
    257–258
Nitrous oxide, use for general anesthesia,
  344
Nonbacterial cystitis, 25
Nonnarcotics, for treating postoperative
  pain, 351–352
Nonsteroidal antiinflammatory drugs
  (NSAIDs), cyclo-oxygenase
  inhibitors, 350
Nortriptyline, for treating interstitial
  cystitis, 298–299
Nuclear medicine, 376–377
Nurse anesthetists, 339–340

O

Obesity, and urinary leakage, 388
Obstetrical trauma, total incontinence
  following, 36
Obstetrics and gynecology, training of
  specialists in, 50–51
Office visit, description of, 357–358
Outpatient diagnostic studies,
  373–377
Ovaries, 10
  cysts of, pain due to, 27–28
  masses in, 76
Overactive bladder, 31–33
  defined, 103
Overflow incontinence, 33–36
  in the elderly, 140–141
Oxybutynin (Ditropan)
  for treating irritable bowel syndrome,
    305–306
  for treating urge incontinence, 123
Oxytrol patch, for treating urge
  incontinence, 124

P

Pacemaker, bladder, for treating urge
    incontinence, 167–168
Pain
  during anesthesia, morphine for,
    343
  in interstitial cystitis, 277
  postoperative
    management of, 348–353
    relieving, 336–337
  urological problems causing, 16–17
Patient-controlled anesthesia (PCA), for
    pain control, 349
Paxil, for treating interstitial cystitis,
    298–299
Pelvic examination
  in evaluating urge incontinence, 115
Pelvic floor
    muscles of, 21
    spasms of, 20–23
    in urethral syndrome, 279–280
    physical therapy, in interstitial cystitis,
    296
    prolapse of, 37–44, 177–222
      blockage due to, 137, 158
      case description, 177–180
      defined, 180–183
      effect of, on infection, 243
      in the elderly, 166, 168–172
      identifying during physical
        examination for stress
        incontinence, 76
      after menopause, 323–324
      symptoms and solutions to
        problems with, 15–44
Pelvic inflammatory disease (PID),
    28
Pelvic pain, 271–307
Pelvic pain syndrome, 304–305
Pelvic surgery
  overflow incontinence following,
    35
Penicillin, for urinary tract infection,
    260
Percutaneous nephrostomy tube
  for kidney blockage, 377–379
  for ureter injury management, 219

Perimenopause
  phase of menopause, 314
  symptoms of, 316–318
Perineum
  anatomy of, 231
  view of, 9, 182
Persistent incontinence, in the elderly,
    150
Personal hygiene, and urinary tract
    infections, 238–239
Pessary
  defined, 199
  for managing cystocele, 171
    figure, 200
  for managing uterine prolapse, 169,
    178, 199–202
Physical changes, in vaginal atrophy,
    320–321
Physical examination
  for evaluating interstitial cystitis,
    288–289
  for evaluating pelvic-floor prolapse,
    193–194
  for evaluating stress incontinence,
    75–76
  for evaluating urge incontinence,
    115
Physical therapy
  for elderly women, 165–166
  for managing interstitial cystitis,
    295–296
  for managing irritable bowel
    syndrome, 305
  for managing stress incontinence,
    81–82
Physicians
  characteristics a patient evaluates in
    selecting, 53–54
  types of practice of, 57
Physiology, of the female pelvis,
    3–13
Plasmids, bacterial resistance to
    antibiotics mediated by, 264
Postcoital antibiotic prophylaxis, 252
Postmenopause, 314
Post-void residual
  in prolapse, 195–196

Post-void residual (*cont.*)
   measuring
      in evaluation of incontinence in the
         elderly, 153
      in evaluation of interstitial cystitis,
         289
      in evaluation of urge incontinence,
         115
      with ultrasound, 359–360
Pregnancy, urinary tract infection
   during, 268
Prelief, dietary supplement, for managing
   interstitial cystitis, 294
Preparation for surgery, medical
   clearance, 338–339
Prevalence
   defined, 383
   of urge incontinence, 105
   of urinary incontinence, 383–384
Prevention
   of urinary tract infections, 250
      estrogen creams for, 330–331
      non-antibiotic, 252–254
   of yeast infections, 266
Prions, potential for transmitting in
   foreign grafts, 94–95
Private practice, comparison with
   hospital-based practice, 58
Progesterone, 315–316
   combination with estrogens, 328
Progestins, side effects of, 332
Prolapse
   lifetime risk of surgery for, and re-
      operation rate, 385
   recurrent, 219–220
   urethral, in the elderly, 157
   after vaginal delivery, 387
   See also Cystocele; Enterocele; Pelvic
      floor, prolapse of; Rectocele;
      Uterine prolapse
Prompted voiding, 165
Propantheline (Pro-Banthine), for
   treating urge incontinence,
   126–127
Prophylaxis, after urinary tract infection,
   252, 264–265
Propofol, for sedation in surgery, 342

Protein in the urine, as an indication of
   kidney problems, 116, 289
Proteus mirabilis
   resistance of, to nitrofurantoins, 264
   urinary tract infections caused by,
      237
Prozac, for treating interstitial cystitis,
   298–299
Psychological problems, and urinary
   incontinence in the elderly,
   147–148
Public Health Service, Agency for Health
   Care Policy and Research, 382
Pubococcygeus muscle, strengthening to
   manage stress incontinence,
   80–81
Pubovaginal sling, for stress incontinence
   surgery, 91–99
Pyelonephritis, 236
   treatment, 266–268
Pyuria, defined, 233

Q

Quality of life, impact of urge
   incontinence, 107–108, 385
Questions, in a history to evaluate stress
   incontinence, 71–74

R

Race, and urinary leakage, 389
Radiation cystitis, 24–25
Radiation therapy, total incontinence
   following, 36–37
Radiologists, training of, 373–374
Rectal examination, for evaluating
   incontinence in the elderly,
   151–152
Rectocele, 41
   defined, 183
   figure, 42, 192
   repair of, 208–210
      figure, 209
   symptoms of, 189
Rectum
   injuries to, during rectocele surgery,
      220–221
   structure of, 13

Recurrent infection
  of the kidneys, 268
  of the urinary tract, 251–252
    vaccines for preventing, 254
Regional anesthesia, 345–348
Reinfection, of the urinary tract, 236
Renal scans, to evaluate kidney function, 376–377
Residency, 47
  training in the hospital, 57
Resistance, of bacteria to antibiotics, 263–265
Retrograde urethrogram (RUG), 371
Risk factors
  for pelvic-floor prolapse, 178
  for stress incontinence, 70–71
  for urge incontinence, 106–107
  for urinary incontinence, 386–389
  for urinary tract infections after menopause, 324

S
Second opinion, suggestions about, 55
Sedation
  from antidepressants for treating interstitial cystitis, 299
  before entering an operating room, 340
Selection of medications, 125–126
Selective-serotonin reuptake inhibitors (SSRIs)
  Duloxetine, for treating stress incontinence, 84–85
  for treating interstitial cystitis, 298–299
Selectivity, of antibiotics for urinary tract infection, 255
Self-catheterization, 366
  intermittent, in the elderly, 158–159
  after prolapse surgery, 215
  after pubovaginal sling surgery, 99
Self-medication, for urinary tract infection, 251–252
Senile urethral syndrome
  defined, 319
  local treatment for, with hormones, 330

Senility, and incontinence, management techniques, 133
Sensitivity, to estrogen, in the female urogenital tract, 315
Sensitivity testing, for bacterial response to antibiotics, 248
Sexual activity, as a risk factor in urinary tract infection, 17–18
Sexual desire, postmenopausal, 325
Short-acting medications, comparison with long-acting medications, 122–123
Short-term incontinence, reversible, 142–150
Side effects
  of anticholinergic medications, 121–122, 128–129
  of antiinflammatory medications, 300
  of fluoroquinolones, 259
  of ketoralac, 350
  of narcotic medications, 349
  of nitrofurantoins, 258
  of oxybutynin, 123
  of progestins, 332
  of tolterodine, 124–125
Sleep cycles, change with age, 111
Sling, location of attachment in surgery, 97
Sling kits, for pubovaginal sling insertion, 96
Small intestine, prolapse into the vagina, 41
Smoking, and menopause, 315
Sodium bicarbonate for treating interstitial cystitis, 297
Sodium pentosan polysulfate (Elmiron), for treating interstitial cystitis, 300–301
Solifenacin (Vesicare), for treating urge incontinence, 125
Sonogram, for evaluating incontinence in the elderly, 153
Specialization, medical, advantages and disadvantages of, 46
Specificity, of antibiotics for urinary tract infection, 255

Spermicides, effect on lactobacilli
    colonization, 242
Sphincter
    stress incontinence and response of, 68
    structure and function of, 7–10
    urinary, effect of estrogen on, 319
Spinal anesthesia, 345–348
    case description, 336–337
    figure, 346
Staphylococcus saprophyticus, urinary
    tract infections caused by, 237
Stent, to manage ureter blockage after
    prolapse surgery, 219
Steroids
    effects of, on urinary tract infections,
        245
    for treating interstitial cystitis, 297
Stool impaction, incontinence caused by,
    in the elderly, 149–150
Stress, pelvic-floor spasms due to, 22
Stress incontinence
    abdominal surgery for, 88
    comparison with urge incontinence,
        104
    in cystocele, 188
    in the elderly, 137–140, 168–173
    and gender, 386
    after menopause, 322–323
        prevalence of, 384
    after pessary insertion, 202
    after prolapse surgery, 213–214
    urinary, 29–31, 63–100
Submucosa, of the urinary bladder, 5–6
Subspecialties, medical, 47–48
Succinylcholine, for muscle relaxation in
    surgery, 343
Sufentanyl, use in surgery, 341
Sulfa-based antibiotics, 256–257
Sulfamethoxazole, for treating urinary
    tract infection, 257
Suprapubic tubes, for catheterization,
    162–163
    after surgery, 172
Surgery
    anesthesia during, goals of, 338–340
    bladder, overflow incontinence
        following, 35

for fistula repair, 217
for interstitial cystitis, 302–304
for prolapse, 202–221
relationship with recurrent infections,
    19–20
for repairing leakage and bladder
    descent, 15–16
for stress incontinence, 87–100,
    208
    case, 63–64
    in the elderly, 168–172
for urge incontinence, 129–130
for uterine prolapse, 178–180
Surgical specialties, list, 48
Symptoms
    of bladder prolapse, 188–189
    of interstitial cystitis, 275–278
    of pelvic-floor prolapse, 186–192
    of vaginal atrophy, 320–321
Synthetic materials, for pubovaginal
    slings, 95–96

T
Tamoxifen, binding to receptors on
    the breast and the uterus,
        315
Testosterone, production of, in
    menopause, 315
Tests, office-based, 358–373
Tetracyclines, for treating urinary tract
    infections, 262
Thiopental, historic use of for induction
    in surgery, 341
Timed voiding
    to manage functional incontinence,
        141–142
    to manage stress incontinence, 80
    to manage urge incontinence, 121
Timing, frequency of urination at night,
    110–112
Tolterodine (Detrol and Detrol LA), for
    treating urge incontinence,
        124–125
Toradol (ketoralac)
    for pain relief after surgery, 337
    for treating acute pain, 350
Total incontinence, 36–37

Transcutaneous electrical nerve stimulator (TENS), for treating interstitial cystitis, 301–302

Treatment
of interstitial cystitis, 292–304
of irritable bowel syndrome, 305–306
of pelvic-floor spasms, 22–23
of prolapse, 198–221
of stress incontinence, 78–100
of urge incontinence, frequency, and urgency, 117–130
of urinary incontinence in the elderly, 154–168
of urinary tract infections, 250–270
of urological disorders after menopause, 325–329

Trichomonas, vaginitis caused by, 242

Trimethoprim-sulfamethoxazole (TMP-SMX), for urinary tract infection, 257

Trospium (Sanctura), for treating urge incontinence, 125

Tubo-ovarian abscess, 28

Tumors, urethral, 157–158

U

Ultrasound
for diagnosing overflow incontinence, 36
for evaluating the extent of bladder emptying, 77, 289
for evaluating urinary tract infections, 249
for identifying an ovarian cyst, 27–28
kidney
for diagnosing kidney infections, 18
for identifying functioning before and after prolapse surgery, 219
before surgery for prolapse, 196
as an office procedure, 359–360
pelvic, for evaluating prolapse, 197

Unresolved infections, of the urinary tract, 236, 251–252

Ureters
injury to, during prolapse surgery, 218–219
structure and function of, 3–5

Urethra
appearance of, normal and in stress incontinence, 67
catherization of, indications for, 363–364
changes with aging, 134
injury to, in pubovaginal sling surgery, 98
normal and post-traumatic, 11
structure of, 7

Urethral dilatation, indications for, 364

Urethral diverticula
figure, 244
surgery to remove, 243
voiding cystourethrograms to identify, 369–371

Urethral syndrome, 278–279

Urge incontinence, 31–33, 101–130
comparison with stress incontinence, 64–66
in cystocele, 188–189
in the elderly, 140
due to bladder spasms, 153
treating, 167–168
hormones for treating, 331
after menopause, 323, 331
after prolapse surgery, 214

Urgency, change in, with menopause, 322

Uricept, antiinflammatory agent for treating interstitial cystitis, 300

Urinalysis, 246–248
to evaluate incontinence in the elderly, 152
to evaluate prolapse, 194–195
to evaluate urge incontinence, 115–116
to identify infection in interstitial cystitis, 289
in an office visit, 358

Urinary cytology, to identify urinary cancer, 116

Urinary incontinence
causes of, 28–37
sling surgery for stress incontinence, 99–100
hormones for treating, 331–332

Urinary retention
    after prolapse surgery, 214–215
    after pubovaginal sling surgery, 98–99
    as a side effect of anticholinergenic
        medications, 128
Urinary tract
    female, figure, 235
    infections of, 17–20, 225–270
        complicated, 236–237
        complicated, defined, 233–234
        evaluating, 156
        versus pelvic muscle spasms, 20–23
        uncomplicated, 233–236
        uncomplicated, recurrent, 250–251
    after menopause, 319–325
Urine output
    diversion of, from ureteral injury, 218
    excessive, in the elderly, 148–149
Urodynamic testing
    for evaluating incontinence in the
        elderly, 153
    for evaluating prolapse, 197–198
    for evaluating stress incontinence, 78,
        116
    in the office, 371–373
Urologist's office, visit to, 355–379
Urology
    compared with gynecology, 48–49
    training for specialists in, 49–50
Uterine fibroids, 26–27
Uterine prolapse
    defined, 183
    figure, 40
    postmenopausal, 318
    symptoms of, 189
Uterus, 10

V
Vaccines, against recurrent urinary tract
    infection, 254
Vagifem, for vaginal application of
    estrogen, 329
Vagina, 10
    bladder prolapsed into, figure, 182
    organs that fall into, 180–183
    tears in, during childbirth, 208–210

Vaginal-approach surgery, for stress
        incontinence, 91–94
    to correct prolapse, 203
Vaginal atrophy
    estrogen cream for, 330
    after menopause, 320–322
Vaginal delivery
    pelvic-floor prolapse following,
        183–184
    stress urinary incontinence following,
        30, 68–70, 75, 387
Vaginal vault prolapse, postmenopausal,
    318
Vaginal weights, for physical therapy in
    the elderly, 166
Vancomycin, for treating C. difficile
    infection, 265
Vasopressin, effect on kidneys, 127
Vesicoureteral reflux, 243–245
Vesicovaginal fistula, defined, 36,
    68
Viral cystitis, 25
Voiding cystourethrogram (VCUG),
    369
Voiding diary
    for evaluating incontinence in the
        elderly, 153
    for evaluating interstitial cystitis,
        289–290, 294–295
    for evaluating stress incontinence,
        77–78
    for evaluating urge incontinence,
        116
Vomiting, from anesthetics, 345

W
Water, intake of
    in stress incontinence, 74
    in urge incontinence, 113
Web sites, HealthGrades.com,
        training record of physicians,
        47
White blood cells, in the urine,
        determining, 116, 246–247
Women's Health Initiative
    data on estrogen, 313

recommendation on oral estrogen, 326
type of estrogen used in, 327

X
X-rays
  for evaluating prolapse, 196–197
  in the office, 366–373

Y
Yeast infections, antibiotic-induced, treating, 265–266

Z
Zelnorm, for treating irritable bowel syndrome, 305
Zoloft, for treating interstitial cystitis, 298–299